Praise for *Pet Care in the New Century*

"Thoughtful, groundbreaking, and often inspirational, Amy Shojai's *Pet Care in the New Century* is an important work that everyone who cares about pets and the future of veterinary medicine must read."
— Gina Spadafori, nationally syndicated pet-care columnist and author of *Dogs for Dummies* and *Cats for Dummies*

"Wow! After thirty-one years of practice, I am amazed that a person can create a book that covers all aspects of modern veterinary care. This book will prove to be an invaluable resource for companion animal lovers, students, and the profession. I am in awe that Ms. Shojai has been able to pull so many people together in this work."
— Robert A. Taylor, DVM, seen on TV's *Emergency Vets*

"Amy Shojai delivers cutting-edge medicine with more flair than Emeril Lagasse, presenting the amazing array of astonishing advances in veterinary medicine. If you have a pet with heart disease, cancer, kidney failure, or any other serious medical condition, this easy to comprehend book is a credible place to start your research. Shojai continues to rank among the most authoritative and thorough pet reporters."
— Steve Dale, syndicated newspaper columnist of *My Pet World* and host of the radio programs *Animal Planet Radio* and *Pet Central*

PET CARE
IN THE
NEW CENTURY

Cutting-Edge Medicine
for Dogs and Cats

Amy D. Shojai

NEW AMERICAN LIBRARY

New American Library
Published by New American Library, a division of
Penguin Putnam Inc., 375 Hudson Street, New York, New York 10014, U.S.A.
Penguin Books Ltd, 80 Strand, London WC2R ORL, England
Penguin Books Australia Ltd, Ringwood, Victoria, Australia
Penguin Books Canada Ltd, 10 Alcorn Avenue, Toronto, Ontario, Canada M4V 3B2
Penguin Books (N.Z.) Ltd, 182–190 Wairau Road, Auckland 10, New Zealand

Penguin Books Ltd, Registered Offices: Harmondsworth, Middlesex, England

First published by New American Library, a division of Penguin Putnam Inc.

First Printing, November 2001
1   3   5   7   9   10   8   6   4   2

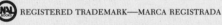 REGISTERED TRADEMARK—MARCA REGISTRADA

LIBRARY OF CONGRESS CATALOGING-IN-PUBLICATION DATA:
Shojai, Amy, 1956-
Pet care in the new century : cutting-edge medicine for dogs and cats / Amy D. Shojai.
p. cm.
ISBN 0-451-20443-3 (alk. paper)
1. Dogs—Diseases. 2. Cats—Diseases. 3. Veterinary medicine. I. Title.

SF991 .S552 2001
636.7'089—dc21   2001032627

Set in New Caledonia
Designed by Eve L. Kirch

Printed in the United States of America

For all the pets of the new century—

May this book give loving owners
The tools they need
To make informed, educated,
Quality-of-life choices
For all the pets who touch their lives.

And especially for Seren, who keeps me sane—

May you never need this book!

CONTENTS

4. A Brave New World 72

PART TWO. HEALTH AND BEHAVIOR CONDITIONS A TO Z

Aggression 87

Anemia 95

Anorexia 100

Arthritis 102

ACKNOWLEDGMENTS

Countless people—and their special pets—made this book possible with their expertise, help, and inspiration. Most especially my husband, Mahmoud, keeps me focused on the important stuff; my cat Seren reminds me to make time for play; and my furry muse, Fafnir, never leaves my heart. I am blessed with a supportive, caring family, and can never thank them enough.

My colleagues from the Cat Writers Association and the Dog Writers Association of America never fail to inspire and impress me with their professionalism and support. I'd especially like to thank Janine Adams, Darlene Arden, Sally Bahner, Beverly Caldwell, Susan Conant, Debbie De Louise, Kathy Joiner, Kathy Keely, Karen Lawrence, Lynn Miller, Carvi Shamsid-Deen, Carol Shenold, Cheryl Smith, and Gina Spadafori for sharing a few of their expert sources and helping me send out the call for "miracle pet" stories. I am touched by your generosity and proud to call you my friends and colleagues.

Heartfelt appreciation goes to the more than a hundred veterinarians and pet owners who allowed me to report their ground-breaking therapies, as well as share their uplifting stories of pet health success. I must also thank the countless veterinary schools and specialty colleges who put me in touch with these experts and pet owners, most particularly the American Veterinary Medical Association; Tania Banak of the University of Wisconsin-Madison; Chris Beuoy of the University of Illinois; Margaret Combs of Tufts University; Jeffrey S. Douglas of Virginia

Tech and the University of Maryland; Pat Edwards of Louisiana State University; Lea-Ann Germinder of Western Veterinary Conference; Cheryl May of Kansas State University; Lynn Narlesky of the University of California-Davis; Charles E. Powell of Washington State University; Helma Weeks of the University of Pennsylvania; and Derek Woodbury of the American Animal Hospital Association.

Most of all, very special thanks to Lisa Sigler for all your help, way above and beyond the call of duty! The wide range of experts you suggested from the American College of Veterinary Internal Medicine and American Academy of Veterinary Surgeons helped give my book wonderful credibility—I am in your debt.

Grateful thanks to Ellen Edwards, my editor, who had the vision to choose *Pet Care in the New Century* and the patience to make it happen. And as always, my deepest gratitude to my agent, Meredith Bernstein, who does all the really hard stuff so I can live my pet-writing dream.

Finally, this book wouldn't be possible without all the cats and dogs that share our lives—and the loving owners dedicated to providing the best care possible for their furry family members. Without you, this book would never have been written.

PART ONE

21st Century Medicine

CHAPTER 1

How We Care for Pets in the New Century

Pet popularity is at an all-time high. Today nearly 60 million households in the United States keep cats and dogs. According to a 1999–2000 survey by the American Animal Hospital Association, 84 percent of pet owners consider their cats and dogs their children, and they would go to any lengths to save their pet's life. In a single year this "pet generation" increased annual pet care spending by $1 billion—to a whopping $23 billion in 2000. The trend will certainly continue into the new century.

This dedication toward pets isn't surprising. Young professionals who delay marriage and/or children tend to lavish affection on their pets. And the emotional attachment to pets continues when they marry and start families. Children raised in families who cherish pets learn from an early age to love and care about cats and dogs, and that affection continues for the rest of their lives.

At the other end of the spectrum, older people relish the interaction and unconditional love offered by dogs and cats. During a time when people may lose spouses or other family and friends who are close to them, pets can fill the void and fulfill an intrinsic need to be needed. The responsibility of caring for another living creature keeps them connected to life. In fact, research has shown that pets are good for human health. While we may not have admitted it in the past, our love affair with pets has become a very public one.

The importance pets play in our lives is immeasurable. Consequently, the health of our cats and dogs has become more important than ever before. Not surprisingly, we have come to demand the same level of expert medical care for our pets as we expect for ourselves. That has brought about a major shift in the way veterinarians treat animals, and how people address pet care needs.

Every veterinarian offers basic care, such as vaccinations, spay and neuter surgery, and flea control, and many veterinarians can diagnose and treat a wide array of health problems. In recent years, researchers have also made amazing new discoveries in specialized areas of veterinary medicine, and pet owners can now take advantage of exciting treatments that can lead to miraculous cures. These treatments can greatly improve a sick animal's quality of life, and often add months or even years to the time the pet and owner can share together.

Yet many pet owners don't think to ask their veterinarian about advanced care options until their dog or cat has received a devastating diagnosis. And few local practices are equipped to provide cutting-edge innovations—the new century medicine—that today may save the pet's life when routine methods fail.

Pet Care in the New Century provides vital and exciting information about the most innovative, up-to-the-minute treatments that are available, tells you where specialists are located, and suggests how to take advantage of care that is offered on a limited basis through specialized research programs and veterinary practices.

Over the course of the twentieth century, cats and dogs have moved from the barnyard into the family room, from being considered work animals to being prized companions. Pets are no longer considered "replaceable." Consequently, today's pet lovers want the most current, highest quality care for their pets that they can possibly get.

NEW CHOICES IN CUTTING-EDGE MEDICINE

Cutting-edge veterinary care offers modern techniques that go "beyond the basics." New research has led to new diagnostic tools, new surgical procedures, new prevention options, and new uses for existing or novel drugs. These innovative veterinary options not only save lives but also extend a pet's longevity and improve the overall quality of life.

New century medicine for pets can be categorized in four major ways:

- **Wellness care** maintains and promotes pet health and longevity, from birth through old age. Treatment ranges from immunity boosters to arthritis-preventing food supplements (neutraceuticals), and even gene mapping that predicts (and so, can help us prevent) devastating inherited diseases. New methods of promoting general pet health will enhance or even replace the current standard for basic pet care.
- **Chronic care** targets ongoing health problems to enhance the quality of life. Increased longevity means more pets develop age-related problems. A new generation of screening tests can now detect problems earlier. Innovative therapies such as new diets and unique drug-delivery systems can ease—and even reverse—the effects of diseases like diabetes and Alzheimer's-like conditions. Today, veterinary medicine aims to keep senior pets happy and active throughout their golden years.
- **Acute care** involves treating deadly diseases or traumatic injuries, with tools such as CT scans and heart bypass machines. Acute care techniques include surgery that reconstructs the body. Treatments range from drugs for pain to organ transplants. Acute care saves the lives of pets whether they are struck by cars or afflicted by cancer.
- **Behavior care** modifies objectionable behavior. New strategies include innovative training tools, an evolution in training techniques and philosophies, and drugs that address chemical imbalances in the brain. Problem behavior is the number one reason why pets are given to shelters or "put down." Promising new therapies that reverse these behaviors will enhance the owner-pet bond and save pets' lives.

Pet owners who become familiar with the most up-to-date options will have all the facts they need to make the best health care choices for their pets, and that will in turn enhance their relationship with their veterinarian. Informed owners are the best veterinary clients. After all, you live with your pet every day, and you know better than anyone when your pet feels under the weather. Veterinarians will tell you that owners are essential partners in maintaining their pets' good health.

General-practice veterinarians remain the backbone of pet health. They also represent the first line of defense in recognizing problems that need specialized attention. Says Dr. Maura O'Brien, a veterinary surgeon in Los Angeles, "Our clients want to know their options, want more advanced treatments if they're available, and want referrals to specialists." Today, pet owners can collaborate with their general practitioner and with veterinary specialists from a wide range of disciplines.

You can do more for your pet's health and happiness than you think, whether you have a puppy or kitten, an adult cat or dog, or a geriatric pet.

Wellness Care

In the last decade, veterinary medicine—like human medicine—has emphasized wellness care. Rather than waiting for illness or injury to strike, a host of preventive options are available to keep pets healthy.

In the 1970s, pets typically achieved single-digit lifespans. Today they commonly reach the mid- to late teens. "This is my thirtieth year in practice, and I can remember seeing a six-year-old dog thirty years ago, and saying wow, this is a geriatric dog," says Dr. Robert Taylor, a veterinary surgeon in Denver. "That's not even considered middle aged now!" Better care will allow dogs and cats in the new century to live even longer, healthier lives.

"Things like improved nutrition, prevention of infectious diseases with vaccines, and even leash laws that keep pets safe have really helped to cut back on young to middle-aged problems," says Dr. David S. Bruyette, an internist in Los Angeles. Veterinarians have also become more attuned to the nutritional needs and physiological changes in senior animals, says Dr. Korinn E. Saker, a clinical nutritionist in Virginia. "That has helped in some regard to increase longevity of our pets," she says.

Today's wellness care goes beyond prevention therapies such as heartworm protection or flea control. It emphasizes early detection at regularly scheduled health exams. That's because pets age so much faster than people do. "Going from nine to ten years in a dog is like going from eighty to ninety in a person," says Dr. Bruyette. "There's a lot that happens in a twelve-month period. If you can pick things up earlier, then the chance of successful treatment is certainly much better."

Senior wellness programs recommend twice-yearly physical exams. Once-yearly screening tests provide early detection of age-related diseases.

Chronic Care

Chronic care benefits any pet that needs long-term medical attention. For instance, some kinds of allergic skin diseases can be controlled with the right food. Pets with diabetes or congenital heart conditions get relief with drugs or components of food that act like drugs (called neutraceuticals). In chronic care situations, the treatment must continue for weeks to months, and sometimes for the rest of the pet's life. Medicines can now be compounded into flavors and doses that are convenient for the owner to give. That means that pets welcome the medicine rather than hide from their owner, or spit out the pill. The stress of medicating a chronically sick pet can sometimes cause as many problems as the illness itself, so new ways to relieve stress are a great benefit.

Veterinarians recognize that the increased lifespan of pets has led to a corresponding increase in age-related disorders. "Ultimately, as they move into their senior years, we start to see a lot of cancers, kidney problems, heart problems, and other 'old age' problems," says Dr. Bruyette. That means that senior pets need both acute care therapies to save their lives, and chronic care therapies to maintain their health and quality of life.

Today geriatrics is a huge area in veterinary medicine, although it is not yet a specialty. Some practices are heavily built around the older pet. "The pet population mirrors the demographics of the human population—both definitely have been getting older," says Dr. Bruyette. "Even if veterinarians haven't focused on senior care, 40 to 50 percent of their patients are probably over the age of seven. So pet care professionals are emphasizing therapies that slow age-related deterioration, and placing importance on the early detection of diseases in the senior pet."

Every owner dreads the thought of losing a pet to age or infirmity. Cutting-edge medicine that's available today—and breakthroughs on the horizon—may allow pets to live twenty years or more.

Acute Care

Emergency medicine has never been better. Acute care treats injuries or illnesses that strike suddenly. For instance, transfusion medicine supplies blood products—and even artificial blood—to pull the dog through the initial crisis of being hit by a car. Ultrasound-guided surgery allows a swallowed needle to be removed from the cat's throat. Lasers and new drugs stop the progression of paralysis from a back injury.

Kittens and puppies and young adult pets tend to suffer more often from trauma—broken legs from falls, shock from car accidents, bite wounds from fights. That's because they're more active and exposed to outdoor risks more often than sedate, older stay-at-home pets. Today, surgery offers everything from dental work and broken-bone repair to cosmetic reconstruction of tissue damaged by fire or lost to cancer.

Acute care relies on state-of-the-art diagnostic tools. Ultrasound and other imaging techniques allow veterinarians to "see" what's wrong, so they can plan treatment. That may include a drug "patch" applied to the skin to control pain, or noninvasive laproscopic surgery using lasers. Acute care can even fix damaged body parts like bone joints and tendons, replace worn-out corneas in the eye, or trade sick kidneys for healthy ones.

Behavior Care

Behavior was long thought to be the territory of dog trainers, but veterinarians now recognize that behavior has a place in veterinary medicine, due in large part to the emerging emphasis on "holistic" or total patient care for their clients. The behavior of a cat or dog cannot be separated from its physical well-being, and more and more veterinarians recognize the need to educate themselves and their clients regarding behavior issues. Otherwise, owners end up putting pets to sleep. "Behavior problems are the number one terminal illness in cats and dogs," says Dr. Ian Dunbar, a behaviorist and dog trainer in California.

An integrated, three-pronged approach to the field of behavior includes evaluating the animal's physical condition, behavioral makeup, and relationship with the owner, says Dr. Myrna M. Milani, a behaviorist and ethologist in New Hampshire. In the past, a great deal of what veterinarians characterize as "owner noncompliance" with giving medicine may have resulted from overlooked behavior issues. "Can you imagine injecting insulin in a dog that tries to bite you every time?" asks Dr. Milani. Ideally, a veterinarian today not only treats the diabetes but also addresses that aggression, and takes steps to enhance the pet-owner relationship needed to cure the pet.

USING THIS BOOK

Pet Care in the New Century covers every aspect of pet care, from birth to old age.

Chapter 2 describes the latest advances in diagnoses and treatment, and how past successes continue to pave the way for future innovations. You'll learn about the different veterinary specialties, how the doctors attain their degrees, and what kinds of treatment they provide. Usually your veterinarian will refer you to the specialist who's best suited to treat your pet's problem skin, cloudy eyes, cancerous tumor, or aging heart.

A frank discussion of the ethical issues raised by cutting-edge veterinary research and pet care is covered in Chapter 3. Should pets be used in medical experiments? What if animal research benefits people, but not pets? How much is too much to spend? Where do organ donors come from? When should we draw the line at preserving a pet's life? These questions are emotionally charged, and though there are no easy answers, Chapter 3 will help you figure out what's best for you and your pets.

Chapter 4 covers some of the most important aspects of molecular medicine, from DNA research and gene mapping to genetically engineered vaccines and diagnostic tests. This fascinating subject is complicated, but offers incredible promise for better health for our cats and dogs today, and in the future.

The heart of the book, and the section you may find most useful, is Part 2, a complete A-to-Z listing of many health and behavior conditions, arranged alphabetically for easy reference. You may want to scan the Contents to decide which problems you'd like to read about first. This part of the book provides brief descriptions of each condition, and compares the "standard" treatments with cutting-edge options.

In each of the A-to-Z chapters, either the researchers who developed the treatment, and/or specialists who offer these therapies, explain how the treatment works and which pets are prime candidates for being helped. Many veterinary specialists across the country are performing these cutting-edge therapies. So if you're interested in finding a veterinarian to help your pet, you can certainly start with the experts I've quoted, but you may also be able to find a specialist in your own backyard.

Throughout the book you'll find countless break-out boxes with interesting bits of information. How can a scent stop your cat from clawing the furniture? Do dogs benefit from glasses? When did behavior medicine become a specialty? Also, you'll find many boxes with details about innovative treatments, new medicines, and even predictions for the future.

Look especially for Modern Miracles, heartwarming stories of real dogs and cats that have had miraculous cures. Applaud Gordon the Pit Bull's new winning attitude. Celebrate Floppy-cat's diabetes cure. Cheer for Molly's lifesaving brain surgery, Peter's restored hearing, and Kazie's new hips. If you're like me, you'll wipe away some happy tears reading these joyful stories that also offer hope for other pets.

Appendix A offers a comprehensive list of veterinary universities, including contact information and website addresses. These universities publish information about current research programs, the scientists involved, and how your pet can participate in groundbreaking studies at low to no cost.

More veterinary specialists are available today than ever before. Appendix B describes the organizations, called "colleges," that board-certify these doctors in a variety of specialized areas, such as dermatology (skin conditions), dentistry, surgery, and internal medicine. Most specialty colleges also list their members by location on their website. Therefore, the contact information for these specialty colleges located in the last half of Appendix B will allow you and your general practice veterinarian to find a nearby specialist.

Websites for veterinary health associations and pet research foundations often list special care options that are available, such as new genetic tests. You'll find contact information for these organizations in Appendix C.

Medical conditions and terms can seem complicated. I've made every effort to explain technical information clearly and simply, and to place it in an understandable context. It may be important for you to tell your veterinarian the specific name of a medicine or treatment, or to know where the research can be found, and that's why I've often included both a technical word and its definition. A glossary in Appendix D helps define some of the scientific terms.

The credentials of the experts quoted in each chapter are mentioned there only briefly. Unless otherwise noted, all the "Dr." designations refer to veterinarians. You can turn to Appendix E, "Source Notes," for a chapter-by-chapter listing of these experts with more detailed information about what they do and where they practice. You or your veterinarian can contact them through the university or clinic with which they're associated to see if your pet might benefit from their specialty.

I hope you'll find this book not only entertaining, but also an essential resource for health care information that will benefit you, your pet, and your veterinarian. Today, pet owners can choose from a wide range of exciting health care options, all of which share one common goal—to provide health care for pets that goes beyond the basics. Pet owners, and their cats and dogs, have never had it so good.

CHAPTER 2

Building on Success

Veterinary medicine builds constantly on the success of the past. Until 1951 the American Veterinary Medical Association (AVMA) did not recognize specialty practices. Today, more than twenty specialty colleges provide advances in pet care and certify veterinarians in all sorts of fields. Partnered with general practice veterinarians, board-certified specialists provide cats and dogs with the latest in today's medical advances.

Not only veterinarian expertise but also modern medical tools make diagnosis and treatment safer and more accurate than ever before. Imaging techniques that show problems inside the body ensure that the right treatment is prescribed without resorting to debilitating exploratory surgery. Advances in tools such as endoscopes and lasers allow surgeons to perform less invasive operations that heal faster with less pain.

Keeping pets healthy has never been easier. Our understanding of the role of good nutrition in maintaining a pet's health is greater now than ever before, and prevention treatments, such as vaccinations and flea medicine, have been significantly improved. Today, health maintenance for pets not only prevents disease, but also improves the quality of life for aging dogs and cats by keeping them pain-free and engaged in life, so they can continue to enjoy the bond they share with their human family.

New drugs stand at the forefront of modern veterinary care. Pharmacists are now compounding drugs into convenient flavors and delivery systems so that pets not only accept but actually beg for the medicine that makes them well.

Behavior medicine has made great strides as well. Today, cat and dog behavior is better understood than at any time in the past, and that has brought about an evolution in training. Now owners are taught how to deal with "normal" animal behaviors and solve problems. There are even drug therapies to treat pet brain disorders, which often cause crippling psychological problems and were once untreatable. Drugs and retraining, alone or together, save the pet-owner bond, and frequently the pet's life.

Many stunning advances in surgical options for cats and dogs are following on the heels of human medicine. Limb-sparing operations allow cancer victims to keep their legs. Others, like cruciate ligament knee repairs that reconstruct the joint, are unique to veterinary medicine. Physical therapy has also been borrowed from humans, especially from sports medicine, to help pets recover more quickly from invasive medical procedures.

All of these are coming together to provide the best health care science has to offer. Cats and dogs are the big winners.

VETERINARY SPECIALTIES

More and more veterinary specialties are emerging. There are about twenty specialty boards, often referred to as "colleges," which certify veterinarians above and beyond the general-practice degree. The American Board of Veterinary Medical Specialties (ABVMS) and the American Veterinary Medical Association (AVMA) publish professional standards that must be met in order for a veterinarian to be certified.

University teaching hospitals have traditionally offered the most advanced veterinary care. There are twenty-seven schools and colleges of veterinary medicine in the United States (see Appendix A for a full listing and contact information.) Grants, educational funding, and the teaching environment often make advanced technology more affordable at these institutions. "In general, Tufts University School of Veterinary Medicine acts as a referral institution for the surrounding veterinarians," says Dr. David Ruslander, a radiologist at Tufts. "We are able to take the medicine to the next level, whereas veterinarians in general practice just don't have the same resources or personnel available."

However, a growing number of private practices are also hiring veterinary specialists. "These referral centers are getting larger and larger, and may have a couple of surgeons, with an internist and cardiologist and ophthalmologist, for example," says Dr. A. D. Elkins, an orthopedic surgeon in Indianapolis. "That's better for the pet and better for the owner." Today, Dr. Elkins says, nearly every metropolitan area has a group of specialists that is able to treat cancer, conduct noninvasive procedures with lasers or laproscopic technology, and even perform the microvascular techniques necessary for organ transplants. "It's amazing what's available," he concludes.

Fascinating Facts! Veterinary Trends

By the year 2020, 70 percent of veterinary practitioners in the United States will be female.

Veterinary Training

Veterinarians typically study for eight to ten years before they receive their doctor of veterinary medicine (DVM) or *veterinariae medicinae doctoris* (VMD) degree. A first year of specialty training, called an internship, includes rotations through many disciplines, so that students can decide on their specialty. Following internship, the veterinarian becomes a resident and studies for three to seven years at a veterinary school or qualified referral practice, focusing on that specialty.

Alternative medical disciplines, including acupuncture, chiropractic, and herbal therapies, have gained popularity, both with pet owners and veterinarians. The American Holistic Veterinary Medical Association was founded in 1982 by Dr. Carvel G. Tiekert. Although in many instances these techniques have been incorporated into mainstream veterinary care, they have not yet become "boarded" specialties.

Veterinary specialists can take additional years of training in an even more specific area, called a subspecialty. For example, neurology is a subspecialty of internal medicine, and radiation therapy is a subspecialty of radiology. A similar certification process applies for those who wish to become subspecialists.

Not all specialties pertain to cat and dog medicine. For instance, the American College of Poultry Veterinarians and American College of

Zoological Medicine are specific to more exotic patients. But most of the boarded veterinary specialties offer great benefits to our pets.

As veterinary medicine continues to advance, new specialties and subspecialties are needed. Completion of three to seven years of full-time training in an accredited residency program is usually required, and many of these brand-new specialties have not been around that long. Therefore, the AVMA has established four specific requirements, at least one of which must be met before it will endorse a new specialty. They include: ten years of active service in the specialty, significant publications, sufficient training, being the head of that specialty-type program, and working primarily in that specialty or a closely related area. (For details about the various veterinary specialties, see Appendix B.)

Fascinating Facts! For Cats Only

In 1995, the American Board of Veterinary Practitioners introduced board certification in feline practice. More than 250 cats-only clinics have opened practices in the last decade.

Mobile Specialties

Specialists also travel to general veterinarians' offices. "There are already hundreds of stand-alone veterinary hospitals in every city, and every general practice has an operating room, anesthetic equipment, and radiologic services," says Dr. E. B. Okrasinski, a surgeon based near Seattle. "It just seemed intuitive to me that it wasn't necessary to create my own hospital." He began his mobile surgical practice in 1992.

A mobile specialist eases the burden on pet owners who would otherwise have to travel long distances to reach a referral practice. Plus, the pet remains under the care of the veterinarian the owner knows best, and the general veterinarian remains intimately involved in treatment. "They're a very critical part of the case," says Dr. Okrasinski. "They know the animal and the clients very well, and they'll be the doctor who sees the pet for the remainder of its life."

Dr. Okrasinski's practice, equipped to do any of the referral surgeries, has been well received in the Puget Sound area—he serves nearly ninety hospitals. He has become so busy, he now performs primarily orthopedic and cancer surgeries. Due to demand, operations are scheduled three or more weeks in advance. The cost for a mobile specialist is comparable to that at a referral practice.

"Most major metropolitan areas have specialists offering this type of service, because it does work so well for so many different reasons," he says. "Here in the Seattle area there are veterinary cardiologists, internists, radiologists, and neurologists with at least a portion of their practice being mobile." The system expands the services that the local veterinarian can provide. For example, a traveling cardiologist will bring along sophisticated color-flow Doppler ultrasound equipment to conduct echocardiography studies on patients.

"A multidiscipline referral practice and a mobile specialized-care practice complement each other quite well. I think we'll see more of both in the future," says Dr. Okrasinski. Multidiscipline referral centers provide emergency and critical care, while mobile practices take specialty services directly to practitioners. "It's driven by the desire to be service-oriented, both to the patient and to the referring doctor as well," says Dr. Okrasinski. "And it's a way for veterinary medicine to provide the whole spectrum of care."

Continuing Education

Like human medicine, veterinary medicine continues to evolve and improve as scientists understand more about pets' physical and emotional health, and as new diagnostic tools and treatments become available. Veterinarians can't just graduate and treat animals for forty years based solely on that early training. They are required to continually update their training with ongoing education courses.

Shared information among specialists and general practitioners keeps members of the profession abreast of the latest developments. Besides the wide range of professional journals that publish the results of research, each of the specialty colleges provides newsletters and sometimes websites with the latest information, as well as contact information through which to reach other professionals. Symposiums sponsored by the various veterinary specialty colleges, as well as the American Veterinary Medical Association (AVMA) and American Animal Hospital Association (AAHA), offer the best way for general practice and specialty veterinarians to learn from their colleagues, says Dr. Elkins. AAHA is an international organization of more than 17,000 veterinarians.

ADVANCES IN MEDICAL TOOLS

Some of the most exciting medical advances for dogs and cats have been made in the tools used to detect and treat illnesses. A look at these instruments shows why they have helped lead the advances in better care.

Ultrasound

"By far the biggest advance in diagnostic capabilities in veterinary cardiology is use of ultrasound, or echocardiography," says Dr. Mark D. Kittleson, a cardiologist at University of California-Davis. M-mode (time motion) echocardiography, the oldest form of the procedure, was introduced to veterinary medicine in the late 1970s. It provides information about a very narrow target of tissue, and the two-dimensional echocardiography provides a wide overall view of the heart. It is ideal when assessing the relative size of the heart chambers and thickness of the cardiac walls. Doppler echocardiography, the newest form, detects how blood flows throughout the heart.

In echocardiography, sound waves are bounced off the heart muscle and surrounding tissues, the echoed signals are processed, and this information is then displayed in a visual or auditory format, reports Dr. John D. Bonagura, an internist at University of Missouri. Ultrasound has largely replaced cardiac catheterization, which was used in the past. That procedure, which is very involved and invasive, requires anesthetizing the pet and placing catheters directly into the heart to inject dyes that show up on X-rays or angiocardiograms. "Echocardiography gives us the capability to put a transducer on the chest and look at cardiac anatomy and heart function noninvasively," says Dr. Kittleson. "With Doppler ultrasound we can actually look at blood flow within the heart and identify congenital and acquired abnormalities. It's a lot better and a lot more fun these days."

The technology, although expensive, has become more widely available. "All the veterinary cardiologists—about ninety of us now in the U.S.—have fairly high-end-level machines and do cardiac ultrasound," says Dr. Kittleson. Until very recently, the machines typically cost in the $150,000–$200,000 range, so most general-practice veterinarians don't have them. But within the last five to ten years, prices on ultrasound machines have come down. Says Dr. Kittleson, "A veterinary practitioner these days can get a very good machine for $20,000 to $30,000."

CT and MRI Imaging

In neurology and neurosurgery, which involves the brain, spinal cord, and nervous system, the biggest advances in the past several years have all stemmed from using computed tomography (CT) and magnetic resonance imaging (MRI) to better "see" the brain. CT was first used to scan a human brain in 1972, and many experimental studies on laboratory animals soon followed. By the early 1980s, CT scans were being used for pets. "With that has come an ability for us to identify a large number of brain problems, anything from brain tumors to abscesses and different types of infections," says Dr. Richard LeCouteur, a neurologist at University of California-Davis.

CT and MRI are more sensitive than X-rays in identifying abnormalities in complex parts of the body. The main advantage is the ability to remove bones from the picture, which otherwise obscure a clear view of the target. "Another advantage is the fact that these imaging techniques are based on digital information," says Dr. Jeryl C. Jones, a radiologist. "Computers can manipulate this digital information to enhance our ability to see very subtle changes in soft tissue or bony structures." Brain studies using CT are done with or without contrast, while spinal contrast and thoracic (chest) and abdominal CT usually use contrast medium—that is, injecting a dye like iodine to help tell different structures apart. Iodine has a high atomic number, so it absorbs lots of radiation, which shows up in the test by making the vessels opaque.

In small animals, CT or MRI are most commonly used to diagnose diseases of the brain, spine, nasal and sinus cavities, and middle ear, says Dr. Jones. Less commonly, they are used to detect muscle or skeletal diseases, respiratory problems, and masses on the heart. "A quick rule of thumb is, if it moves, bleeds, or is made of bone, it is better imaged with CT," says Dr. Beth Paugh Partington, a radiologist at Louisiana State University. Innovations in MRI may make thoracic imaging easier in the near future, she adds. CT and MRI imaging are mostly available in veterinary schools and secondary private referral centers. Dr. Jones says CT scans typically cost from $100 to $400, and MRI scans range from $300 to $1,000.

CT uses an X-ray source and detector to take pictures of an object's internal structure from 180 to 360 different directions, and then "reconstructs" that object through computer projections. Because it takes only two seconds to scan each "slice," CT offers a more accurate picture of moving portions of the anatomy (i.e., in the chest/abdomen region moved by breathing and heartbeats) than MRI.

New and improved variations of the technology continue to appear. "Our spiral CT scanner is similar to other CT scanners except it's a very fast machine," says Dr. David Ruslander. "We can do a CT scan on an entire dog or cat patient within ten minutes, and the detail is much better than with other CT scanners." This state-of-the-art CT scanner is equal to or better than the technology currently available at many human hospitals, he says. The machine also includes "pinpoint technology," which directs a needle to remove samples for tests, or to inject medicine into a specific area.

One of the newest and most exciting innovations, the CT-guided brain biopsy system, offers an extremely accurate noninvasive method to diagnose brain disorders. "We use the CT scanner to guide a special needle into the center of any type of brain lesion or mass," says Dr. LeCouteur. The needle extracts small pieces of tissue that can be examined under the microscope, cultured, or tested in other ways. "The real beauty is, the whole procedure can be done through a little hole that's only an eighth-inch in diameter, and a skin incision that's only about three-quarters of an inch long."

Magnetic resonance imaging (MRI) was first used to scan a human wrist in 1977, and the first human brain MRI followed in 1979. Veterinary MRIs weren't used experimentally until the late 1980s. Today, the technology has become increasingly available, and more and more applications are being discovered.

MRI images are similar to CT, but unlike X-rays, they involve no radiation. The image comes from recording radio-frequency signals given off by the tissue. "The principle of MRI is that a spinning asymmetrical charge has a magnetic field associated with it," says Dr. Partington. While CT and X-ray imaging refer to "density" of tissues—bone shows up white on the images because it's denser than muscle tissue—that does not apply with MRI. Instead, body structures are defined by degrees of signal intensity. Each part of the body, from bone to skin or lungs, gives off a different amount of radio frequency. On an MRI image, areas that are bright or white have increased signal intensity, and those that are dark or black have decreased intensity, says Dr. Partington. The MRI offers unsurpassed soft-tissue detail. "There currently is nothing better for brain, spinal cord, and joint imaging," she says. However, while CT takes seconds to scan a "slice," the MRI takes three to seven minutes per imaging sequence, and may take a total of forty-five to sixty minutes for a complete scan.

Testing for Animal Poisons

The API 2000 LC/MS/MS system (liquid chromatography tandem mass spectrometry) offers the "gold standard" in forensic testing for the presence of chemicals like poisons in tissue or other body samples. The $200,000 machine is part of the Cornell University College of Veterinary Medicine's Analytical Toxicology Laboratory, and is on indefinite loan to Cornell from PE Biosystems of Foster City, California. The LC (liquid chromatography) component of the technology separates chemicals in a complex mixture, like a blood or urine sample. Then these separated chemicals are transferred to the tandem mass spectrometer for detection and confirmation. The new system also incorporates an "ion spray" LC/MS interface developed by Cornell that allows even hard-to-identify chemicals to be distinguished.

Endoscopy

The term "endoscopy" means "looking within," and the technique is another noninvasive way to examine the internal structures of a pet's body. The respiratory, digestive, and urinary tracts, as well as some areas of the abdomen or chest, can be viewed with an endoscope.

Before the method became available, the stomach and intestines were most commonly examined by having the pet swallow a contrast medium, like barium, and then taking pictures with X-rays. Exploratory surgery was often the only way to gain a true diagnosis.

Today, the fiberoptic endoscope and the video chip endoscope produce images of the internal body structures on a viewing screen, via a tiny incision. The fiberoptic endoscope is the older of the two, and can transmit light (including lasers) through optical fibers. The newer video chip cameras are less fragile, produce better images, and tend to be more versatile. In either case, the veterinarian inserts the long tube of the endoscope into the appropriate part of the body and literally sees what's going on.

This tool also can be used to take tissue samples and perform biopsies from deep inside the body. In addition, the endoscope can be used to find and retrieve foreign objects such as inhaled grass seeds or swallowed toys that have lodged in the respiratory or digestive tract.

Arthroscopic procedures, long used in human and equine joint repair, are today used to help cats and dogs. The instruments are inserted into three small incisions, rather than requiring a large, invasive opening. The arthroscope contains a chip and a light, and an image of the joint is transmitted to a video screen. The veterinarian can view the joint and decide if there are lesions, loose fragments of cartilage, foreign bodies, or infection. All these procedures cause little trauma, so the pet has less pain and returns to normal much more quickly.

Fascinating Facts! An Inside View

The next evolution in endoscopic technology may do away with the long, flexible tube. An experimental model for humans employs a camera-containing capsule that, once swallowed, travels naturally through the digestive system, taking pictures along the way. The capsule is slightly larger than an antibiotic pill and covered with a nondigestible coating. One end of the capsule is clear—a window—to let light in, and holds a camera with a fixed, wide-angle lens powered by a tiny battery. Dr. Paul Swain of the Royal London Hospital directed the initial tests on the camera capsule, which eliminates the need for pushing wires and cables inside the body. Of course, the capsule cannot be guided, stopped, aimed, or backed up for another view, like current endoscopic tools.

Laser Technology

Medical lasers have been commonly used only since the early 1980s. "With veterinarians as well as physicians, the biomedical laser was a tool in search of application," says Dr. Kenneth E. Bartels, a professor of laser surgery at Oklahoma State University. "The laser advantage, basically, is that it will seal blood vessels, lymphatics, and nerve endings, so you don't have as much hemorrhage or as much inflammation or pain," he says. However, because surgical lasers use photothermal energy—heat—healing takes longer than an incision with a scalpel. But lasers are able to vaporize tissue in a very controlled and gentle way that offers a strong advantage.

Lasers are often used in dermatology and skin cancer therapies. Veterinary ophthalmologists have developed ways to treat glaucoma, or to use lasers to spot-weld retinal detachments back in place. In addition, laser energy can be shot through special fibers to reach deep within the body without requiring invasive surgery.

Although the carbon dioxide laser is quite common, varieties of special lasers such as the diode laser and the Nd:YAG laser (neodidium yutridium aluminum garnet laser) are also available. Each type uses a different wave length of energy, which is absorbed by tissue in different ways and offers specific benefits. For instance, a diode laser can be put through a silica fiber less than half a millimeter in diameter and two meters long and administered through an endoscope. "If you can see it through a scope, you can get a laser fiber to it," says Dr. Bartels.

Laser technology also helps diagnose illness. A new hematology (blood) analyzer at the University of Pennsylvania Veterinary Hospital uses light and lenses to magnify objects that cannot be seen with the naked eye. A blood sample passed through a stationary laser beam produces a "scatterplot" image that represents the size and complexity of the various blood cells. Lasers allow clinicians to distinguish among cell types by their size as well as their complexity. Various conditions produce characteristic scatterplots, so the clinician can tell if the pet is ill, under stress, or even receiving steroids.

Early on, veterinarians purchased laser units on the secondary market—that is, they bought equipment previously used for humans. "They were huge and very expensive, and a lot of them had to be water cooled. The first one in 1987 was about the size of a Volkswagen," says Dr. Bartels. Today, the price has come down, and the lasers themselves are better suited to veterinary practice. "Four years ago there were a couple dozen lasers out there in practices and academic institutions," he says. "Today there's probably more than 800. It's been an explosion." A number of companies, such as Luxar, Ceramoptic, Millennium Lasers, and Veterinary Alliance, now market lasers for veterinarians. Competition has dropped the cost of laser units from about $150,000 to $50,000 or less. Practitioners typically charge $25 to $125 for a laser procedure.

Modern Miracles: Eye-Opening Experience

Red's eyes began to water excessively, so Marilee Woodrow of Springfield, Oregon, thought the little Japanese Chin must have airborne allergies. Red had come from Japanese Chin Rescue the year before with a number of health problems that the organization had addressed one by one, before Marilee adopted Red. So when his weepy eyes didn't clear up, she had her veterinarian examine him.

Dr. Martha DeWees of the McKenzie Animal Clinic in Springfield discovered that Red had entropion, a congenital defect of the eyelids that causes them to turn inward so that the eyelashes abrade the eye with each blink. Red's entropion affected just the lower eyelids. "It was good timing that the veterinarians of the practice had just returned from a seminar on laser surgery the week before," says Marilee. Dr. DeWees offered to have Red's entropion corrected when the CO_2 laser equipment arrived at their office. Since Red was the first "demo dog," there would be no charge.

The laser surgery involves making a series of X-shaped laser cuts on the lower lid, and involves no stitches. The laser basically evaporates the tissue in the X pattern, which acts to gently pull the lower lid down and out to a normal configuration.

"Red came through with flying colors!" says Marilee. The very next day he seemed back to normal with no sign of discomfort or pain. "He's never been one to give kisses," says Marilee, "but that week, for the first time since he was rescued a year ago, he was feeling so much better, I got nose kisses and he gave my husband and me hand washings—quite a big step for him! We're so happy about that!"

Telemedicine

Remote-access diagnostic procedures were first pioneered in the late 1970s with the launching of Cardiopet by cardiologist Dr. Larry Tilley. Electrocardiography, a noninvasive diagnostic tool used to study the heart and its surrounding tissues, previously was available only at veterinary teaching hospitals and at a handful of referral practices. Cardiopet made it possible to perform electrocardiography over the telephone in the convenience of a local veterinary clinic. Information translated via the phone was evaluated by the machine at the other end, and the printout was faxed back to the originating veterinarian along with an evaluation by the cardiologist. "This innovation drastically expanded the diagnostic field of cardiac medicine in pets," says Dr. Tilley.

Today, telemedicine has expanded with the aid of the Internet and digital cameras, says ophthalmologist Dr. Paul A. Gerding, Jr., at the University of Illinois. Diagnostic images like X-rays have been sent digitally for a number of years. But now even standard photographs of a dog or cat patient can travel from computer to computer, no matter where the pet is.

"Obviously you can't do cataract surgery over the Internet," says Dr. Gerding, "but we can now help a private practitioner to diagnose a problem in the eye by examining the image sent."

ADVANCES IN HEALTH MAINTENANCE

Veterinarians agree that preventing disease is much easier than curing it. Important advances have come from the science of nutrition. Dogs and cats require a balanced diet to keep them healthy, and their needs change as they age or become ill. Today, nutrition is an essential part of the total care package.

Nutrition

Good health starts with what the pet puts in his mouth. On the simplest level, a "good diet" builds a healthy pet, while a bad one can cause disease in virtually every body system. Food scientists today create diets that not only support "normal" health but also compensate for disease by using nutrition to manipulate the way the body works. For instance, skin function in allergic pets can be enhanced with omega-3 fatty acids. The immune system can be boosted with neutraceuticals—food supplements that have a medical action. Some types of diabetes can be controlled by delaying digestion with a high-fiber diet.

New research has now shifted from providing minimum nutritional requirements to developing optimum nutrition.

Many studies are now being conducted at the cellular level, to better understand what cells do or don't do in certain situations. "For the better part of the 1900s, animal research has been at the cellular and biochemical level," says Dr. Steven Hannah, a food scientist at Ralston Purina. At this level, nutrition scientists recognize that animals don't just need food, they need protein. And they don't just need protein, they need twenty amino acids, the chief building blocks of protein, in the right ratio to each other.

Once we understand what occurs on the molecular level, science must then come full circle. Researchers must pull back from the microscope and apply their new knowledge to the whole animal. "Because no system in the body, no cell in the body, works in isolation of the rest of the body," says Dr. Hannah.

New research will allow diets to be designed on a case-by-case basis, keyed to the individual pet's unique needs, environment, and predispositions. Even the desires of the owner will be considered.

Once scientists formulate a new nutritional theory, they seek to test it on real cats and dogs through "feeding trial studies."

"In the past, most food studies were conducted on reproducing females because that was felt to be the most demanding life stage," says Dr. Dan Carey of the Iams Company. These studies defined success by measuring weight gain and growth rate. "Of course, that cut out all the males and spayed females," says Dr. Carey, "so although the studies were important for that time, they didn't address a large percentage of the pet population."

Modern feeding trials designed for various groups of animals offer a clearer picture of what's needed when, for instance, a dog or cat grows old or has a weight problem. "We've found that a higher protein level in foods is extremely important, especially in old animals," says Dr. Grace Long, a veterinarian at Ralston Purina. "In order to support a healthy immune system, and keep things working right, older pets actually have a higher requirement for protein than a younger animal."

"Nutrition has directly improved pet health and enhanced longevity over the years by coming up with life-stage diets," says Dr. Korinn E. Saker, a nutritionist at Virginia-Maryland College. These diets address the needs of pets at various times during their lives, from "growth and reproduction" (puppy/kitten or pregnancy) to "maintenance" and "all life stages." In the past few years, diets designed for "senior" pets also have appeared. "That's heightened pet owner awareness to the actual nutrient needs of their pets," says Dr. Saker.

As with their own foods, owners read pet food labels to make informed decisions about what to feed their dogs and cats. But pet food labels are complicated and hard to understand. This continues to be an area of concern for owners and veterinarians alike. "The pet food labels today are often very misleading," says Dr. Nancy Irlbeck, a nutritionist at Colorado State. "They are truthful, very correct, and within the letter of the law—but creatively misleading," she says. Discussions to resolve these concerns currently involve academics, government regulators, veterinary associations, pet food company officials, and pet owners. It is hoped that simplifying labels will allow pet owners to more clearly understand what's in the food and make the best nutritional choices for their dogs and cats.

Besides overall improved nutrition, probably the biggest advance in nutrition has been the therapeutic diet, says Dr. David S. Bruyette, an internist in Los Angeles. A better understanding of the body's natural metabolic pathways—the way calcium and phosphorus work together at the molecular level, for instance—allows nutrition scientists to design diets that help the system maintain health and heal imbalances.

"We don't look at foods as drugs or cures," says Dr. Long. "They're just to help in the management of health conditions." Therapeutic diets are not used as a substitute for other treatments, but as an adjunct. They are truly therapeutic diets available only from veterinarians who determine which type of diet is most appropriate. Today, there are diets for kidney problems, and diets for diabetics designed to help regulate blood sugar. Other diets help manage cancer, liver disease, skin disease, digestive problems, pancreatitis, obesity, and even heart problems. "We're definitely fine-tuning animal requirements at the different physiological levels," says Dr. Irlbeck. "I think we'll see more and more of it as preventative and as treatment."

Of course, in order to benefit the dog or cat, the animal must eat the food. "We believe we can get the nutrition right on any of the diets, but it's a matter of developing diets that are palatable," says Dr. James H. Sokolowski, a veterinarian with Waltham USA. A battery of feeding trials are conducted to measure palatability—pet acceptance of the food—and digestibility, as well as effectiveness.

Prediction: Neutraceutical Help

"We'll better understand and use supplements, particularly antioxidants and oxidated stress-related supplements, for pets in different life stages," says Dr. Korinn Saker. "In the next five to ten years, I predict we'll have really useful products available that are used on a regular basis."

Vaccinations

Some of the most important medical achievements in the last century have occurred in the area of virology (study of viruses), resulting in treatments that prevent early death and allow cats and dogs to live longer, healthier lives. First came vaccinations for distemper and rabies, and then protection against feline upper respiratory viruses. Veterinary virologists identified a number of new diseases during the 1960s, including feline leukemia virus (FeLV) and feline infectious peritonitis (FIP). In 1967 Dr. William D. Hardy Jr. demonstrated that FeLV was contagious among cats, and that it was responsible for various cancers and other diseases. In 1978 canine parvovirus, a devastating and often fatal disease, was first recognized. In 1987 Dr. Niels Pedersen and his veterinary research group at University of California-Davis reported they'd isolated a feline immunodeficiency virus (FIV), similar to the human HIV or AIDS virus. More recently, researchers have identified a new virus in dogs similar to the feline leukemia virus. In many cases, tests that identify the presence of both infected and carrier animals have been developed alongside the discoveries of these emerging diseases.

The past decades have witnessed the development of highly reliable vaccinations. "The vaccines are very effective now, and we probably don't have to give them as frequently," says Dr. David S. Bruyette. For decades the policy has been to give every vaccine available every single year, but that's changing, says internist Dr. Dennis Macy. Today veterinarians recognize that pets should be vaccinated only against those agents for which they are at risk, and risk factors vary from pet to pet.

Part of the change in policy reflects concern that excessive vaccination may cause more problems in some pets than no vaccination at all, especially when given as "combination" shots. New recommendations include risk assessment to determine which vaccinations should be given as well as how often. "People should still bring pets in annually for an exam," says Dr. Macy, "and they probably should receive one or two vaccines each visit, but not seven or eight at once." Some of the new vaccines protect for three years or longer.

One hot-button issue concerns the form of the vaccine—"killed" products versus "modified live" vaccines. Vaccines work by prompting the immune system to create protective cells, such as antibodies in the bloodstream or other components at the cellular level (cell-mediated immunity). Modified live vaccines use the actual virus that's been inactivated so it stimulates immunity but reduces or eliminates the potential

to cause disease. But some diseases, such as rabies, can't be safely inactivated, and so a killed virus is used—the infectious portions of the virus
have been inactivated. Such killed vaccines need help stimulating immunity, though, so a component called an adjuvant is included that
helps the body recognize the antigen—the disease portion of the virus.

"We used to think killed products were safer, but to be effective you
have to have the adjuvant," says Dr. Macy. "An adjuvant is kind of the
Hamburger Helper of the vaccine world—it extends the antigen." But
killed products tend to enhance only one arm of the immune system,
antibody immunity. Even more problematic, the adjuvant has been
linked to a variety of life-threatening reactions in cats and dogs.

There are also inherent problems with modified live virus vaccines.
They are very good at stimulating both cell-mediated and antibody immunity. But modified live vaccines for rabies, feline leukemia virus, and
canine distemper can cause the disease they meant to prevent. "That's
very similar to what happened with polio in people," says Dr. Macy. "All
the cases of polio in the United States last year were vaccine-induced.
Some people's immune system cannot even handle the attenuation
[weakened form] of the virus that's contained within the vaccine. The
same thing occurs for canine distemper. So there has been a push
toward safer vaccines for both humans as well as veterinary medicine.
And that means the more genetically engineered products."

Genetically engineered vaccines are clearly safer than other vaccines. They are also more effective because they tend to enhance both
cell-mediated and antibody protection. Currently, these vaccines are
available for canine distemper and feline rabies.

ADVANCES IN MEDICATIONS

New medications are also used in wellness care, acute care, chronic
care, and behavior care. Some medicines are used for only a brief time
to reverse acute conditions. For instance, anemic dogs benefit from an
artificial blood transfusion when whole blood isn't available. Products to
prevent fleas and heartworms, on the other hand, have been designed
for lifelong use on dogs and cats, and are part of a general health maintenance program. Chronic care patients may require lifelong drug
therapy to control conditions such as epileptic seizures, thyroid imbalances, diabetes, or heart disease.

The last ten years have seen the advent of angiotension-converting-enzyme, or ACE, inhibitors, for treatment of heart diseases in pets. These drugs help prevent sodium and water retention (common in congestive heart failure), dilate the blood vessels to control blood pressure, increase heart output, and improve exercise tolerance. "Diuretics are still the mainstay of treating patients with heart failure, whether they be dogs or cats, but the ACE inhibitors have come along and helped us stabilize those patients," says Dr. Mark D. Kittleson, a cardiologist at the University of California-Davis. Diuretics relieve the fluid accumulation in the lungs and other tissues that accompanies heart failure.

Drugs not officially approved for animals but commonly used by people are often prescribed for dogs and cats. One example is cancer drugs—nearly all chemotherapy used to treat cancer in cats and dogs are human medicines. In order for the medicine to be approved for specific use in pets, the appropriate controlled studies must be performed—and that means lots of time and money, the lack of which delays and even prevents the use of potentially life-saving treatments. Therefore, the Animal Medicinal Drug Use Clarification Act provides for the legal off-label use under certain specific conditions. Off-label means treating pets with drugs that are not approved for that purpose, and legal only when done with the informed consent of the pet owner within a valid client/veterinarian/patient relationship. Two of the newest and most exciting areas of drug therapy for cats and dogs, which are often prescribed off-label, address behavior problems and pain management.

Pain Management

In the past, it was believed that cats and dogs didn't experience pain in the same way as people, and certainly not as intensely. Pets were rarely offered pain medication following medical procedures because veterinarians believed the discomfort would prevent the pet from reinjuring himself during the recovery period.

That theory has been turned upside down in the past five years. Today's thinking recognizes that dogs and cats do indeed feel as much pain as people—they simply don't express it in the same way. "We now realize that anesthesia and pain management is a more complicated process than just immobilizing the patient and creating an unconscious state with an anesthetic," says Dr. William Tranquilli, an anesthesiologist at the University of Illinois. Besides ethical considerations, alleviating pain has been shown to improve the rate of a pet's recovery.

Growing interest in veterinary pain management may prompt the creation of a new veterinary subspecialty in the future. To better understand the mechanisms of pain and how best to offer relief, Pfizer Animal Health, along with the University of Tennessee, University of Illinois, and Colorado State University, have created regional pain centers at their respective veterinary schools. The Companion Animal Pain Management Consortium, a combined effort launched in early 2001, supports research on key issues. "A coordinated effort will allow us to make faster progress with multicenter studies, and generate data quicker," says Dr. Tranquilli. The regional pain centers will also be a consulting resource for veterinarians across the country.

Owner Information Sheets

In April 2000, Pfizer Animal Health was the first animal health company to provide pet owners with medication information sheets written in an easy-to-understand format. They are similar to patient Prescribing Information Sheets commonly distributed with human pharmacy prescriptions, which were introduced in 1970 and became the standard for all human medications by 1995.

Owner Information Sheets provide a clear explanation of what the medication treats, how it should be given, common side effects and what to do if they occur, when to call the veterinarian, and where to find more information. Pfizer worked with the FDA to develop the information sheets with the goal of promoting the safe, effective use of products so pets receive the maximum benefit. The innovative sheets debuted with prescriptions of Rimadyl (carprofen), prescribed for the relief of arthritis pain in dogs. Pfizer plans to add Owner Information Sheets to their major animal pharmaceuticals in the future.

Compounding Pet Prescriptions

In the beginning the doctor wrote the prescription and the pharmacist prepared, or compounded, the medicine on an individual basis for the patient. Pharmacists kept all the necessary ingredients and mixed up the proper combinations on an as-needed basis. "Compounding is the foundation of pharmacy," says Alton Kanak, a Houston pharmacist, "but over the years, modernization has resulted in most medicines being manufactured." Mass production of pills, liquids, injections, salves, and ointments in a wide range of strengths has been driven by a demand for convenience, and this has changed the face of pharmacy. Today, the giant pharmaceutical companies provide the lion's share of prescription medications.

"A resurgence in compounding started about ten to fifteen years ago when [the medical community] found there was a void in specialized items that you couldn't get in manufactured products," says Kanak. "Veterinarians especially have a limited formulary of drugs made for animals in the dosage form and strength that they need," he adds. That means veterinarians must often scale down or up dosages from manufactured strengths, especially for the off-label use of human medicines. For instance, a cat dosage of a standard-size form might be an eighth of the pill, while a horse or giraffe dose could be several bottles of tablets. Also, pets that are already sick rarely benefit from the added stress of being force-fed pills or liquids they dislike. "Owners wonder if it's worth it to risk getting bitten, or putting the pet through so much," says Kanak. "And you don't always know if she really swallowed the pill."

The compounding pharmacist takes the veterinarian's prescription and creates the proper dose for the individual pet, often in a flavor or form—such as fish-flavored paste—that the pet takes like a treat. The dose is made to fit the patient, rather than the patient made to fit an already-prepared dose.

Specialized equipment and access to the drug chemicals are required. "None of the chain pharmacy stores do compounding," says Kanak. "The specialty remains a very limited practice within the independent pharmacists."

Few pharmacists are equipped to compound prescriptions. Compounding is no longer taught in pharmacy school, and there are only a few major training centers in the United States. One of the largest is Professional Compounding Centers of America (PCCA), located in Houston. Another, National Association of Compounding Pharmacists, offers a three-day training period, access to all their formulas, and the opportunity to consult with their PhD researchers and pharmacists.

Today, you don't need to have a compounding pharmacy in your city to benefit from the expertise. Most prescriptions can be filled with a phone call from the veterinarian and shipped directly to the pet owner. Standing orders for ongoing medication can be filled on a monthly basis, for convenience. "Controlled drugs require the pharmacist to have the original prescription in hand," says Kanak, "but we can fill the prescription on the basis of a faxed signed prescription as long as we receive the original in the mail."

Compounding pharmacies also fill prescriptions via the Internet, he says. Shipping takes one to two days, as requested.

Depending on the particular prescription, compounding may be more or less expensive than manufactured medicine, and offers options that otherwise are not available to veterinarians and their clients. "If an animal will be on the medicine for the rest of his life, compounding a large quantity cuts the price down drastically," says Kanak.

ADVANCES IN BEHAVIOR MEDICINE

Behavior drugs intended for human use have had a huge impact in veterinary behavior medicine. Behavior modification and training, and the science behind them, remain relatively new, and reflect the modern acceptance of pets as part of the family.

"Thirty to forty years ago, we would never have known if pets had [behavior] problems because someone was always home, or the pet was out on the farm," says Dr. Karen Overall, a behaviorist at the University of Pennsylvania. "How would you know if your dog had separation anxiety if someone was always home?" Those animals that did cause problems were likely killed or dumped, she adds.

Today, pet owners are strongly motivated to solve a variety of behavior problems that have become evident in recent decades. When pets spent their lives outdoors, inappropriate elimination and clawing or chewing of furniture were not problems. But cats and dogs that spend the majority of their time at home alone while owners are at work can develop all kinds of destructive or self-damaging behaviors from boredom or stress. "We tend to see more problems associated with energetic dogs who get anxious or play too roughly because most people don't need the pet dog they have," says Dr. Overall. "I really don't need three Australian Shepherds, given that I have no sheep—so I have to try to meet their needs [in other ways]."

A groundswell of interest from pet owners and veterinarians alike has prompted more continuing education courses and behavior specialty programs. People now realize they need a diagnosis before they can treat a behavior issue, just as they need a diagnosis to treat a physical condition.

Part of this process, of course, is learning to recognize "normal" dog or cat behavior so the owner can spot a deviation from this norm. As with physical problems, behavior issues are best addressed early on. Delay only allows the problem to become entrenched. Veterinary behaviorists look at every angle; they may run diagnostic tests of the brain with CT, MRI, PET, or SPECT scans, or perform a blood chemistry analysis before designing a treatment plan.

Dr. Myrna M. Milani, a behaviorist and ethologist in New Hampshire, says that our thinking about behavior training has developed in tandem with new research on the brain over the last decade. "Prior to that time the feeling was you couldn't change the brain," she says. More recent studies have shown that the brain is really quite plastic. "Behavioral modification can rewire the brain," she says, "and positive and negative experiences can alter brain chemistry."

Dogs and cats that behave improperly often do so because the correct neural pathways in the brain have not been created. These pathways are created by experience and practice, so new routes can be forged—new behaviors learned—even later in life. In other words, with the proper knowledge, you *can* teach an old dog (or cat) new tricks.

Behavior Drugs

Drug therapy has proved to be extremely helpful in changing poor behavior. In some cases these drugs are the only way to help the pet. More often, though, drugs are used in combination with more traditional behavior-modification techniques. They are meant for temporary help rather than a "magic bullet" that cures a given problem. Unfortunately, the very success of these drug treatments makes it tempting to just give pills to the dog or cat rather than work to help the pet overcome the problem that prompted the bad behavior in the first place.

"People have the sense that a little pill or injection works like a magic wand that makes a behavior problem go away," says Dr. Ian Dunbar, a dog trainer and behaviorist in California. He says some people view their pets as a kind of VCR, available for companionship and entertainment whenever they want. When they don't want it, they want the dog to "turn off."

Dr. Overall agrees that relying solely on drugs to cure bad behavior is a mistake. "There is, unfortunately, no substitute for hard work that will involve the entire family in a behavior-modification plan," she says. "Clients and practitioners seeking 'quick-fix' solutions will doubtless be disappointed." Misuse of a drug won't cure the problem, and may blunt or mask the behavior without changing the cause. It's like giving an itchy pet cortisone shots to stop the scratching, and ignoring the fact that she's crawling with fleas.

Getting owners involved is important for another reason. Pets cannot tell us when they begin to suffer from the side effects of medication, Dr. Overall explains, so owners must be aware of potential problems and stay alert for changes that indicate an adverse reaction. Most behavioral drugs are metabolized through the kidneys and/or liver, and can have side effects that impact the heart. Other drugs may interact with behavior medications, too. So dogs and cats must have a full physical evaluation (as well as behavioral workup) before drugs are given, to ensure that their liver, kidneys, heart, or other body systems are able to handle the medication. Many behavioral drugs must be used for six to eight weeks before any change can be expected. In certain conditions, the pet may require medication for the rest of his life.

Only a few drugs used to treat pet behavior problems have actually been tested and licensed for use in dogs and cats—and therefore, care must be taken. How new drugs are used makes the difference between successful treatment and resorting to the tried-and-true, and final, option of euthanasia.

What About Hyperactivity?

True hyperactivity is rare in cats and dogs, but in some cases, stimulant drugs can be effective. This "paradoxical effect" means that the stimulant actually calms down the true hyperactive patient, whereas it would do the opposite in a clinically normal animal. Drugs like Ritalin, often prescribed for hyperactivity in human patients, haven't been widely used in pets, but may offer hope. If the drug makes the hyperactivity worse, though, that means the pet wasn't truly hyperactive and would be best treated with behavior therapy, a new diet, and increased exercise.

ADVANCES IN SURGERY AND REHAB

Chronic illness, injury, or sudden problems such as kidney failure require state-of-the-art technology and skill. Today, surgeons can fix a wide range of orthopedic (bone) problems that cause crippling disorders. They can also repair malformed organs and return pets to full health.

But surgery is only the first step toward a complete cure. Physical therapy and rehabilitation now routinely follow surgery, and return convalescing pets to full mobility more quickly than in the past. Now surgical practices often include swimming pools, massage therapists, and rehabilitation experts for their pet patients.

Surgery

The aging population of pets has meant an increase in many medical conditions that are common to geriatric cats and dogs. The advent of advanced tests has also increased the number of diagnoses.

Over half of veterinary surgery cases are orthopedic procedures, dealing with bones and joints, says Dr. A. D. Elkins. Most are done on dogs, who seem to have more injuries and congenital orthopedic problems than cats. Years ago, dogs were put down because hip problems left them in such pain. Today, those dogs benefit from hip and knee reconstructions, hip replacements, and ligament repair.

Dr. Elkins says surgical techniques and information change so quickly that the specialized surgeons have begun to subspecialize. "There's a fellow in Houston who only does hip replacements, and we have people who do almost nothing but arthroscopic procedures," he says. "We used to stay fifteen to twenty years behind the human health care professionals, but that's not the case anymore. We're able to scope their abdomens; noninvasive surgeries can be done; tumors can be removed; we even do spays through the laproscope."

Veterinarians have performed open-heart operations ever since Dr. George Eyster at Michigan State began experimenting with the procedure in the late 1970s. Since that time techniques have been greatly refined and improved, and are now performed with a high degree of success in dogs. Open-heart surgery remains limited to only two veterinary centers in the country—Colorado State since 1993 and University of Pennsylvania since 1999. "We do approximately one case a month, and we're hoping to increase that, because the need out there potentially is tremendous," says Dr. E. Christopher Orton, a surgeon at Colorado State. He is very selective in choosing dogs that qualify, and there has been up to a four-month wait to be accepted.

"We're struggling to find good treatment options for some [types of] heart disease," says Dr. Daniel Brockman, a surgeon at University of Pennsylvania. "For example, heart valve replacement is commonplace in people with leaking heart valves. And leaking heart valves are very common in small animals, especially very small dogs." Unfortunately, tiny dogs don't do well on the heart-lung bypass machine that pumps and oxygenates their blood while the heart is stopped. Therefore, they are not good candidates for valve replacement. "That's a huge population of patients that could potentially benefit from having open-heart surgical procedures done for whom we haven't worked out the best operation," he says.

Surgery isn't limited to orthopedics or the heart. "We do many other things in neurology and neurosurgery these days," says Dr. Richard A. LeCouteur. Neurosurgery covers a wide range of procedures, from operating on spinal cord tumors and slipped disks to taking biopsies of muscle to diagnose disease. For instance, nerve conduction velocity (NCV) studies, long an integral part of a human neurological evaluation, are now also used with cats and dogs. Under anesthesia, small electric needle electrodes applied to the nerve being studied prompts an impulse from the muscle or nerve, and the reaction is measured and recorded. In people, NCV measures are routinely used to evaluate carpal tunnel syndrome, nerve injuries, and neuromuscular diseases among others. The same applies to dogs and cats, although humans typically don't require anesthesia. However, Dr. Anne M. Sylvestre of the Ontario Veterinary College at the University of Guelph has completed a Morris Animal Foundation study that shows noninvasive electrodes instead of the invasive needles can be successfully used while the pet is awake. That eliminates the added stress of anesthesia on the already sick pet.

Reconstructive surgeries, from skin grafts to dental procedures, are now possible for pets with traumatic injuries. "In the springtime when kids hit balls with bats, the dog tries to grab the ball out of the air and gets hit in the head with the bat," says Dr. Paul Orsini, a surgeon and dentist at the University of Pennsylvania. "You get broken teeth, broken bones of the face, or a broken jaw." Reconstruction of the jaw, as in people, requires screws and plates, along with intra-oral appliances similar to orthodontics, to fix the teeth together and stabilize bone fractures.

One of the most amazing surgical treatments now available in veterinary medicine is organ transplantation. "The first kidney transplantation program was pioneered at the University of California-Davis around 1987," says Dr. Lillian Aronson, a surgeon at the University of Pennsylvania. When she started her residency there, transplantation was still rarely done, but complications were beginning to be understood and reduced, and the success rate began to improve.

In 1993, a transplant case was performed about once every two or three months. "By the end of my residency we were doing a case a week with a waiting list," says Dr. Aronson. "At that time Davis was the major center for transplantation for the veterinary patient, so we had feline patients from all over the country, and even outside of the country." Once Dr. Aronson's residency was complete, the University of Pennsylvania expressed interest in becoming the "East Coast center" for transplantation. Dr. Aronson helped launch the program in 1997, and today a number of veterinary teaching hospitals and a few referral practices offer transplantation.

Modern Miracles:
Fritz's Broken Heart

More than a decade ago, a veterinarian listening to Fritz's heart heard a murmur. "I didn't think much about it, and just let it go," says Fritz's owner, Bill Luedeke of New Paltz, New York. But then, in January 1999 at the age of thirteen, the tricolor Beagle developed heart failure. At the dog's advanced age, Bill was told, not much could be done other than keep Fritz comfortable for as long as possible.

Then an intern working at Bill's veterinary clinic mentioned he'd heard about an innovative heart surgery at Colorado State University that might help Fritz. Dr. Joel Edwards, a cardiologist at the Albany County Veterinary Clinic, ran some tests on Fritz at the request of Dr. E. Christopher Orton, at CSU. The results were forwarded to Dr. Orton to diagnose Fritz's condition and to determine if the dog was healthy enough to be a candidate for the program.

"In Fritz's case everything seemed to be fine," says Bill. Everything, that is, except his heart. The tests showed that unless something was done, Fritz would not survive another month. Bill called Dr. Orton and made an appointment.

Bill immediately drove Fritz out to Colorado—he was too sick to travel by plane in the cargo hold. "The trip took thirty hours," he says. Fritz remained with Dr. Orton for three weeks following his heart-valve transplant, in which a mechanical valve replaced the wornout valve that was failing. Bill stayed with Fritz for the first week through the February 2 surgery, but then had to go back home and wait for the doctor's call.

"They said if Fritz made it through the first couple of days after the surgery, everything would be okay," he recalls.

"The people at Colorado State couldn't do enough for Fritz and me," says Bill. "Everyone was wonderful, and I thought I was in the Twilight Zone, they were so nice. Dr. Orton is a phenomenal man."

Once the artificial valve was in place, Fritz made a full recovery. He'll need to take Coumadin, a drug that helps prevent blood clots from forming in his mechanical heart valve, for the rest of his life. "Sometimes the little stinker finds the pill and spits it out, so I have to outwit him," Bill says jokingly. Fritz's heart continues to be monitored by local veterinarians who report the dog's progress to Dr. Orton. "The local veterinarians are Dr. Orton's hands and eyes, since he can't be here," Bill explains.

The surgery turned back the clock for Fritz. Today the little dog acts like he's five or six years younger than his true age. The bill was $4,000 for the surgery, and around $7,200 total when the driving and plane expenses were added. Bill says he didn't think twice about the money. "It's what we do for our friends."

Physical Therapy

Performance horses have long benefited from physical therapy that helps them recover from injuries or surgical procedures. But not until fifteen years ago did these techniques become a reality for dogs and cats. "In 1986, I began to notice there were many postsurgical recovery situations where the animal would do well, and then begin to falter or have problems during recovery," says Dr. Robert Taylor, a surgeon in Denver. "I became interested in providing postoperative rehabilitation and physical therapy to improve and augment the surgery we were performing on animals."

Today, many veterinary surgical centers include physical therapists on staff. "Physical therapy allows everybody to contribute to the ultimate success of the animal's life," says Dr. Taylor. "Owners become involved in some of the rehabilitation, so they feel more connected and feel like they're part of the solution. And the animals benefit from the added attention and enhanced quality of life—it's another part of the bonding experience."

Many of the same techniques created for human athletes have been adapted to dogs and cats. Massage and muscle stretching, muscle stimulation with E-Stim (electrostimulation), or treadmills and whirlpools are available. Swimming is often used to rehab dogs, and specialized heated pools with adjustable jets create a resistance against which the pet swims to help speed recovery.

One of the newest developments in rehab is the underwater treadmill, says Dr. Darryl Millis, a surgeon at the University of Tennessee. Many dogs feel severe pain for several weeks following surgery and refuse to swim because it hurts too much. Even water-loving dogs tend to be fearful of water in the veterinarian's office. They thrash so much they're in danger of hurting themselves. "But with the underwater treadmill, you just open up the door, and they walk into an empty holding tank that looks kind of like an aquarium," says Dr. Millis. "You seal the door and pump the water in. The water rises slowly underneath their feet and they're much less fearful. It provides an opportunity to begin using the limb in a buoyant situation, so they're not bearing as much weight on the joints or their limbs." The water, warmed to 85 to 90 degrees, soothes sore muscles, and walking on the underwater treadmill doesn't force them to stay afloat. "It's a little bit lower impact exercise than swimming," says Dr. Millis. "They just walk very slowly initially and build up pretty rapidly." The therapist controls the amount of water—up to four feet deep—and the speed at which the treadmill runs.

The University of Tennessee unit, the first of its kind, is based on a human unit used by the UT football team. There are windows on all sides so the therapist can watch the dog's body in action—and so the dog can see where he's going.

The underwater treadmill helps dogs recover much more quickly than older methods, says Dr. Millis. "As an example, a client brought in her dog with a pretty bad forelimb lameness, and as a surgeon, I said the dog needed surgery. But the owner wanted to exhaust all conservative options before doing any surgery." He agreed to try the dog on the underwater treadmill, thinking it wouldn't hurt the dog and surgery could be done later. He thought they'd wasted their time. But after two to three weeks of three times weekly underwater treadmill work, the dog dramatically improved. Dr. Millis documented the improvement by trotting the dog across a force-plate in the floor hooked up to a computer that measured the weight the dog placed on each leg. "Just one session increased weight bearing about ten percent," says Dr. Millis. To put this in perspective, studies of pain relief medication hope for an average of 5 percent improvement. "That dog now works forty minutes twice a day, two days a week, on the underwater treadmill—and he still hasn't had surgery," concludes Dr. Millis.

The therapy has been so successful that nine more underwater treadmill units have been ordered by veterinary facilities, and Dr. Millis and Dr. Taylor predict they will soon become a mainstay of veterinary rehabilitation.

Modern Miracles:
Wolfie Wins Again

When Wolfie first came to live with Ann Buckley of North Attleborough, Massachusetts, he wanted nothing to do with her. For her part, after living with "perfect little Casey," Ann says the comparison between the two Brussels Griffon dogs made Wolfie's standoffish behavior seem even worse. The black Casey and red-gold Wolfie took about six months to adjust to each other, and then they became inseparable, says Ann.

After Wolfie became infatuated with obedience training, he fell in love with Ann. "The transformation was amazing," she says, and their partnership turned Wolfie—short for Wiffelwood's Sundemon—into both an American and Canadian obedience champion. The little dog even made it into the Dog Hall of Fame in Chicago. "From then on, he was never more than about twelve inches away from me, wherever I went," says Ann.

One Friday night several years ago, when he was nearly six years old and in peak competitive condition, Wolfie suddenly screamed and keeled over. Ann hadn't a clue what was wrong. He'd been fine during their training sessions that week, and had been playing happily with Casey only minutes before. Now suddenly, Wolfie was paralyzed from the waist down. He was so scared, he dragged himself halfway under the bed before Ann could reach him.

For the first time since she could remember, Ann separated the two dogs as she rushed Wolfie to the emergency room. "He only had deep pain sensation left, and couldn't control his bladder," she says. "I held him up under his tummy, and his poor back legs swung back and forth like Jell-O."

The veterinarians told Ann that he was in such bad shape, euthanasia was a consideration. Another option was to give the dog cortisone for the inflammation and hope for the best. "The only other choice was back surgery, the laminectomy," says Ann, "so I rushed him to Tufts University, fifty miles away. I drove in the dead of winter to get him there."

Wolfie received a series of tests, including a myelogram, in which dye injected in the spinal cord contrasts on an X-ray to reveal the injury. But the myelogram was inconclusive, and not even back surgery, performed soon afterward, revealed what was wrong. "They don't know what caused the injury," says Ann, "but said it could have been a spinal infarction—kind of a blood clot [that] lodges and settles there." The laminectomy and tests cost about $1,800.

Wolfie spent several days in the hospital, and when he came home, he was vomiting and had diarrhea. Ann took him back to the local veterinarian, but fluids injected beneath the skin to counteract the dehydration didn't seem to help. She rushed him back to Tufts. "They told me if I'd gotten there an hour later, he wouldn't have made it," says Ann. Wolfie was bleeding internally. Tests showed he was having an acute pancreatitis attack, a condition often associated with fatty foods. His kidney function was at about 20 percent, he had liver problems, blood clotting problems, and was severely dehydrated.

Wolfie wavered between life and death for the next twelve days, kept alive only by tubes running in and out of his tiny body. "On Friday, I almost decided it was time to say goodbye," says Ann. "I didn't want him to go through more pain." But he'd received a transfusion of plasma, a component of blood, just the night before, and the veterinarian suggested Ann wait another few days to see if he'd respond.

On Sunday, Ann was amazed to find that he was like a whole new dog. He wanted his dumbbell and his Hall's cough drops (his favorites), whereas before he wouldn't even look at them. "I knew then that he had it made," says Ann.

Wolfie came home with Ann the following Wednesday. After a slight relapse with pancreatitis three weeks later, he went on a special bland diet and has had no other problems. He required physical therapy to regain the full use of his rear legs after the back surgery. "He'd lie on his back while I peddled his legs like riding a bike, six to seven times a day," says Ann. "For a month or two, we regularly visited a friend's swimming pool. We put his front feet up on a kick board while he swam by kicking his back legs. It took a while, but now if you throw a ball for him to chase, you can't tell anything's wrong," she says, though his back end does sway when he stands still and his rear right side is a bit weaker than the other. "His rehab brought us even closer," she says.

Wolfie's injury and illness forced his early retirement from competitive obedience, but Ann keeps him occupied with walks and games. She credits the little dog's winning attitude, and the strong bond between them, for pulling him through. "This guy loves life more than any dog I've ever known," she says. The total bill for Wolfie's health crises ran in excess of $6,000. "I took out a five-year loan and am still paying it off," says Ann, "but it was well worth it."

Today, Wolfie has the energy of a dog half his age. "We have had so much fun these past four years—he loves to make people laugh!" Ann says. "He was my diamond dog in the rough, but he's shined for years. And I thank God every single day for allowing this miracle boy to live."

A WINNING COMBINATION

Today, veterinary medicine embraces a wide range of disciplines. Many are brand new. Others are old therapies with new twists. Veterinary specialties expand the quality of care available to pets and their owners. The general veterinarian, veterinary specialists, and the latest medical techniques combine to make an unbeatable team that maintains and restores cat and dog health better than ever before.

CHAPTER 3

Ethics and New Century Medicine

There have always been strong ethical concerns about pet medical care. The complicated issue raises questions on many levels, and there are no easy answers. Pet lovers often line up on opposite sides of the fence to passionately argue their opinions. The argument becomes even more heated when medical care goes beyond the basics.

Most ethical questions tend not to have one right answer. They fall into a gray area where pro and con arguments must be weighed and the greater good–lesser evil chosen. What is right for one pet may be wrong for another.

Countless new therapies, diagnostic procedures, and treatments are touted to provide great benefits for cats and dogs. Yet it often takes years for researchers to prove the effectiveness of a new approach. Innovative techniques that are not yet universally accepted may be worth a try, however, when traditional methods have either failed or hold little promise.

Even more important than the possibility of prolonging life is the quality-of-life issue. A longer life filled with pain, stress, or discomfort isn't necessarily a better life.

When evaluating potential benefits, pet owners must ask themselves and their veterinarian if the procedure will enhance the quality of the pet's life, and secondarily, if that life will be prolonged. Treatments should enhance rather than detract from the cat or dog's enjoyment of simple day-to-day pleasures, says Dr. David S. Bruyette, an internist in

Los Angeles. Part of this evaluation should include whether or not the pet—or the owner—will be able to tolerate what could potentially become lifelong daily medication. For example, organ-donor recipients must take daily antirejection drugs for the rest of their lives. A cat that becomes hysterical when pilled would likely be a poor candidate for a transplant simply because of the emotional stress of receiving the medication.

Also, critical judgment is needed when evaluating the potential benefits of any new procedure, drug, or therapy. Getting FDA approval for drugs can be enormously expensive, and often cats and dogs are offered the benefits before the new medication has finished FDA trials. Clinical trials funded or sponsored by universities, pharmaceutical companies, or health research foundations review the research proposals and require some sort of proof of potential benefit prior to endorsing them. Don't hesitate to ask about the studies of any treatment being considered for your pet.

"Some people like to make a splash, and there's just a lot of hand waving about potential benefits, but not proof," says Dr. Gail Smith, an orthopedic surgeon at the University of Pennsylvania. "There are some studies being done now to show that the claims that were made fifteen years ago are not really valid." Dr. Smith believes veterinarians should look more at past records to determine what should be done in the future. "I'm not saying you should suffer inexorably waiting for the proof," he says, "but you have to know that some things can cause you harm. Just like in human medicine, don't hesitate to get another opinion."

THE BOND

Many ethical questions about pets would never come up if not for the strong bond we share with our dogs and cats. Once a pet becomes a "family member," she is no longer a nameless, faceless piece of property that can be easily replaced if care becomes too expensive or time-consuming. "One of the characteristics of domestication is the ability to have relationships with species other than your own," says Dr. Myrna M. Milani, an ethologist practicing in New Hampshire. "Humans are the most domesticated species out there, so it's only natural we would do this. To say that it is aberrant for us to want to have this relationship is like saying it's aberrant for us to be human—that's what makes us human."

Some people are amazed that anybody would waste their time or money on "just a dog" or "just a cat." Nearly every pet lover has at some point been advised by others to abandon their misguided attachment to their pets, and instead champion a worthier cause—such as starving children or the environment.

Yet studies of the human-animal bond have shown that children who learn empathy toward animals tend to feel it toward people, too. They recognize that "different" isn't "wrong." Learning to treat a dog like a dog and a cat like a cat, recognizing that each species has its own physical and behavioral needs, and that animals are not little fur-covered humanoids, goes a long way toward developing a recognition and tolerance for all creatures that are different, including different people.

Behaviorists speculate that just as puppies and kittens have a socialization period during which they "learn" to accept other species, humans also have a similar window of opportunity. The pathways in the brain for various functions are forged early in life. Early positive contact with pets forms the necessary brain circuitry to "turn on" the switch that makes it possible for a special connection with an animal. Miss that window of opportunity, and the door slams shut, says Dr. Milani. The "pet potential" probably exists in everyone, but not everybody develops the ability to connect with animals.

"In domestic cats and dogs, it's seven to twelve weeks, and I think in people it's very young, too," says Dr. Milani. People who miss that opportunity as young children can learn as they grow older, but may never have that deep sense of "oneness" with animals.

Dr. Leo K. Bustad was one of the earliest to recognize the benefits of the human-animal bond. More than twenty years ago, he helped establish the Delta Society, an organization dedicated to celebrating and promoting pet-people partnerships, including training and certification of a variety of service animals that benefit human health. Dr. Ian Dunbar, a behaviorist in Berkeley, California, believes that Dr. Bustad's vision has had a huge impact on how we train, care for, and interact with animals, and even on how people treat each other. Through the 1980s Delta funded more than $300,000 of research on the dynamic between humans and animals. Due in large part to these efforts, federal laws have been passed protecting the relationship between pets and their elderly or disabled owners, or families residing in public housing. Additionally, state regulations barring animals from health-care facilities are being loosened to allow animal-assisted activity and therapy programs.

The wonderful work done by dogs and cats that act as surrogate eyes, ears, or hands for their disabled human partners has long been recognized. Dogs and cats have always assisted people in a wide range of capacities, as herders, guardians, and hunters. Today's service animals are following in that tradition, with a different work assignment. For example, modern cats and dogs learn to "alert" their owners—that is, give a warning of impending medical events such as seizures and migraines—so they have time to seek help. Pets can detect changes in their owner's breathing or heart rate, allowing them to help head off blackouts, and even heart attacks. Some dogs have "sniffed out" skin cancer. Apparently cancer smells different than other kinds of skin sores, and more than once, a pet's fanatical sniffing has pestered his owner into seeking medical care. Such pet-human partnerships are most effective when they acquire a deep emotional attachment.

People with stress-related conditions such as high blood pressure can especially benefit from a pet. Petting a cat or dog, or simply having one in the same room, lowers blood pressure. People living with pets visit the doctor less often, and recover more quickly when they are ill. Heart attack victims living with pets statistically survive longer than those without pets.

People who are partnered with service animals, senior citizens living with cats or dogs, and children suffering from a variety of problems who have a pet all benefit both physically and mentally from this "pet effect." Pets help people connect with other people. An elderly person stays more involved in life in order to care for a beloved pet, when she might not make the effort for herself. Pets help normalize relationships. Disabled children who withdraw from peers often respond when a pet becomes the focus and bridge between them and other kids. Injury victims who are reluctant to endure painful rehabilitation will push themselves when therapy involves throwing a ball for a dog. For many people, a connection with pets is vital. "It's what we need to feel whole," says Dr. Milani. That's resulted in a sea change in nursing and rehab facilities that now routinely incorporate pets into therapy.

This new relationship has greatly influenced animal training philosophy as well. Attempts are being made to establish standards in an industry in which anyone can claim to be an expert. In March 1998 the Task Force on Humane Dog Training was formed. It involves trainers, veterinarians, applied animal behaviorists, animal welfare experts, and veterinary behaviorists in the effort to create guidelines for humane dog training. Later that same year, following the Association of Pet Dog Trainers' annual meeting, an assembly nearly twice the size of the task force met to create the first draft of the guidelines. The final standards will be available soon.

Modern Miracles: A Pocketful of Love

DebbieLynn barely survived a horrible car accident, and today lives in Beverly Hills, California, suffering from side effects caused by drugs intended to keep her alive. She lives with a kaleidoscope of disabling health problems, from migraines and secondary hemophilia that could cause her to bleed to death, to heart irregularities that leave her breathless. She's lost most of her hearing and has no peripheral vision left. Despite these problems, DebbieLynn runs her own business and has a full, rewarding life because of her partnership with a two-pound pocket-size furry angel named Cosette.

After her accident and recovery, DebbieLynn began to search for a canine companion that would fit her new lifestyle and health limitations. Her lungs are down to 22 percent capacity, so the doctors wanted a dog that wouldn't shed. Plus, the dog needed to be tiny, two and a half pounds or less. It took her eighteen months to find the perfect Yorkshire Terrier.

Cosette arrived in December 1996. "She started trying to help me, and I wasn't sure exactly what she was telling me," says DebbieLynn. The doctor suggested she have Cosette trained and certified as a service dog. That way she could accompany DebbieLynn everywhere, even to the hospital. Delta Society recommended a trainer, and after four months the little dog was certified. "Cosette had such a thirst for knowledge, she kept wanting to learn more and retained everything she was taught," says DebbieLynn.

Today, Cosette alerts DebbieLynn to a migraine about seven minutes before it hits, as well as to changes in her heart rate so she can take medicine and head off fainting spells from lack of oxygen. "I've not blacked out since she's been alerting me," she says. Cosette also acts as a hearing-alert dog and tells her when something or someone approaches from her peripheral blind spots. And if DebbieLynn is bleeding, Cosette knows how to find the pressure point, apply pressure, and stop the bleeding.

Cosette, who turned four years old in August 2000, has improved DebbieLynn's quality of life in countless ways. Cosette even inspired DebbieLynn to create two e-commerce businesses that cater to pet lovers—Cosette's Closet and Cosette's Choice. "She has saved my life nine times by dialing 911," she says. "I can't imagine how I ever got by without her."

WHEN THE BOND BREAKS:
DEALING WITH MISBEHAVIOR

Treating the root of behavior problems has become both an economic and an ethical issue for veterinarians. Bites and other injuries from pets are estimated to cost as much as $25 million per year. Insurance premiums that cover dog bites alone total more than $1 billion annually. Animal welfare organizations estimate that between 15 million and 20 million pet dogs and cats are put down each year for behavior problems. That number doesn't include the pets put to sleep in private veterinary practices; an estimated 15 percent of pets seen by veterinarians are put down for behavior problems.

Experts believe this epidemic can be stemmed only by rethinking behavior issues and making them an intrinsic part of routine veterinary care. "Behavioral medicine provides the clinician and practitioner with the opportunity to be more than an executioner," says Dr. Karen Overall, a behaviorist at the University of Pennsylvania.

Dog Training

Prior to the advent of behaviorists, dealing with behavior problems fell mostly to dog trainers, many of whom had learned their trade while training dogs for the military of the 1940s and 1950s. The military used a classical conditioning model: dogs were taught to associate punishment with undesirable behavior and rewards (or cessation of punishment) with positive performance, until obeying a command became almost instinctual. For instance, Pavlov used classical conditioning to train dogs to associate the ringing of a bell with food. It was no longer a choice—the dogs simply reacted to the trigger by salivating at the ringing tone.

Military dog training was based on the notion that the dog is your adversary in the training field, and you must dominate him before he dominates you. The training process became an extremely rigorous test of temperament, very physical, almost brutal. "The idea was to make sure poor temperament would show up in early training rather than on the battlefield or in the trenches," says behaviorist Dr. Ian Dunbar. "So if they're going to break, break them when it's not important."

Those that didn't break became useful work animals for the military, protecting and guarding property or prisoners, tracking and rescuing soldiers, attacking or capturing the enemy—even carrying messages behind enemy lines. Military dogs parachuted into battle alongside soldiers, and fought to the death to protect their handlers. Trained dogs obeyed commands without question at all times, especially during the bombs and bullets of combat, or they risked both their own and soldiers' lives.

"These methods applied to pet dog training, of course, are totally unsuitable," Dr. Dunbar adds. "I think that was the lowest point in dog training history."

Applied animal behavior emerged as an independent discipline in the 1960s, but not until the 1970s did animal behaviorists, pet therapists, and behavior consultants become popular. The theory of operant conditioning and reward training put forth by Leon Whitney and Ed Beckman set the stage for an evolution in dog training. Operant conditioning deals with relationships among stimuli, responses, and consequences—the dog learns that what he does is critical to what happens next.

The traditional coercion methods relied on waiting for the dog to make a mistake, then using leash-jerk corrections and physically positioning the dog. With the new protocol, the dog was encouraged to want to perform the task on his own.

Dr. Dunbar urges owners to see pet dog training from the dog's point of view, and to make it fun by using food as lures and rewards. "Training should be efficient, effective, easy, and enjoyable, or pet owners and the dogs won't do it," he says. He considers pet dog training to be a completely different field from training for professional field trials and competition work. "The training of pet dogs encompasses not just teaching basic manners—come, sit, stand, roll over, walk on leash—but a major part includes the prevention and treatment of behavior and temperament problems."

In 1994, Dr. Dunbar founded the Association of Pet Dog Trainers (APDT) to educate trainers and dog owners, offer networking among member trainers, and encourage the use of positive reinforcement training methods. The Association has grown to over 3,000 members in the United States, and similar organizations have been established around the world. APDT also seeks to establish standards and professional level certification for pet dog trainers.

Some of the newest training tools reflect this evolution in training philosophy. The "Halti" and the "Gentle Leader" head halters offer much better alternatives to the cinch-type choke or correction collars that can injure a pet if used incorrectly. "These head collars work to prevent and help fix many behavior problems, and the Halti is dirt cheap," says Dr. Overall. Gentle Leader costs more at $30 but includes a great deal of informational and instructional material that helps with behavior training. The halter fits over the dog's face and, with gentle guidance, gets even giant-size dogs to go where they're guided—no jerking necessary.

The more traditional slip or "choke" collars must be fitted appropriately and used correctly. A quick jerk-release directs the dog's actions. But if fitted wrong, the collar won't release the pressure, so a pet owner can easily hurt the dog by accident. Toy dog breeds are particularly prone to collapsing tracheas and can be permanently damaged by a jerk to the neck.

Electronic collars—those that deliver a remote-controlled low-impulse shock to correct poor behavior—are even more controversial. Many ethicists object to their use altogether, and even proponents agree that only professional trainers are qualified to use electronic training tools.

Other training techniques teach pets to recognize a desired behavior by linking the action to appropriately timed verbal praise, sound signals such as a clicker training tool, or "cookie" (food) rewards. Whether you use a head halter, a clicker or verbal command, or cookie power, the major part of training involves teaching the dog *to want to comply*. " 'If you sit, Fido, I'll open the door.' Or 'If you sit, I'll put your leash on.' 'If you sit, I'll throw the tennis ball,' " says Dr. Dunbar, "so then the dog says, 'I love this sitting thing!' " Dr. Dunbar says teaching the dog the meaning of the word "sit" is only 5 percent of the training; 95 percent of training teaches the dog, "Why do it?"

"Training is a way the two of you learn to dance together in a very individual and exquisite choreography," Dr. Dunbar adds. "You learn to lead and follow each other's lead—and you don't invite someone to dance by jerking on their necklace or necktie!"

Prediction: Self-Training Pets

In the next decade there will be a tremendous revolution in "auto-shaping," says Dr. Dunbar. Rather than coercing the animal to perform, or punishing him for bad behavior, trainers can "shape" desirable actions by rewarding the pet when he naturally performs them. The dog sits and is rewarded, and learns that he can make the trainer reward him by performing that "good" behavior. That knowledge shapes a natural behavior into one the dog wants to do, so he sits when the doorbell rings instead of barking and running around like crazy. This method requires a knowledgeable trainer and can be time-consuming and labor-intensive.

Instead, computerized errorless learning management systems may someday allow the dog to train himself, and eliminate annoying problems like house destruction, house soiling, and noisiness. "There will be no punishment in training whatsoever," says Dr. Dunbar. "No shock, no leash jerk, no shouting, no nastiness—just reward-based electronics." Veterinary clinics, humane societies, animal behaviorists, and dog trainers will likely have these autoshaping devices and set up centers where owners can bring pets, then come out with a trained dog. Dr. Dunbar is saddened by the trend, because it loses the human element. But he adds, "You really add efficiency and effectiveness, a tremendous asset when we're talking pet dog training."

When Training Fails

Dog trainers and handlers often consider deviation from their standard of "normal" behavior to be a product of the owner's mismanagement of the dog, i.e., King wasn't disciplined strongly enough or was corrected too strongly. Training certainly does affect how a pet behaves or misbehaves, and sound training practices offer good tools for managing and resolving these problems. But according to Dr. Overall, lack of proper training is not usually the primary reason why a dog or cat misbehaves. Most misbehavior is quite simply an abnormal response to everyday life, or a way for the pet to deal with an abnormal social system. Also, some pet behavior problems are rooted in abnormal brain chemistry. "Disorders of serotonin metabolism underlie many severe behavior problems," says Dr. Overall.

Because of the surge in interest, veterinarians are becoming much more precise in diagnosing and treating behavior problems, especially as practitioners of this relatively new field begin to define a common vocabulary. This helps behaviorists across the country remain "on the same page" when discussing cases. "Behavior can be both an event and a process," says Dr. Overall. You can't divorce a particular behavior from the external events or from the internal responses of the individual animal.

Behavioral problems are often caused by a combination of factors. Diagnosis and treatment are further complicated because cats and dogs cannot describe why they act out. Diagnosis becomes a matter of linking "probable" causes to a particular event associated with the behavior. A particular drug, for instance, might cause one dog to show signs of anxiety while another dog might not be affected at all. Growling isn't necessarily bad—for example, it can be normal while playing. Context is important in determining if the behavior is a problem or a normal reaction to the environment. Growling isn't a disease. It is a sign of a potential problem, just as diarrhea is a sign of a wide range of potential health issues.

So the veterinary behaviorist becomes in large part a "pet detective" who relies on a description of how the pet acts, the events surrounding the behavior, the way the pet owner reacts, and the pet's overall physical health. A true "behavior problem" is defined as one that has no known physical or physiological cause.

In many cases, the dog or cat behavior is entirely appropriate to the circumstances. The cat or dog gives fair warning, but we don't recognize the signals, and our subsequent reaction actually escalates the aggression or anxiety. For instance, staring at a dog or cat is considered a challenge and can aggravate behavior problems. A cat's flattened ears warn you to back off, or she'll claw or bite. And not all wagging tails are friendly—dogs may use fast, jerky, high-held wags to signal an imminent attack. Veterinary behaviorists can help owners learn to recognize dog and cat language and so avoid triggering inappropriate behaviors. They also can offer behavior modification programs that help pets learn to better handle events that potentially may prompt problems.

Psychoactive drugs can help treat pet behavioral problems, but Dr. Milani says they tend to treat the symptom, not the root cause. "If you don't make the [right] changes in the animal's environment or the relationship with the owner, they're going to be on the drugs for the rest of their life."

Many ethical concerns surround behavior care. What constitutes appropriate treatment? Who is qualified to treat the animal—a trainer, a behaviorist, a veterinarian? When and what kind of training tools are appropriate? And is drug therapy necessary, or used as an easy fix?

Behaviorists agree that a combination approach works best. Drugs should be merely one step in a well-thought-out program of modifying behavior, evaluating the pet-owner relationship, and enhancing the environment.

Modern Miracles:
Caesar Takes the Stage

Four years ago, Todd Bachl found the dog of his dreams in two-and-a half-year-old Caesar. "I'd always thought Aussies were cool, and my friend put me in touch with a rescue group where I found Caesar," he says. The two were soon fast friends. Todd had always enjoyed outdoor sports, and he looked forward to sharing his passion for sports with the red merle Australian Shepherd.

"About a month after I got him, I took Caesar along to watch a couple of friends play softball," says Todd. As they walked by the field, with Caesar on a leash beside him, Todd was amazed when the dog suddenly went nuts. It took several weeks for him to make the connection, but once he did, the problem was obvious: Caesar freaked at the sound of the bat striking the ball—whiffle ball, softball, or baseball, it didn't matter.

Todd was disappointed that Caesar couldn't share his passion for baseball, but he wasn't terribly concerned until that fall, when seasonal thunderstorms began to rumble. He soon discovered that thunderstorms set the dog off as well. Then, after they'd been together two or three months, the smoke alarm went off. Caesar got so scared that he urinated on Todd's couch. Todd felt he had to do something about Caesar's behavior.

Todd contacted local veterinarians and trainers near his Groton, Connecticut, home, and was advised the dog's problem stemmed from extrasensitive hearing. "So they had me break balloons—that didn't work," says Todd. "It just made him afraid of balloons, even when they don't pop." Finally he received a referral to Dr. Myrna Milani, a behaviorist in New Hampshire. In April 1999 they began consulting by e-mail and telephone. Their first phone conversation lasted two hours. Dr. Milani's first suggestion was to crate-train Caesar, and the second was to switch from using a choke collar to a Gentle Leader training halter. In different ways, both tools seemed to offer the dog the sense of security he lacked, and Caesar adapted very quickly. "He had to have been crated as a puppy, because I just open the door and say 'kennel time' and he goes in," says Todd.

Todd says Australian Shepherds tend to do best when they have a job to perform. "During a thunderstorm, Caesar didn't know what to do, and he'd try to climb me or destroy the house," he says. "But if you put him in a kennel, or on the Gentle Leader—or give him a Frisbee to carry around and make him work and think—then that takes his mind off the noise so he can't worry!"

Caesar even conquered his fear of the crack of the bat and noise of the crowd, after a friend suggested that Frisbee competition with the dog might be fun. "The first competition, Caesar had stage fright and ran," says Todd, "but now he knows he's the star and he works the crowd just like a spotlight switches on. We do Frisbee shows at a local baseball field. Just two years ago, Caesar couldn't be anywhere near the field!"

After fifty e-mails and a half-dozen phone consultations with Dr. Milani over a four-month period, Todd was satisfied that Caesar was 100 percent improved. Finally he met Dr. Milani for the first time. "We met and talked for about three hours one Saturday morning," he says. She was impressed with both Caesar's progress and Todd's commitment to the dog.

Todd can't say enough about the Gentle Leader and crate training. "Caesar is incredibly attached to me, and I work with him every day. We're inseparable and go everywhere together," he says. "He's not perfect with everything—fireworks are horrible. But he tries really hard."

ORGAN DONORS: A LOVING LEGACY

As organ and tissue transplants become part of veterinary medicine, ethical questions must be addressed. Among these is: Where do donors come from? In the case of kidney transplants, the answer is straightforward since donors have one kidney to spare. No pets are killed to harvest an organ and save another animal's life. In fact, because most donors are either laboratory animals or shelter rescues, part of the "deal" is that they are adopted by the owner of the recipient pet and get a permanent home.

Other organ transplants are fraught with ethical uncertainty. No veterinarian wants to sacrifice a healthy animal. Dr. Clare Gregory's team at UC Davis is attempting to use partial-liver transplants in dogs, which may allow both recipient and donor to live normally, since similar techniques have been used in humans. "I'd certainly be interested in doing a heart at some point," says Dr. Lillian Aronson, a surgeon at the University of Pennsylvania. "But we certainly wouldn't euthanize a patient to save another. It would have to be a situation where the owner said, I want my animal to help another animal."

Growing Organs

Scientists had previously grown patches of skin or cartilage, but entire organs were another matter until researchers led by human surgeon Dr. Anthony Atala, at Children's Hospital and Harvard Medical School in Boston, rebuilt a bladder from cells grown in a laboratory. Since then, man-made bladders have been transplanted into six dogs, and Dr. Atala hopes the technique, once perfected, will help people who have bladder problems caused by cancer, injury, or birth defects. Current options involve using tissue from the intestines or stomach to reconstruct a patient's bladder, but those transplants create problems in the body's salt balance and can lead to cancer.

Dogs were chosen because their bladders are shaped similarly to people's. Researchers grew bladder cells in lab dishes from a tiny piece of bladder from each dog, and after four weeks there was enough to put together a new bladder. To give it the right structure, a hollow biodegradable fabric-mesh sphere was covered inside and out with the bladder cells, then bathed in special nutrient fluid maintained at body temperature. After transplantation, the new bladders gave the dogs normal function for the eleven-month period of the study.

Grafts and Tissue Donors

Other than kidney transplants, the only routinely performed donor procedures involve grafts. Here again, how the grafts are obtained raises questions. "We do not euthanize any dogs or cats to make them donors. Most of my animal donors come from research institutions," says Dr. Helen Newman-Gage, owner of Veterinary Transplant Services. These animals, already scheduled to be "sacrificed" at the end of the research trial, thus contribute in another positive way. Some institutions keep cats and dogs as laboratory models for the benefit of human research, says Dr. Newman-Gage. "When they have to euthanize an animal, if they allow us to recover the bone graphs, corneas, or other tissues, it helps them feel that their dog has not died completely in the service of humans, that it's gone also to help other animals."

Dr. Newman-Gage admits this can be a sticky ethical situation. "Some of our donors come from animal shelters, healthy dogs and cats that can't be adopted for one reason or another, and will be euthanized anyway. So after they're euthanized, sometimes they call us," she says. It helps the shelter workers to know that the animals haven't died in vain, and that in some small measure their lives are making a difference to other pets and their owners.

Dr. Newman-Gage would like to pursue the possibility of receiving donations directly from pet owners whose pets must be euthanized because of some trauma. She sees a correlation to human donation, an area where she worked for many years. "That would take a tragedy and turn it into something positive for not only the recipients but also the donors," she says. "It's the only tiny little bit of positive light in a very dark place for most families; it's such a sad time." Some pet owners might be comforted by the idea that a part of their beloved pet lives on in the recipient.

Modern Miracles:
Yogi's Gift of Life

Yogi, a six-year-old smoke Persian, had always been healthy, so when he began vomiting frequently and losing weight, Alan Mazzetti of Newark, Delaware, became concerned. In late 1997, Alan was told Yogi was in the end stages of renal (kidney) failure. "The type of kidney disease he had was terminal," says Alan. "They told me it couldn't be stopped or reversed." The veterinarian recommended a diet change to relieve the strain on his sick kidneys, supplements and medications, and fluids to keep him hydrated. "It worked for several months, but then he started to nose-dive," says Alan.

When Yogi was first diagnosed, Alan searched the Internet for everything he could find out about kidney disease. He found a website on feline renal failure that talked about transplantation—and listed the University of Pennsylvania program. "I never thought a transplant was realistic, or that anybody would actually do that for a pet," he says.

Alan learned the program was just getting off the ground, and there was a waiting list. "But by April I knew Yogi was on his way out, no matter what I did for him. He was in and out of the hospital, more and more miserable. I couldn't let him hang on, I had to do something."

He called the university and spoke with Dr. Aronson, who agreed to see Yogi. "He was near death when they got a hold of him," says Alan. "He was severely anemic, he was walking in circles." They gave him a blood transfusion, and he immediately perked up. Dr. Aronson explained that Yogi's odds weren't good because he was so sick. Plus, the surgery would cost $5,000. But Alan kept lobbying her to do the surgery. Dr. Aronson agreed to keep Yogi and run tests to see if he was a suitable candidate for a kidney transplant.

Finally his surgery was scheduled for June 3, 1998. In the meantime, Alan visited with the little orange longhaired cat named Fritz who would donate his kidney. Fritz would go home with Yogi and Alan, and have a home for life.

"The surgery took way longer than usual," says Alan. "I figured he had died, and I was vowing to never be religious again." Yogi had some internal bleeding during recovery and required a blood transfusion, which delayed his recovery, but otherwise he was fine.

Within several days of the surgery, Fritz came home and fit right into the family. "You have to worry a little bit with a cat who's spent his whole life in a cage," he says, "but Fritz is very sweet and has a great personality, and gets along with everybody."

They kept Yogi an extra week to be sure he was okay, and then he came home on June 29. The surgery, tests, and hospitalization cost $7,000. "I put down $1,000, then paid off the bill over time," says Alan. "It was worth it, because Yogi's been home and he's been fine ever since."

Yogi must take cyclosporin and prednisone, antirejection drugs, every twelve hours for the rest of his life. The medication and blood tests to monitor his kidneys cost about $400 a month. But Dr. Aronson told Alan that as long as he gets the medication, Yogi can live out a normal lifespan, so he's careful to be very vigilant.

"When he was sick, it was such a slow decline I didn't really notice until he was really, really sick," says Alan. "Now he's more active and more robust than I remember him being since he was a kitten. He's totally healthy in every measurable way."

WHAT PRICE HEALTH

It is that mystical, unbreakable bond more than anything else that prompts the cat or dog owner to pay dearly, and without hesitation, to save their pet's life or make it more comfortable. Some people who love pets never question this reflex while others believe that spending a small (or large!) fortune on the family pet is a poor ethical choice.

Cost is a factor for routine pet care, and specialized treatments are even more pricey. "For instance, chemotherapy drugs are the same drugs used in people, so we pay the same price," says Dr. William G. Brewer, Jr., an internist at Auburn University.

How much is too much? $500? $5,000?

How do you budget love?

No one would argue that a choice between funding health care for human family members should have priority over pets. Yet pet lovers are often offered helpful advice on "better ways" to spend those funds so they won't throw money away on their cat or dog. After all, they're told, it's "just a dog." Or they point out that the cat was a stray, it's not like she's an expensive show cat—and they can always get another one.

Nonsense! People rarely suggest that we should skip that dinner out, or the weekend at the lake, and spend the money on a worthier cause. And no one suggests we should "replace" a human family member who grows infirm. In the past, pet lovers often had to deal with amazed disbelief or even anger from those who were unable to understand their devotion to their furred family members. Today people tend to be more tolerant of how others may choose to spend their affection and discretionary funds. "There's a lot of disposable income," says Dr. Kenneth E. Bartels, a professor of laser surgery at Oklahoma State University. "People have a right to spend it how they want—whether they spend it on golf or on their cat."

Pet lovers today must ensure that their choices to offer beyond-the-basics care are based on their own individual sense of what's right and wrong for them and their pet. "It's terribly important for people who love animals to know that advanced care options exist. They are possible," says Dr. Richard A. LeCouteur, a neurologist at the University of California-Davis. "People can make for their pets whichever decision they wish, but they first of all have to be informed of the possibilities."

More than cost, the most important ethical consideration involves quality of life. "It isn't worth it if they're going to be sick or if the treatment makes [the pet] more uncomfortable," says Dr. Maura O'Brien, a surgeon in Los Angeles. "You don't want them to live longer if they'll be in pain. That's not worth it." The ultimate goal is that treatment helps the pet maintain a happy, enjoyable relationship with her owner and continues to be able to do "normal" pet things at home.

Pet Insurance

A heart-wrenching dilemma arises when treatment is possible, but the owner can't afford the expense. Clinical trials and experimental treatments at many research institutions are priced at half or less of the actual cost to the facility; a few are funded by grants or subsidized by the university, and are free. Treatment that is not experimental, though, can run many hundreds of dollars—for radiation treatments for cancer, for example—and up to several thousand dollars for involved treatments that include complicated surgery or diagnostic tests.

Thankfully, most university veterinary hospitals and specialty practices sympathize with pet lovers—they truly want what's best for the pet, too—and make every effort to arrange reasonable payment plans. Although the cost for advanced medical care for cats and dogs runs far less than comparable human treatments, funding necessary care can place a financial burden on a committed pet owner. According to the American Veterinary Medical Association, Americans spend over $12 billion annually on medical care for their pets. The figure doubles when general pet care costs for food, cat litter, and other nonmedical care items are added. Two-thirds of Americans take their pet to the veterinarian more often than they see their own doctor.

Wellness care for puppies and kittens, and chronic care for old age, represent the costliest health periods for pet owners, according to Sue Prelozni, vice president of business development for Pet Assure, a health care program for cats and dogs. "Humans have HMOs, but pet owners have nothing comparable," she says. Pet Assure, founded in 1996, offers a 25 percent discount on any veterinary care for pets—regardless of health status, age, or species. Ferrets, monkeys, and birds, as well as cats and dogs, benefit from the program.

The Pet Assure service is limited to about 2,100 participating veterinarians in 750 practices located across the country. Prelozni says, "We're the wellness factor. Enrollment helps reduce the cost of vaccines, spay/neuter surgeries, and other routine care. But for catastrophic coverage, pet owners would want to consider pet insurance."

In 1980, with the support of 750 independent veterinarians, Dr. Jack

Stephens founded the oldest and to-date largest health insurance provider for dogs and cats, Veterinary Pet Insurance (VPI). He believes insurance gives pets a better opportunity to get the service they need, by offering a way to pay a portion of the cost.

The insurance is much different from that for humans where the doctor typically files the insurance and receives the payment, and later bills the patient for the difference. With pet insurance, the owner pays the entire cost directly to the veterinarian, then the owner submits receipts to the insurance company to be reimbursed for a percentage of the expense. "We don't tell the veterinarian what to charge," says Dr. Stephens. "But we do have a fee schedule so it controls our cost." The percentage covered varies depending on the cost charged by the veterinarian. "Depending on your geographic location, there could be a 1,000 percent difference in fees from one veterinarian to another," says Dr. Stephens.

Since the first pet insurance company was launched, many more have come on the scene (for a complete list, see page 61). Dr. Stephens thinks that's a good thing. "It's all about choice," he says. "Consumers having more choices and more competitors validate the need for the service."

Premier Pet Insurance, one of the newest, was founded by Tom Kurtz in 1999 and has a current enrollment of about 12,000 pets. It adds another 1,000 a month. Pet Assure has an enrollment of about 50,000 pets. And in 2000, the grandfather of pet insurance, VPI, had an enrollment of 200,000 and was growing about 17 percent each year.

Some carriers are available only in certain states, but many are nationwide. Depending on the carrier, it may participate only with listed network veterinarians (similar to some human HMOs); others allow a choice of any practitioner. A variety of plans covers everything from puppy/kitten care to old pet conditions or even cancer. Typically, the basic plan covers accidents and illnesses. Routine care—vaccinations, spay/neuter surgeries, teeth cleaning, and flea treatments—requires additional coverage.

For example, VPI coverage addresses more than 6,400 health conditions, from dermatitis and vomiting to abscesses and ear infections, as well as diagnosis and treatment for liver disease, diabetes, pancreatitis, and cancer. Most preexisting conditions are disallowed, so you have to buy the insurance before the pet develops the problem. Some insurers decline to cover inherited conditions. In other words, if your dog is a

Pet Insurance Companies

Premiums, plans, and coverage varies:
contact the company for complete information.

American Pet Care Plan (1987)
7904 E Chaparral Rd., #470
Scottsdale, AZ 85250
800-755-7387
480-483-6245

Petshealth Insurance Agency
  Inc. (1997)
PO Box 2847
Canton, OH 44720
888-592-7387
330-492-3948

National Pet Club (1994)
7771 W. Oakland Park Blvd.,
  Ste. 141
Sunrise, FL 33351
800-PET-CLUB
954-781-0989
www.pet-club.com

Pet Protect Inc. (1997)
830 Anchor Road Dr.
Naples, FL 34103
888-738-7873
941-403-4100
www.pethealthinsure.com

Pet Assure (1996)
10 S. Morris St.
Dover, NJ 07801
888-789-7387
973-537-9889
www.petassure.com

Preferred PetHealth Plus Pet
  Owners Association (1995)
PO Box 636
New Haven, IN 46774
888-424-4644
219-749-4426
www.pethealthplus.com

Pet Care Plus (1997)
4270 Aloma Ave., Ste. 124-34J
Winter Park, FL 32792
800-645-2939
407-658-1961
www.petcare-plus.com

Premier Pet Insurance Group
  LLC (1999)
9541 Harding Blvd.
Wauwatosa, WI 53226
877-774-2273
414-453-7443
www.ppins.com

PetPlan Insurance (1989)
777 Portage Ave.
Winnipeg, MB R3G 0N3
  CANADA
905-279-7190
www.petplan.com

Veterinary Pet Insurance
  Co. (1982)
4175 E. La Palma Ave., Ste. 100
Anaheim, CA 92807
800-872-7387
714-996-2311
www.petinsurance.com

breed known to be predisposed to developing hip dysplasia or cataracts, those conditions would not be covered. Dr. Stephens says VPI has filed with state insurance boards for approval to offer an additional "hereditary coverage" that would address some forty-eight conditions. "Premium costs for certain breeds like a Bulldog would run higher than for a mixed breed animal," he says.

Unlike human insurance, pet insurance typically covers more experimental treatments for pets. "We don't get into whether it should or shouldn't be done," says Dr. Stephens. "If it's in the best interest of the pet and the veterinarian's doing it, we cover it." VPI has always covered "alternative" therapies like acupuncture, as long as treatment is prescribed and performed by a veterinarian. They've routinely paid for state-of-the-art procedures like kidney transplants, cataract surgeries, heart valve replacements, and limb sparing for bone cancer under their basic medical policy.

Industry estimates currently put coverage at about 5.3 percent of all pet households in the United States. That's changing as pet owners become more aware of the care that is available, and want to make more treatments possible for their pets. Owners today are often faced with life-and-death choices based on affordability. With insurance, those decisions are easier to make.

Modern Miracles:
Ronald McDonald House for Pets

In September 1999, Carmel Travis of Pullman, Washington, opened "The Lucas House," named in memory of her fifteen-year-old Sheltie. "It is a place for people to stay while their pets receive veterinary treatment at the Washington State University Veterinary Teaching Hospital," says Carmel. Pets may stay with their people at the Lucas House between treatments, and companion pets are also welcome to keep the owner and ill pet company.

"Staying at Lucas House helps reaffirm that what they are doing for their companion animal is very normal," says Carmel. Often pet owners must travel great distances to reach specialized care at a university facility. Renting a hotel room can be impersonal, and the hotel may not allow the owner to keep the ill pet with them. Lucas House provides a family-type setting where both the pet and the owner can relax and spend time together while receiving advanced medical care.

Carmel typically hosts one family at a time, and has had at least one guest every month since she opened. Rates start at $25 a night. The facility offers a four-room basement apartment with a private entry, located on three tree-filled acres. "It's a very peaceful, relaxing setting," says Carmel. Lucas House is the first veterinary-respite facility in the country— but it won't be the last.

Dr. Carolyn Henry, an assistant professor of oncology at the University of Missouri, has spearheaded an effort to create a similar respite facility as a part of the School of Veterinary Medicine. The idea was prompted in late 1999 while Dr. Henry was treating a very special dog. Barkley, a 155-pound Great Pyrenees, was receiving radiation for osteosarcoma (bone cancer) under her care. "His owner [Sally] drove him back and forth from Kansas City for his treatments," says Dr. Henry. "Then Sally broke her ankle and that made travel even more difficult for her."

It isn't unusual for people to travel long distances for therapy. During this same period, a client flew with her cat to the University of Missouri from Atlanta for treatment of a mouth cancer. "She didn't have a rental car to get back and forth from the hotel to the clinic, and the hotel didn't want her to keep the cat there," says Dr. Henry. "She was all by herself in the hotel in a strange city, while her cat was clear across town with us. I kept wishing we had somewhere nice these clients could stay so it wouldn't be such a hassle for them."

That December when, at eight years old, Barkley was finally released from his pain, his owner told Dr. Henry she wanted to do something as a tribute to her dog. About the same time Dr. Henry learned about Carmel Travis's place, Lucas House. The idea for the Barkley House was born.

"Everything just seemed to happen at once," says Dr. Henry. She talked to the dean and then with Sally and with other anonymous donors. So far they've collected $15,000 to get the project off the ground. The next step will be to find an architect to bring the vision to life. They hope to be operational by 2002.

Dr. Henry envisions a houselike building that contains five rooms to accommodate dog patients and one for cat patients, with a big common area like a family room. "I want to get folks out of the waiting room and into a more comfortable environment where they can talk with other people who are going through some of the same sorts of things that they are," she says. Veterinary students will also have the opportunity to talk with these clients and learn how to better help them. "I'd definitely see counseling and emotional support programs being included," says Dr. Henry.

The Barkley House will be built on university property within walking distance of the veterinary clinic. That will allow even critical patients to spend time with their owners, knowing that medical help is only minutes away. Dr. Henry says ill pets do better in the presence of their owner. "Owners do better as well," she adds. "In reality, a lot of my patients are terminal, and I don't see much sense in separating them from the owners. You want them to have more time with their family."

ANIMAL EXPERIMENTS

One of the most difficult ethical issues concerns the validity of testing new treatments on animal subjects. The mere idea raises the specter of ghoulish experimentation, bizarre trials with questionable applications, or the prospect of inflicting needless pain and suffering on innocent beasts.

The truth is more complicated. Different experimental models prompt minor to more serious concerns, depending on the circumstances, goals, and outcome of the experiment. One example is the dog and cat colonies maintained by many of the major pet food research facilities. The animals basically eat for a living, taste-testing countless new formulations. These animals tend to have a home for life at the facility, and a percentage of the animals are adopted as pets into family homes. Other facilities maintain colonies of animals for the sole purpose of perpetuating certain disease characteristics, for research purposes. However, the expense of dog and cat colonies in a laboratory setting makes this option uncommon.

Animal welfare proponents have raised the ethical yardstick, and through their questions, they have brought a new awareness to the scientific community. Animal experimentation saves both human and pet lives, no question. But researchers have become cognizant of the concern, and realize that if not legally, then at least morally, they will be held accountable for the way in which subject animals are handled.

PET RESEARCH

Researchers who investigate new treatments and diagnostic procedures may be boarded specialists in a private referral practice, at universities, or in commercial settings. In nearly all instances they find the dogs and cats for their studies through referring veterinarians. By the time the new advance is tested on a pet, most of the dangerous bugs have been worked out.

Early studies may be done on laboratory animals, or on a small number of dogs or cats obtained from kennels. "In veterinary medicine we just don't have the research dollars to fund huge colonies of dogs in laboratory settings," says Dr. Smith. "A dog costs $6.75 a day just to board in the laboratory, so if you have a hundred dogs and a two-year project, that's lots of money." In nutrition, funding often knocks the "little guys" out of the research arena, says Dr. Nancy Irlbeck, a clinical nutritionist at Colorado State University. "They don't have the financial backing to do the necessary studies and research that is needed for a new product," she says.

Researchers have learned that creating injuries or disease conditions in the laboratory answers many but not all their questions, and often does not apply in the real world. An artificially created injury, such as cutting the spinal cord, does not represent natural injuries where the cord is crushed. Laboratory animals infected with a virus won't react the same way as pets exposed to the neighbor's sick cat. Natural infection and injury pose different questions, such as how do natural immunity and exposure impact the disease's progression, whereas lab animals in a sterile environment won't have the same exposure challenges or immune status.

"You're really answering different questions," says Dr. Richard B. Borgens, a researcher at Purdue University. "In a guinea pig or a rat, you can ask very precise questions about how does this treatment affect the anatomy." But that fails to address real-world considerations. From these experimental models, researchers develop treatments to fix the problems they've artificially induced, but they may not have the same applications in a natural setting. And yes, these laboratory animals are typically sacrificed—killed and opened up for examination—at the end of the experimental trials to measure the success of the treatment.

Hurting these animals in order to determine a cure does raise major ethical concerns, but the methods used today allow researchers to minimize or even eliminate the kind of distress that laboratory animals typically experienced in the past. "The tools that we have to work with and the knowledge we have about pain have developed and evolved over these last twenty years," says Dr. William Tranquilli, an anesthesiologist at the University of Illinois. Today, more humane treatment has become the rule, not the exception, in animal experimentation.

The injuries or diseases that are induced in rats and guinea pigs are not the same as those that affect cats or dogs—or humans. So after first working out the details in laboratory animals, the procedures with the most promise are moved to dog and cat trials, says Dr. Borgens.

Once the research shows that the new procedure is safe and won't make patients worse, pet dogs and cats may be invited to participate. "You may not have efficacy nailed down, but you have safety, and you can anticipate and explain the risks to prospective clients," says Dr. Smith. "We have to get pet owners to understand, I think, that clinical trials are not Frankensteinian investigation."

Only pet dogs and cats with a naturally occurring disease or injury need apply. Veterinary researchers do not cause cancer in a cat or paralyze a dog in order to cure them. After all, these are beloved family members.

Dr. Barbara Kitchell, a cancer researcher at the University of Illinois, takes animals who have cancer, and offers them a chance to get well—or at least to feel better for as long as possible. "These pets are owned by people who care about them, and therefore, when the people sign a consent form to be part of the cancer research trial, everybody understands that it's a research trial," she says. Dr. Kitchell's team conducts "proof of principle" work that they hope will show how a particular concept will help in cancer therapy.

But using pets in research has limitations. "You really can't learn any more from that pet than you can from a human volunteer," says Dr. Borgens. "You can't sacrifice the animal at the end of the experiment—somebody owns him. And you can't do anatomy on that animal unless he dies of natural causes and he's donated to you."

Universities and referral clinics often send local veterinarians letters and announcements outlining the types of studies being conducted and the types of pet cases they seek. "The vast majority of our practice here are either people who have been referred in by other veterinarians or people who come here for a second opinion on their own," says Dr. Mark D. Kittleson, a cardiologist at the University of California-Davis.

Many veterinarians in private practice participate in cooperative studies with universities. It's a way for pets that live far from a university to benefit from experimental treatments, and it's a way for researchers to accrue more cases and gather more information.

Most research trials limit the numbers of pets that participate, and candidates must meet very specific criteria. The public information offices at the university or specialty college may post information about current studies on their websites. Researchers often speak at various continuing education seminars and veterinary conferences to spread the word among their colleagues.

Typically, an owner must sign an informed consent form for any type of investigational treatment that is open to pet cats and dogs. Particularly in cases of terminal illness—in which the pet will die anyway—such consent may seem unnecessary. But in veterinary medicine the intent to help and not hurt remains paramount.

How Studies Are Designed

"Most of the time, somebody gets an idea and then decides to pursue it," says Dr. Dale E. Bjorling, a professor of surgery at the University of Wisconsin. Other times, a study may be prompted by a medical research foundation. "For instance, the Morris Animal Foundation has funded a lot of the work that's been done at Purdue," says Dr. Borgens.

Clinical trials are designed to answer specific questions about the safety and effectiveness of a proposed idea. Although considered "experimental," such trials will have already been proven safe through preliminary tests, and are considered of potential benefit to the patient. In many cases, experimental treatments are reserved for pets whose condition has not been helped by standard treatments or who, for whatever reason, cannot undergo conventional therapy.

The quality of the investigation's design, the way data is collected and interpreted, and the numbers of patients that actually complete the trial all have an impact on the validity of the study. Clinical trials are required for FDA approval of new drugs. The trials may be performed by one person or school, or by a group of researchers in the pharmaceutical industry; by veterinary clinicians in private practice; by veterinary researchers at universities; and by federal regulators. These trials are performed in stages, and each typically takes months or years to complete. Studies are expensive to perform, and some promising treatments never receive sufficient funds to launch the necessary trials.

Clinical Trials, Phase by Phase

Phase I Clinical Trials are initial safety trials, often done on normal cats and dogs, or sometimes on critically ill pets (such as cancer patients) with little to lose.

Phase IIa Clinical Trials are pilot studies conducted after safety has been established in Phase I trials. Pilot studies generally use small, se-lected populations of pets—perhaps fifteen or twenty dogs—and are the first step in proving the effectiveness of the treatment.

Phase IIb Clinical Trials, sometimes called "pivotal trials," are con-trolled studies in a representative group of animals. "Control" refers to the percentage of animals that don't get the treatment at all, and receive only a placebo—a pretend treatment such as a sugar pill. The control group is then compared to treated animals to judge the true effect of the new therapy. In a double-blind trial, both the patients and the re-searcher are kept in the dark about who receives the placebo and who receives the experimental treatment.

Phase IIIa Clinical Trials come after safety and efficacy have been proven in preliminary studies. They are usually aimed at obtaining spe-cific information that the pharmaceutical company believes to be im-portant for drug labeling requirements. Once this trial is completed, a New Drug Application is submitted to the FDA for approval.

Phase IIIb Clinical Trials are done after the new protocol has been submitted for regulatory approval, but before approval has been granted, or the product offered to the public.

Phase IV Clinical Trials take place after the product is available for purchase, to determine even more details about safety and effective-ness, to compare the product with other drugs or treatments, to study possible interactions, and the like. This is when "adverse reactions" are identified and risks assessed.

Pets Helping People Helping Pets . . .

Research in human and pet medicine drive each other onward, and in the best instances they create mutual benefits. Sometimes the break-through comes on the human side and then is adapted to veterinary medicine. For instance, the limb-sparing technique used today for dogs was adapted from those devised for teenagers with osteosarcoma. Con-versely, Colorado State conducts research in the natural progression of this bone cancer in dogs, funded by the National Institutes of Health and the National Cancer Institute. Researchers hope to be able to apply what they learn about this canine bone cancer to humans with osteosar-coma, since the disease progresses similarly in both species.

Similarly, Dr. Debbie Knapp at Purdue has studied bladder cancer in dogs. She has found that a drug called piroxicam (Feldene) helps fight transitional cell carcinoma (cancer) in dogs. "Transitional cell carcinoma of the bladder in the dogs is very similar to the invasive form of the disease in people," says Dr. Ruthanne Chun, a cancer specialist at Kansas State University. As a direct result of Dr. Knapp's breakthrough with dogs, the drug has entered human trials at an Indiana hospital, says Dr. Chun.

Diagnostic tools can be equally effective in both humans and animals, says communications specialist Charles E. Powell. Washington State University Veterinary Teaching Hospital medical image center owns the only magnetic resonance imaging machine (MRI) that is built to accommodate large animals such as horses and cows. "It is of such quality that our machine is actually shared by the local human hospital," says Powell. "Every day human beings come to the veterinary hospital in Pullman, Washington, for diagnosis."

Patented Procedures?

Unlike human medicine, veterinary practice allows people to patent certain medical techniques. A well-known example in veterinary surgery involves the Tibial Plateau Leveling Osteotomy (TPLO) technique invented by Dr. Barclay Slocum, an orthopedic surgeon in Oregon. TPLO repairs cruciate ligament injury, a common problem in dogs, with a patented surgical restructuring of the knee.

Colleagues in orthopedic surgery agree that Dr. Slocum's innovations are often brilliant. However, some are concerned and frustrated by his tight control over the procedure, which disallows independent investigation of the technique. Dr. Slocum requires practitioners to pay to attend his course to learn the procedure, and they must agree to certain confidentiality conditions before they are granted a license that allows them to perform TPLO.

Show Me the Money

The fact that medical research on pets has applications in human medicine is a double-edged sword when it comes to funding and final development of the product. As more and more development companies merge, they become less willing to fund research on anything except products with the potential to earn millions of dollars for the company.

For example, Dr. Dennis Macy, an internist at Colorado State University, would like to be able to offer a plague vaccine for cats. "In terms of public health, it's far more serious in the Western U.S. than rabies, and yet there is no vaccine," he says. But the vaccine manufactures aren't interested because only 5 percent of the U.S. population would need the vaccine. "These conglomerate companies won't bother with a $5 million a year product," says Dr. Macy. "It must be $50 million a year or they won't bother to investigate or develop it. As a result of that management decision, the cats and dogs are the losers. And people are losers because 25 percent of human plague cases come from cats."

Most of the money for large-scale veterinary research is ultimately intended to benefit people, says Dr. Borgens. For example, enormous funding pours into research of the feline immunodeficiency virus (feline AIDS), a lentevirus very similar to HIV. "Most of the FIV vaccine stuff is being funded as a model for strategies that could be utilized in human vaccines, because we can do it more ethically in cats than in human models," says Dr. Macy. "Even though dogs and cats may be the 'guinea pigs' to get a particular drug or treatment approved, it ultimately will not be officially available for their use," says Dr. Steve Withrow, a cancer specialist at Colorado State University. The scientists don't go out and market the products and make them available—the development companies do. And their eyes remain on the market where the most money is to be made. "It's not worth their time and effort to go through veterinary licensing issues," says Dr. Withrow.

The process frustrates many dog and cat researchers, who see these promising therapies snatched away as soon as the study advances to human trials. If they're lucky, years down the road, after the human treatment has been approved and marketed, it can then be used again in pets—but only as an off-label product not officially sanctioned for veterinary use. Dr. Borgens suggests that veterinarians—and pet owners—need to put pressure on companies to make these treatments available to them. "They need to be part of the solution," he concludes.

MAKING ETHICAL CHOICES

Cutting-edge medicine makes modern miracles possible. But other considerations must be addressed as well. Can owners financially afford the treatment? How much is too much? If they have the money, can they provide the necessary home care that's needed for a complete recovery for as long as the animal needs it?

Owners often struggle to answer ethical questions about animal experiments that are distasteful to them, yet might save a stricken pet's life—or benefit human health in the future. When making decisions for our pets, there is no doubt that quality of life must be our first consideration. Where to draw that ethical line is a question that each owner must answer for his or her particular pet.

The bond we share today with our cats and dogs has no parallel in human history. We love our furry family members and want desperately to do right by them. When you make a decision from the heart that is based on the best information available to you at the time, it cannot be wrong.

CHAPTER 4

A Brave New World

Genetics, DNA, gene maps, gene therapy—it all sounds like science fiction, and altogether too complicated to understand. Nevertheless, molecular medicine has become a reality. Rather than searching for causes of diseases arising from outside of the body, the new medicine looks for causes of disease at the most basic level—in the genes. By understanding what happens in normal cats and dogs, and what can go wrong, researchers are discovering ways to prevent genetic diseases and cure existing ones.

Breeders of purebred dogs and cats have been doing this for years. Much of the groundwork for today's new century medicine can be found in the pedigrees—genetic records—of families of the various breeds. With each answer found, new questions arise, especially ethical considerations in this brave new world. For example, if you had the opportunity to clone your beloved pet, would you?

Today, the canine and feline genetic codes are being mapped. Causes of diseases have been found and tests developed that have literally wiped out certain health conditions in our pets. Questions are being answered that will improve the health of present-day pets and those yet to be born. It is an incredible time to be alive!

MOLECULAR MEDICINE

In the past, medicine treated people—and their dogs and cats—in a similar way. Signs or symptoms were evaluated, a diagnosis identified the problem, and then treatment addressed the cause—or more commonly, attempted to relieve the symptoms. Drugs and surgery were the mainstays of traditional medicine.

But there are several problems with this medical model. First, traditional diagnostic tools have not always been able to pinpoint the true cause of the problem. That may be because the signs of illness are vague, or are symptomatic of a wide range of problems, or the "bug" is so small or hidden that it's difficult to identify. The veterinarian has had to use her "best guess," which is often confirmed only when a particular treatment improves the animal's health. For example, in the past a dog that suddenly started limping, and had a history of exposure to ticks, might be given a round of antibiotics—and when he stopped limping within a day of this therapy, he would be considered "confirmed" for Lyme disease.

A more serious drawback of this model is that the dog or cat may be very ill or disabled by the time a pet owner notices the signs of illness and seeks a diagnosis. In the case of kidney disease, the organs must lose up to 70 percent of their function before symptoms develop—and once that happens, the damage can't be reversed, despite the best of care.

Molecular medicine creates a shift in the established paradigm with cures at the cellular level. Researchers predict that within a few years, therapeutic genes may replace vaccinations or antibiotic treatments that have been the mainstay of veterinary medicine in the last decade. This new century therapy can be used to treat inherited diseases such as hemophilia and acquired illnesses like diabetes.

Much has been made of the human genome project, and more than 4,000 genetic disorders have been identified in people. Despite this fact, molecular medicine will likely offer even more benefits to cats and dogs.

A genome is the complete set of coded genetic instructions for making any living thing, such as a person or pet. While all cats, for instance, have the same basic set of instructions, each cat has subtle variations that make her unique. The genome consists of long chains of the chemical DNA, coiled up into chromosome bundles inside virtually every cell of the body. Stretches of DNA, called genes, hold instructions that tell the body what to do. A defect in the genetic instructions can cause disease.

Inherited diseases can devastate entire breeds of dogs or cats, especially if a prize-winning breeding animal is a "silent" carrier of a problem gene. "In humans, diseases that are present in more than 1 percent of the population are considered to be frequent," says Dr. Urs Giger, a genetics researcher at the University of Pennsylvania. "We have identified many diseases in the purebred population that appear at a higher frequency than that." For instance, the gene that causes the bleeding disorder called Von Willebrand's disease is carried by 40 percent of Doberman Pinschers. New studies reveal that many less well-known diseases, such as canine cystinurea—a type of bladder stone—are also quite common.

Fascinating Facts! The DNA Fingerprint

Every living thing is made up of strands of genetic material called chromosomes that are strung together like beads on a thread. The order in which they are arranged determines whether the organism is a dog or cat, a Great Dane or Siamese, shorthaired or longhaired, curly-haired or bald. The chromosomes are built from DNA molecules that are formed in a coil-like ladder called a double helix. The exact way that these DNA molecules are arranged is unique in every living organism—that is, the "DNA fingerprint." Just as positive traits are passed on through the parents' genes, errors in the DNA fingerprint that cause diseases can also be inherited.

Dog and cat breeds are ideal for identifying genetic diseases because reputable breeders keep careful records of inheritance and track diseases that may affect their particular breed. They work with researchers to identify and record how often the problems appear within breeds. "Very often the family studies by the breeders will lead to a diagnosis and even a mode of inheritance," says Dr. Giger. Other times a protein, or "marker," that's associated with a disease may be identified. That can point out carrier animals even if the specific mutated gene has yet to be found.

As more and more diseases are discovered to have genetic components, steps are being taken to reduce or eliminate the frequency of a disease. Rather than wait for it to strike, new century medicine can actually predict the potential for disease by identifying the animals carrying the bad gene. This allows each new generation of a breed to further reduce the flaw in the family tree.

Researchers around the world continue to look for the genes responsible for a range of illnesses, from cancer and eye diseases to immune disorders and even behavior problems. For example, a test for progressive retinal atrophy (PRA), a degenerative eye disease very similar to retinitis pigmentosa in humans, was developed in 1995 for Irish Setters. Within two years, use of the PRA test by breeders eliminated the condition in Irish Setters. Molecular medicine can do that, and more.

Kinds of Inheritance

A dog or a cat is the sum of its genes (genotype) as it interacts in a specific environment. The pet's phenotype is the end result of both the genotype and the effects of the environment. There are several ways pets can inherit defective genes that cause diseases. "Most diseases are autosomal-recessively inherited," says Dr. Giger. (An autosome is a non-sex chromosome.) Other modes of inheritance can be sex-linked or polygenic.

- **Simple autosomal-recessive** means that the parents look normal but are carriers of the abnormal gene. Both parents must be carriers to pass the disease on to offspring.
- **Dominant autosomal-recessive** inheritance passes the disease to offspring when only one parent has the defective gene.
- **Sex-linked genes** can be either recessive or dominant, but are always expressed on the X-chromosome. Typically this makes females "silent" carriers, while males show the disease. Hemophilia is an example.
- **Polygenic inheritance traits** are controlled by many different genes that in combination cause the disease condition. In addition, environmental factors influence whether or not the trait is expressed. Hip dysplasia is an example.

Gene Testing for Disease

Research conducted at the Fred Hutchinson Cancer Research Center in Seattle, PennGen Laboratories, the Josephine Deubler Genetic Disease Testing Laboratory at the University of Pennsylvania, the James A. Baker Institute for Animal Health at Cornell University, Michigan State University, and elsewhere has identified the genes involved in many canine and feline inherited diseases. Researchers can often pinpoint the specific mutation and how or why it occurs. With this information, tests can be performed to identify animals suspected of carrying the trait.

Dr. Giger recommends that breeders should check for genetic diseases whenever they can. "Tests performed at the molecular level are extremely accurate and rather simple," he says. Tests currently are relatively expensive, though—anywhere from $50 to $250 depending on the test—but will become more economical as the technology becomes more widely available.

"Some tests are very straightforward," says Dr. Giger. "You can submit a sample for DNA testing in a particular breed, and you can clearly find out whether you're going to spread the disease gene further in the population or not." For instance, dogs can be screened for a wide range of genetic eye diseases through the Canine Eye Registration Foundation (CERF) at Purdue University. "That group has been working since the seventies," says Dr. J. Phillip Pickett, a veterinary ophthalmologist at Virginia-Maryland College of Veterinary Medicine.

When the specific gene is not known, "linkage tests" can still tell breeders a great deal. These tests look for a genetic marker that typically is found together with the diseased gene. Testing for this linkage lets you predict whether the animal has the disease, or is a carrier, even without knowing which gene it is. For instance, linkage tests are used to identify copper toxicosis (similar to Wilson's disease in people) in the Bedlington Terrier.

The final goal in molecular medicine is, of course, a cure. The best medicine for dogs and cats is simply to eliminate genetic disease entirely by selective breeding. But in some instances, such as canine hemophilia, gene therapy offers incredible cures. In simple terms, in gene therapy a "normal" gene is inserted into the defective gene to correct the disorder. Dog and cat health problems that gene therapy will help—and may cure—include: cancer, eye diseases, epilepsy, diabetes, and immune disorders. A recent issue of *Science* magazine described the first successful gene therapy "cure" in two human infants who were born with a rare immune defect called SCID—the "boy in the bubble" disease. The treatment completely restored the function of the babies' immune systems. Pets with similar immune disorders stand to benefit from the human research—and vice versa. "Most certainly gene therapy is the future—or actually, we can now say it is the present for some diseases," says Dr. Giger. "There will be much more to come."

Prediction: Picking Perfect Pets

"Within the next ten years, people will be able to take a puppy or kitten and do a blood test when they're eight to ten weeks old, and know whether or not they're a carrier or actually have a defect," says Dr. Pickett. That will not only allow breeders to avoid perpetuating a genetic problem, but also help owners to provide early preventative treatments. "We may be able to look at the genetic makeup of animals and formulate diets that prevent skeletal abnormalities or genetic-related diseases that we know occur in certain breeds," says Dr. Korinn E. Saker, a nutritionist at Virginia-Maryland College. Twenty to thirty years from now, the neighborhood grocery store may have a kiosk computer where you input specific information about your cat or dog's age, breed, lifestyle and other genetic characteristics, and the computer will spit out a unique diet designed just for that pet, says Dr. Steven Hannah, a food scientist in St. Louis.

Modern Miracles:
Max Foils Fate

Sue Shorey of Millington, Michigan, had always wanted a white cat, and four years ago she chose broad-nosed Max from a friend's barn cats. "He'd run and play, then his hind legs would go out behind him, and he'd have to stop and pick himself up," she says. "I thought it was just kitten play." Other than that, Max seemed healthy and loved to cuddle in Sue's arms.

Soon he developed dark "points" on his face, tail, and lower legs, and Sue realized her white kitten took after his Himalayan daddy. He was extremely loving and playful, but he began to cry when he was handled, and she feared he'd been hurt when a baby gate toppled onto him. Dr. Glen Darrow of Bavarian Veterinary Hospital in Frankenmuth, Michigan, took an X-ray that showed a slightly enlarged liver—and hip dysplasia. "The hip dysplasia seemed to be the reason that his legs didn't move like they should," says Sue.

Sue began to notice more and more problems. The beautiful seal-point baby slept with his hind legs so far forward they were nearly in his ears. His eyes looked cloudy, and his chest seemed sunken. "Finally he could only drag himself around, lost the use of both back legs, and was in terrible pain. My vet sent us to a neurosurgeon an hour and a half away."

Dr. Michael Wolf of Oakland Veterinary Referral Services in Bloomfield Hills, Michigan, did a spinal tap that ruled out infection, but the dye from a myelogram (a specialized X-ray) showed a number of spinal compressions that the neurosurgeon believed were causing Max's pain and loss of mobility. The surgeon was sure he could widen the canal and relieve the compression, says Sue, and because Max was six months old, most of his growing was done, so he should be fine after the surgery.

"It ended up costing a couple thousand dollars before we were through," says Sue. On top of that, the surgery was anything but straight-forward. "The surgeon found all these fibers that had multiplied and wrapped around the spinal column," she adds. The surgeon suspected that Max had a storage disease called MPS VI (mucopolysaccharidosis), a fatal genetic disorder. Within weeks of sending off blood and urine for tests at the University of Pennsylvania, Sue learned that Max's problems were all due to MPS.

The disorder results from an abnormality of a specific enzyme that affects the way carbohydrates are metabolized within the cells. Rather than having a normal recycling process, Max's body stored substances called mucopolysaccharides in the tissues. That caused a variety of problems. Max suffered from nearly all of them, including spinal compression, enlarged organs, cloudy corneas, depressed sternum (chest), hip dysplasia, nonretractable claws, head tremors—even his distinctive broad nose was due to the disease. Sue learned that the disease is carried primarily through the Siamese and Siamese-related lines. "Max was lucky he didn't also have mental retardation that some cats get," says Sue.

That was small consolation. She was told Max wouldn't get any better. Eventually severe arthritis from bone changes might cause the spinal column to actually detach from the hips. He was given less than a year to live.

Sue wasn't about to give up. Max was in the hospital for nearly two weeks and came home just in time for Christmas. "I turned my whole den into a padded playroom, so he could drag himself around," she says. He never once missed using his litter box, and as she massaged his legs to keep them flexible, she noticed he could paddle his rear feet but had no strength. "And one day my husband grabbed his tail and lifted him to his feet—and Max suddenly could walk again!" Slowly, Max taught himself to pull himself into a sitting position to eat and to walk a step or two for treats. "Max got so he'd run up to my husband, swing his butt around, and there'd be barely enough time to grab that tail before Max was off and running."

Carpeted ramps and floors help Max keep his balance, and he has no problems when he's outside hunting bugs. Prednisolone, a type of cortisone that reduces painful inflammation, keeps him moving more easily. There really is no standard treatment for MPS cats, since they all die or are put to sleep very early in life, but Sue's veterinarian supports her in trying to help improve Max's quality of life.

"He wasn't supposed to live twelve months," says Sue. "He wasn't supposed to ever walk again. But nobody ever told Max." He celebrated his fourth birthday on June 30, 2000.

Sue knows Max lives on borrowed time, so she cherishes him while she can. After he was diagnosed with the disease, she learned that children also suffer from this rare genetic defect. So she donated tissue and blood samples to the University of Pennsylvania and Michigan State University in the hope that they might help researchers learn more about preventing MPS. Today, a simple urine screening test for the detection of different types of MPS disorders is available (another form of the disease, MPS VII, can affect cats, mixed breed dogs, and German Shepherds). DNA tests are also available for specific types of the disease.

The X-rays, tests, and back surgery cost Sue well over $3,000, but she says she's never regretted the treatments. "He plays, purrs, washes, and teases other cats. This household revolves around Max—he is my constant companion."

Gene Maps

Researchers have identified more than 364 genetic disorders in dogs and more than 200 in cats, and more are being identified daily, says Dr. Stephen J. O'Brien, a geneticist at the National Cancer Institute in Maryland. Clinical research into feline genetics is relatively new compared to dog studies, but experts believe it's likely that the frequency of inherited problems will prove to be similar.

Creating purebred dogs and cats, however, does not cause genetic diseases, says Dr. Giger. The mutated genes are already there. In a larger population, though, they may be hidden or "silent." They are more likely to show up when a selected gene population, like a particular breed, is limited to a smaller group of related animals. That allows more of these hidden traits to be matched in a breeding with another animal that also has the problem gene, so that signs finally appear in the offspring.

Mapping the canine and feline genome has the same goal as the human genome project. The information will allow us to predict the potential for disease in pets. In dogs and cats, gene mapping and genetic tests go a step further, because breeders are able to plan matchmaking strategies to avoid known genetic problems.

A genetic marker is a short segment of DNA, and gene maps are composed of large numbers of genetic markers. Every individual has two copies of each chromosome, one inherited from each parent. Often there are differences between the two copies. Different copies of the same segment of DNA are called alleles. A genetic marker must have at least two alleles. When the frequency of the most common allele in a population is less than 95 percent, that marker is referred to as polymorphic. A gene map is made by examining the inheritance of alleles of polymorphic markers.

"Gene mapping is important when you don't know what gene mutated to cause the disease," says Dr. Giger. Instead of searching the entire DNA forest for a single gene, a map of existing markers, or links, shines a spotlight on a particular tree or branch, so scientists can narrow the focus. For instance, a researcher may not know the specific gene, but the map has identified a particular chromosome or group of genes that are likely to be involved.

To help the canine mapping process, the Canine Family DNA Distribution Center was established by Ralston Purina, in cooperation with the American Kennel Club Canine Health Foundation. DNA from eight canine families is stored at the center. From there it's distributed to scientists around the world.

Although the canine gene map seems to get more attention, the feline folks are ahead of them, says Dr. O'Brien. "We've got the entire genome pretty much covered with two categories of markers that we invented a few years ago. Our laboratory has been mapping the cat for the last eighteen years." Their work has reached a stage where the feline genome is second only to the human, mouse, and maybe rat genomes in terms of advances and usefulness. "We've got a good comparative idea of the segments that are homologous [parallel] to humans across the entire feline genome," says Dr. O'Brien. So far eighteen inherited canine and seven feline diseases have been attributed to genes homologous to human disease gene mutations.

"The dog people are still trying to figure out which linkage groups are on which chromosome," Dr. O'Brien says. Humans have twenty-three chromosomes, cats have nineteen, and dogs have thirty-nine.

Many are identical but are arranged in various combinations. The dog genome is more complicated to map because the chromosomes are "shuffled" much more extensively than the cat or human. "If you line up the cat and human genome, it only takes about ten scissors cuts to re-arrange the human into the cat or vice versa," says Dr. O'Brien. "But it takes maybe fifty to do the dog."

Many animal diseases serve as good models for diseases in people. "Dogs and cats have probably more medical surveillance than any other species except humans," says Dr. O'Brien. That's certainly an advantage when studying new medications and treatments. "If one does look at dogs and cats with some of the hereditary diseases, and develops new treatments for these genetic diseases, these are probably good models for people," says Dr. Giger.

Dog and cat gene maps will help not only pets, but also humans—and the human genome studies will in turn further help cats and dogs. "All the genetic work in any species will progress more rapidly because of work done on the human genome," says Dr. Steven Hannah, a food scientist at Ralston Purina. Genetic maps of cats and dogs can help scientists identify the genetic error that causes a problem and develop tests to screen for the disease. In pets, these tests will help to plan breeding programs to weed out a defect in a particular breed.

GENETIC ETHICS

In 1998, one year after Dolly the sheep was cloned, an anonymous donor gave $2.4 million to Texas A&M University to clone his dog Missy—and the Missyplicity Project was born. Backers have also funded cat-cloning research at A&M under the name "Operation Copy-cat." The idea of cloning pets generated so much interest that a number of new companies were formed, intent on preserving the DNA of client pets, with the hope of cloning a duplicate at some point in the future.

Harvesting the pet's DNA requires taking tissue samples in a proce-dure similar to a biopsy. The sample goes to a biotech lab for processing. Cells are grown, harvested, and frozen in liquid nitrogen for storage un-til they can be cloned safely and successfully. "Banking" the samples costs from $500 to $1,000, plus a monthly fee, depending on the biotech company. And the cloning procedure itself will (at least at first) cost up-ward of $25,000.

However, even if you could clone your pet, should you?

Geneticists caution that even once cloning is perfected, you can never get your old friend back. With any biological creature, environment and experience play huge roles in the formation of personality. The bond you have with your cat or dog cannot be duplicated.

Double the Love?

For more information on processing, storing, and cloning your pet's DNA, contact:

Genetic Savings & Clone
3312 Longmire Dr.
College Station, TX 77845-5812
888-833-6063
415-383-8531
www.savingsandclone.com

PerPETuate, Inc.
PO Box 1424
Farmington, CT 07034-1424
877-4PERPET
860-674-8404
www.perpetuate.net

Lazaron Biotechnologies
Louisiana Business and
    Technology Center
South Stadium Dr.
Baton Rouge, LA 70803
888-822-8918
225-334-6988
www.lazaron.com

Breeding Good Genes

Selective breeding has made dogs the most diverse species on earth. But in order to maintain and propagate specific behavioral and physical features, closely related individuals must be bred together. Desirable traits are obtained, but inherited diseases are also a consequence.

For instance, a number of significant eye diseases of purebred dogs can be inherited, including glaucoma, cataracts, retinal disease, and eyelid and conformational disorders. Veterinary ophthalmologists agree that certain breeds of dogs require eye conformation standards that are unhealthy for the animal. Eyes set too deep, or those that are too prominent, predispose a dog to lifelong problems such as persistent eye discharge, conjunctivitis, and corneal ulceration, according to Dr. Kirk N. Gelatt, an ophthalmologist at the University of Florida.

Eyelid disorders are also part of several current breed standards and need to be eliminated, says Dr. Gelatt. The normal eyelid opening is a horizontal oval, but selective breeding to create triangular or other abnormally shaped openings can cause lifelong eye inflammation and pain for these dogs. The eyelids, eye opening, "third eyelid" position, eye depth, and skull shape and size are interrelated and are determined by existing breed standards. "We need to update any breed standard that requires abnormal ophthalmic structures to promote a healthy and pain-free eye that is also appropriate for that breed," he says.

Even dogs and cats that are not affected by the disease may be a carrier able to pass on the problem to offspring. Diseases that appear later in life are an even greater problem because the animals may be bred several times and pass on these undesirable traits before they ever become apparent. Gene mapping offers a way to predict these problems, so that arranged breedings can eventually reduce the incidence of these diseases.

Screening for genetic defects has ethical implications for cat and dog breeders, says Dr. Dennis Hacker, an ophthalmologist in California. "If you know a great conformation dog has the gene for PRA [progressive retinal atrophy], do you eliminate him from the breeding program? Not necessarily," he says. Because if you eliminate all the dogs and all the cats that carry a bad gene, you create an even smaller gene pool. "Then you run the risk for a whole lot more genetic problems coming up in other areas, from heart problems, bone problems, joint problems, and on and on," says Dr. Hacker. "So eliminating all these carriers from the gene pool isn't the right answer either." Instead, breeders may need to carefully match carrier animals to clear ones to gradually eliminate a percentage of the disease, yet keep the gene pool as diverse as possible.

NO EASY ANSWERS

Nothing is clear-cut with genetics. Genes do not predict everything, says Dr. Hannah. "Once you get past conception, once the egg and the sperm join, you're pretty much stuck with those genes. The genetic code is everything you could be. That's health, disease, performance, hair coat, everything," he says. "But what you ultimately become is dictated by your environment's impact on what genes are expressed."

In other words, nurture is as important as nature. The way a dog or cat is raised, what they experience, the benefits of socialization and training, the impact of disease exposure (or lack thereof) on their health—all determine how healthy a pet may be.

Genetic research does offer answers, though, that cannot be addressed any other way. It is the ultimate in cutting-edge medicine, and is paving the way for continued medical breakthroughs that will keep pets healthy and happy into the new century, and beyond.

PART TWO

Health and Behavior Conditions A to Z

AGGRESSION

Contrary to popular belief, dog and cat aggression is not the same as viciousness. By definition, viciousness results from a desire to inflict pain on another, and that's a human trait pets don't have. Aggression is simply a component of dog and cat behavior, and is normal within the appropriate context. Aggression is resolved once the animal (1) launches an attack, (2) turns tail and runs, or (3) displays a subordinate position—cries "uncle."

Problems arise when dogs and cats are unable to distinguish a proper context in which to display aggression from an inappropriate one. We expect pets to read our minds, and act like humans with fur. For example, the instinct toward territorial aggression prompts a dog to protect his yard from intruders. That makes sense for a herding dog that must deal with predators that threaten his flock, but it becomes a problem when the dog identifies the mail carrier as a threat. We need to understand what triggers aggressive behavior, recognize the warning signs of impending aggression, and know how to respond to avoid or diffuse the aggression.

Dominance Versus Leadership

In the past, trainers advised owners to dominate the aggressive animal, show the pet you are the boss, and manhandle him into submission. Aggressive dogs fitted with prong collars that pinched, or electronic training tools that offered a "shock" correction, learned to behave, or were put to death in the name of public safety.

Much of that behavior-by-force tradition has fallen into disfavor as we've learned more about dog and cat dynamics. Pet owners are now encouraged to discard lifelong beliefs that no longer apply.

In simplest terms, dominance forces the dog or cat to submit to the owner's will. The pet may actually hate, fear, or resent the owner, and only obeys because he has no choice in the matter. Dominance techniques incorporate punishment—negative reinforcement—to make the bad behavior unpleasant enough for the pet to stop. The reward is cessation of the unpleasantness—like the release of a tightened training collar. A drawback of this approach is that once you've left the house, or the dog is off-leash, he has no reason to obey, because the threat of punishment is absent. Also, the owner must be physically able to dominate the pet, particularly large dogs, or the animal may challenge human authority and the aggression become even worse.

Dr. Myrna M. Milani, an ethologist in New Hampshire, believes the bond between people and pets is crucial. "The only way you can guarantee that a dog is not going to bite," she says, "is to believe one hundred percent that the dog is not going to bite—or be a damn good actor!"

That's because owners can't help but communicate their emotions to their pet, through unconscious body language, tone of voice, and even body scent. Dr. Milani says that when you are afraid, your body pumps out cortisol, a kind of steroid. "To animals, increased levels of cortisol communicate a subordinate position," she says. So even a macho guy flexing a prong collar isn't fooling the dog, who knows he's really thinking, "My God, I hope he doesn't bite me!"

"That's such a silly way to train, if you think about it," says Dr. Ian Dunbar, a behaviorist and dog trainer. "You do nothing to educate the dog. You wait for it to misbehave before training starts, and then you punish it by jerking it or shocking it." Dr. Dunbar prefers reward training that first teaches the dog what you want it to do, then rewards the dog for doing it. "That way the dog doesn't develop the bad behavior to begin with," concludes Dr. Dunbar.

This leadership (rather than dominance) approach requires a confident attitude, combined with a knowledge of animal behavior, and builds on the positive aspects of your relationship with your pet. The owner doesn't coerce, he inspires the pet to *want* to do the human's will. The dog learns that what his "leader" wants him to do results in good things for him. Instead of acting out all the time, he tries to figure out ways to please his owner. For instance, if he stops barking, he gets a treat, or when she sits at the door, she'll get a ride in the car. Rather than fostering resentment or fear, this approach strengthens the bond between people and pets because the dog or cat looks to the owner for approval and permission.

Aggressive behavior can be difficult to unlearn, but it can be done. Pets can fall into the "habit" of aggressive response. They've always growled at other dogs, or lunged at men in hats. But animals can learn to react to these situations in new, more positive ways.

Pets growl and snap for different reasons, and behaviorists have characterized a dozen or more kinds of aggression. For instance, hormones can prompt maternal aggression intended to protect puppies, or even toys and bedding. This type of aggression goes away when the hormone level changes. Play aggression is typical of youngsters who haven't yet learned to inhibit their bite or claws. Pain aggression can be a reflexive response to being hurt, or even in anticipation of being hurt. Each type of aggression must be addressed differently.

"Aggression, like diabetes, is not curable but may be controlled in the majority of cases," says Dr. Karen Overall, a behaviorist at the University of Pennsylvania. You should seek qualified professional advice in any case of aggression, or you risk making the problem worse. An animal attack has severe health risks for the victim and liability issues for you. It can turn into a question of life and death for your pet, should he bite someone and be labeled vicious, or if rabies is suspected. Until help is available, the best policy is to avoid situations known to trigger the aggressive episodes. Don't try to treat them alone.

An owner needs to work hard with a behaviorist to diagnose the problem and to design an individual treatment plan. It's possible to desensitize some pets to the circumstances that trigger the aggression. For instance, dogs that hate men who wear hats can participate in staged situations that bring them in contact with hat-wearing men. Each time they are rewarded in some fashion during the encounter (i.e., given a treat or favorite toy), they are distracted from the aggression and encouraged to associate hat-wearing men with happy, positive outcomes.

Success is defined as modifying the pet's behavior enough that both the specialist and the owner recognize the improvement, and are comfortable living with the pet in this state.

Fascinating Facts! Rage Syndrome

Rage syndrome is a unique pathological form of aggression thought to be caused by a seizure-like episode of the brain. A sudden inexplicable rage causes the dog to attack anything—living or not—with little or no provocation. The rage disappears just as suddenly. Certain breeds are associated with this condition, in particular Springer Spaniels, Bull Terriers, and Cocker Spaniels. Behavior modification techniques don't help in this case, but seizure medications like phenobarbital help some dogs. Complete cures are impossible, and sadly, in cases where the dog presents a danger, euthanasia is the only option.

Aggression Classifications

The first step in diagnosing dog or cat aggression is to examine the context and body language involved. Once the type of aggression has been classified, a treatment program can be designed. Dogs and cats share some types of aggression, while other types are unique to each species.

Status-Related Aggression   Cats usually use the "leave me alone" bite when they want you to stop petting them. You have done nothing wrong, but these cats need to control when the attention begins and ends. Some cats bite and leave, while others simply hold the owner's hand in their mouth. Owners can learn to read the warning signs and stop the interaction by dumping the cat off their lap before she bites, and ignore her unless she behaves. Physical correction rarely works. The cat may view this as a challenge and intensify the aggression. If dumping the cat off doesn't work, interrupt the behavior with an air horn or water pistol. The interruption must occur within thirty to sixty seconds of the beginning of the behavior for the cat to "learn" why it happens. Correction in the first second is ideal. These cats won't be cuddly but may learn to sit quietly on your lap for longer periods.

Dominance Aggression Ninety percent of the pets who display dominance aggression are male dogs that develop the behavior by age eighteen to thirty-six months, which corresponds with canine social maturity. Testosterone makes dogs react more intensely, and more quickly, for a longer period of time. When the dominant aggressive dog is female, the behavior tends to develop during puppyhood. The hallmark of dominance aggression is that it gets worse with punishment. It may be hereditary. Dominance aggressive behavior includes guarding food and possessions (toys or other objects), and redirected aggression, which is defined as follows.

Redirected Aggression In both dogs and cats, this behavior occurs in response to a verbal or physical correction or the thwarting of a desire, in which the victim was not part of the trigger. For instance, the dog can't reach to bite the mail carrier, so he bites the owner instead. Or the cat can't reach the squirrel through the window, and instead attacks your feet. Cats seem to stay hyped up for attack for a long period after an aggressive act is interrupted.

Fear Aggression Dogs that are acting aggressive out of fear tend to bark, growl, or snarl while backing up, shake or tremble during or after the display, bite from behind and then run, or cower and look for escape. Cats flatten their ears sideways, fluff their fur, and turn sideways, or crouch, hiss and claw/bite, and run for cover. There is a genetic component in both shy and aggressive cats, and some cats become aggressive every time they become scared.

Interdog Aggression This behavior is related to social standing and usually affects male-male or female-female interactions. Dogs challenge each other with stares, shoulder or hip bumps and shoves, mounting behavior, or blocking access to food, play, or attention. Older or weaker pets are often victimized. Similarly, intercat aggression is most commonly male-male between whole toms. Cats reach social maturity at two to four years of age, which is when many cats first challenge others.

Territorial Aggression Dogs protect property (house, car) by barking, growling, snarling, and biting no matter who is present. Territorial aggression is made worse by boundary confinements (fences, chains, etc.). The aggression goes away when there's no territory to defend, but these dogs typically identify new territory quickly. In cats, territorial aggression is aimed at other cats or people. Cats mark their "property" with cheek rubs, patrol, and urine marking (spraying or otherwise). Cats may lure others into their territory and then "discipline" the other cat for trespassing. Feline territorial aggression is notoriously hard to correct, and marking behavior is a hallmark of potential aggression. Treatment includes changing the environment, behavior modification, and sometimes drugs. One cat may need to be placed in a new home or segregated from the other.

Predatory Aggression in dogs is extremely dangerous. These dogs silently stalk smaller animals or infants and/or stare at them silently and drool. They may track and stalk bicyclists or skateboarders. High-pitched sounds, uncoordinated movements such as an infant might make, or sudden silences (as happens with prey animals) may provoke an attack. Predatory aggression is similar in cats, with components of stealth, silence, alert posture, hunting postures, and lunging or springing at "prey" that moves suddenly after being still. In cats, predatory aggression varies widely. Some pets have little to no interest, others target even inappropriate objects like an owner's hands and feet, or even the baby (although most cats lose interest once the baby has matured enough).

Protective Aggression is unique to dogs. These animals protect their owners from other people or dogs. Quick moves or embraces may stimulate the aggression. Protective aggressive dogs are not aggressive when their owners are not present.

Idiopathic Aggression is also exclusive to dogs. This is an atypical aggression that arises spontaneously and has no known cause. Most affected dogs are one to three years old, and the behavior is often misdiagnosed as dominant aggression.

Preventing Aggression

Hormones influence aggression to a large extent. Intact male dogs have the most problems with aggression toward other dogs, and neutering decreases interdog aggression in about two-thirds of the cases, says Dr. Overall. It's less clear how neutering affects other forms of aggression. Neutering before twelve months decreases or even prevents up to 90 percent of cat-on-cat aggression. Early-age neutering (at age eight weeks or older) would likely increase this percentage, since aggression is hormone-related.

Heredity plays a large role in shyness and aggression, particularly in certain breeds of dogs. Shyness is an important component of aggression because many animals bite out of fear. "I think you inherit some neurochemical substrate that allows you to be anxious," says Dr. Overall. Other factors like environment and life experience or breed tendency also come into play if that inherited fear gene is expressed as separation anxiety, obsessive/compulsive disorder, or fear aggression. Dr. Overall and her colleagues have submitted a grant to the AKC Canine Health Foundation to study the heritability of some behavior problems. "Not all behavior conditions are inherited," she says, "but many are. And I'm willing to bet that virtually all of the situations that we deal with have a genetic basis." If some of these questions can be answered, reputable breeders may be able to reduce aggressive behavior with targeted breeding.

Of course, a positive environment, life experiences, and training during the pet's formative age have an enormous impact on behavior. Early socialization of kittens and puppies—that is, handling them and interacting with them in a positive manner, and exposing them to positive experiences with other pets, people, and places—programs their little brains to be less fearful, more confident and well adjusted, and better prepares them to learn. For instance, kittens raised without human contact before age twelve weeks don't know how to react to people. If deprived of contact with other cats during this sensitive period, they never develop a normal curiosity toward other cats. Once they grow up, any forced contact with strange cats or with people triggers extreme aggression.

Socialization benefits puppies, too. "Early training and good socialization prevents so many problems, especially the really serious temperament problems like fighting and biting," says Dr. Dunbar. Dog trainers and breeders have taken up the cause in the last ten to fifteen years by promoting "puppy classes" for early dog-to-dog socialization and training. But Dr. Dunbar says you must start early. Starting even at five to six months of age may be "too little too late." Puppies and kittens soak up knowledge at an exponential rate before they're eight weeks old, and training is best begun between eight to twelve weeks.

Today, most cases of aggression arise from misunderstandings between human and pet social interactions and/or miscommunication. Ignoring the dog or cat's clear warning of flattened ears or fluffed fur escalates the pet's aggression. And a pet may misinterpret the human's admiring stare, or a friendly pat on the top of his head, as a threat or challenge to authority, and attack.

However, behaviorists also recognize that a significant amount of aggressive behavior stems from abnormal brain function. Those pets need extra help in the form of drug therapy. For example, benzodiazepines (a class of tranquilizers) help inhibit intercat aggression. The Valium dose is so small that cats can safely stay on it indefinitely and do not act tranquilized at all. The drug has a so-far-unexplained but beneficial side effect—it makes cats friendlier.

Fluoxetine (Prozac) has been used with mixed results to treat canine aggression. Studies from the University of Pennsylvania indicate that many cases of canine aggression are neurochemically related to anxiety, and may benefit from antianxiety drugs. Generally, these drugs are used for only a short time, along with behavior modification techniques, and are not intended for indefinite use.

Fascinating Facts! Early Socialization Studies

In the 1930s, Eileen Karsh, PhD, conducted the first research that found that kittens handled throughout the period between three to fourteen weeks of age grow up better socialized and more attached to people than kittens that are not held until seven weeks of age, or not held at all. The discovery of this "Window of Socialization" revolutionized kitten care.

Modern Miracles:
Gordon Makes Friends

Leslie McDevitt of Erdenheim, Pennsylvania, adopted Gordon, a fifty-three-pound Shepherd/Pit Bull, from a local PETsMART when he was about two years old. "He looked like my Shepherd mix Maggie, and I had to have him," she says. His whimsical one ear up, one down was irresistible. He fit perfectly into her pet family, getting along well with Leslie's dog, Maggie, and her two cats.

Leslie was anxious to show off her new baby at the dog park, where she and Maggie went every day. That's when she learned how fearful Gordon was. He was especially terrified of men. Every time he met a strange man, he'd lunge to the end of his leash and huff to make him go away. "Men coming over to the house, forget it," she says. "We had no more friends." Gordon was so afraid of Leslie's husband that he'd urinate in submission at a mere glance from the man.

"When you have a dog that's been abused and you don't know what's happened to it, and it's so afraid and unhappy, it's totally overwhelming," says Leslie. She hadn't known Gordon would be afraid when she met him. "He was sweet in the shelter," she says. She even introduced Maggie to him to be sure they'd get along. But the shelter was staffed entirely by women.

Because Gordon's aggression toward men stemmed from fear, Leslie felt sure she could change the dog's fearful expectations to positive ones. She'd already seen the benefits of training with Maggie, so she found a professional dog trainer and asked for advice. "He told me to give strange men treats and have them throw the treat on the ground to Gordon," she says. That way Gordon would begin to look forward to meeting men rather than fearing the encounter. "I did that at the dog park, and it worked very quickly," she says.

Now Gordon, Leslie, and Maggie spend time at the dog park without worrying about meeting men. "When Gordon's expectation about seeing a man changed, the [aggressive] behavior went away," says Leslie.

ANEMIA

Anemia refers to a lower-than-normal volume of red blood cells. These cells are one of the major components of circulating blood, and they carry oxygen throughout the body. Anemia can affect a dog or cat of any age or breed. It can occur if not enough red cells are manufactured by the bone marrow, or if too many are lost out of the body (i.e., from bleeding).

Cells of the body do not live forever. As they wear out, they are immediately replaced with new ones. In a dog, red cells live only 110 to 120 days, and in a cat about two and a half months. If cells aren't replaced as quickly as they are lost, anemia results. Puppies and kittens, which have a lower blood volume to begin with, are more seriously prone to anemia than adult animals.

Anemia in pets has a variety of causes. The most typical causes are blood loss from traumatic injury; blood-sucking parasites such as fleas; or a bone marrow disorder, often caused by chronic kidney disease, that interferes with making new red blood cells.

Hemolytic anemia, a less common type, develops from an abnormal immune system that mistakenly identifies the red blood cells as foreign and destroys them. In certain instances kittens may be born with a different blood type than the mother cat. When that happens, kittens develop neonatal isoerythrolysis, a kind of blood incompatibility reaction caused by the immune agents passed to them through the mother cat's milk, which attack the infants' red cells. Dogs may inherit bleeding disorders like hemophilia or Von Willebrand's disease, which result from defects in the blood that prevent clotting.

Blood Types

Although blood from a donor offers lifesaving help, today we know that donor blood may carry parasites or viruses. In addition, all canine and feline blood is not created equal—just like people, pets have different inherited blood types. Giving incompatible blood can have life-threatening consequences.

Antigens, a kind of protein on the surface of blood cells, define a blood type. The immune system responds to a foreign antigen by producing antibodies against it. Like people, cats have very strong antibodies against the wrong blood type, and they attack and destroy the foreign blood the same way they would a virus or bacteria. Consequently, giving an incompatible blood transfusion can quickly kill a cat.

Researchers have identified one feline blood group system made up of three types: feline type A, type B, and type AB. Most domestic shorthair and domestic longhair cats, Siamese and related breeds like Burmese and Tonkinese, and American Shorthair cats have type A blood. About 25 to 50 percent of British Shorthair, Exotic Shorthair, Devon Rex, and Cornish Rex cats have type B blood, as do about 15 percent of Persian and Abyssinian cats. Blood type AB is rare, but has been found in a number of breeds and domestic shorthair cats. When a type B cat receives type A blood, antibodies in the type B blood attack the foreign type A red cells.

Dogs seldom react the same way to incompatible blood. They rarely have naturally occurring antibodies against blood, and must be "primed" to recognize the foreign blood and build antibodies before a problem develops. For that reason, most dogs can receive a transfusion from any other blood group the first time. After that, though, the immune system will recognize the foreign blood if it's given again.

Thirteen different canine blood group systems have been identified, and dogs can be classified as positive or negative for each DEA (dog erythrocyte antigen). An erythrocyte is a red blood cell. The canine blood groups most commonly recognized are DEA-1.1, DEA-1.2, DEA-3, DEA-4, DEA-5, DEA-6, DEA-7, and DEA-8. When a dog has those specific antigens on its red cells, it's said to be positive for that particular group; if the red cells do not have a given antigen, then the dog is negative for that blood group. Some blood types cause more dangerous reactions than others, and the DEA-1.1 group is the worst offender. DEA-1.1 negative dogs should get only DEA-1.1 negative blood, whereas DEA-1.1 positive dogs may get either DEA-1.1. positive or negative blood. An incompatible transfusion can result in both clumping and destruction of the red cells. Usually the reaction is immediate, but it may be delayed up to four days.

Veterinary Blood Banks

Transfusion medicine has made great strides in the past decade, and dogs and cats often require a transfusion as a part of their treatment. Pets belonging to the staff or veterinarian were often kept available as handy donors in case of emergency. In 1989, one of the first blood banks for pets was launched by Angell Memorial Animal Hospital in Boston. Washington State University is home to a transfusion medicine program begun on a grant in 1986 that today provides more than 300 units of blood and blood products for cats and dogs throughout the Pacific Northwest each year. A standard unit of whole blood is 500 cc, or almost 17 ounces, while packed red blood cells and plasma units are smaller. A pet's size and degree of illness determines how much he'll need. A number of blood bank programs run by veterinary teaching hospitals, as well as private commercial entities, are currently available.

Cat donors typically are housed in "closed colonies" to ensure they remain clear of blood-borne diseases that could potentially infect animals receiving the transfusions. Donor programs like the one that serves UC Davis keep cats in the program only for one to three years and then, through a rigorous screening process, find them a new home. "We use Greyhounds rescued from the track," says Charles E. Powell, communications specialist for Washington State University. "They're in our program for a maximum of two years, donate blood no more than twice a month, and then are adopted out. We have a 100 percent adoption rate for these animals." Even while they are donors, the animals are treated to lots of special attention from technicians.

Veterinarians now have easy-to-use canine and feline typing cards to screen for the most problematic blood types in their office. Cross-matching can also be easily done, and although it won't determine the type, it will tell whether a transfusion reaction will occur or not. A drop of serum or plasma from the recipient animal's blood mixed with a drop of blood from the prospective donor will clump when the blood is incompatible.

Artificial Blood

Hemoglobin is the oxygen-carrying component in red blood cells that makes them red. Oxyglobin (Biopure Corp.), released in 1998, is a hemoglobin-based oxygen-carrying solution, a synthetic made from cow hemoglobin. Used to treat canine anemia, it is the only treatment other than a blood transfusion that offers immediate relief.

Stored blood has several drawbacks. It must be refrigerated, then rewarmed prior to transfusion. It requires type matching to avoid transfusion reactions. Plus, donors must be screened to avoid potential infectious agents. Oxyglobin is ready to use as packaged, remains stable at room temperature for up to three years, is compatible with any blood type, and has been purified to remove potential infectious agents. In studies conducted by Biopure, Oxyglobin molecules have been shown to be three times more efficient than natural red blood cells in their ability to deliver oxygen to tissues.

Controlled, randomized clinical field studies conducted by Animal Medical Center in New York, the University of Pennsylvania, Virginia Polytechnic Institute, North Caroline State University, Ohio State University, and Tufts Veterinary School agreed that the Oxyglobin solution was safe and effective. Currently the product has FDA approval for dogs and is undergoing approval for cats.

Synthetic Hormone to Fight Anemia

Kidney disease affects up to 30 percent of cats and 10 percent of dogs older than fifteen. As a result, many also suffer from anemia. That's because the kidneys manufacture erythropoietin, a hormone that stimulates the bone marrow to make new red blood cells. Pets with complications of kidney disease, certain kinds of cancer, or other chronic disease that interferes with the production of erythropoietin can develop life-threatening nonregenerative anemia. Without erythropoietin, the body can't replace red blood cells.

A synthesized form of the human erythropoietin has been available for over ten years, but it is not safe for use in cats. Dr. James N. MacLeod and Dr. John F. Randolph of Cornell University, with a grant from the Winn Feline Foundation, have developed a new synthesized form of feline erythropoietin. Researchers hope further studies will show it will help cats with nonregenerative anemia—that is, anemia caused by the failure to produce new red blood cells.

Fascinating Facts! FIA Culprit Identified

The cause of FIA, or feline infectious anemia, has finally been classified. Researchers have long known that it is caused by *Haemobartenella felis*. They thought the organism was a rickettsial, a kind of intracellular parasitic bacterium. Instead, the organism turns out to be a mycoplasma, a specialized kind of bacteria and the smallest free-living cells known to exist. Research by Joanne B. Messick, a University of Illinois professor of veterinary pathology, not only unmasked the culprit, but also developed a new test to diagnose suspect infections using polymerase chain reaction (PCR) assay, a genetic test. This may also lead to identifying the genes involved in activating the disease, and eventually a vaccine.

Genetic Test for Anemia

Pyruvate kinase (PK) is an enzyme that helps metabolize glucose (blood sugar) into a form that can be used by red blood cells. Without this energy source, red blood cells can't function and are destroyed, a process called hemolytic anemia. Various genetic defects cause PK enzyme deficiency in dogs and cats. Affected dogs typically suffer severe chronic anemia and generally die before they are five years old. Cats more often suffer intermittent anemia, and with care they may have a normal life expectancy.

The University of Pennsylvania School of Veterinary Medicine has developed and established genetic screening tests to diagnose PK deficiency in Abyssinian and Somali cats, and in Basenji, West Highland White, and Cairn Terriers. The blood test identifies affected pets, carrier pets, and clear/normal pets. This helps breeders and pet owners make informed decisions about care and breeding. Test results remain confidential.

ANOREXIA

Pets suffer from anorexia—a profound loss of appetite—when they become physically ill or emotionally stressed. Some finicky cats and dogs develop strong preferences for certain foods and refuse to eat anything else. Other times, stress from a move to a new home, boarding at a kennel, or mourning the loss of a family member can kill a healthy appetite. Cats are especially susceptible to stress from any change in their routine, even a stray cat trespassing on their turf. Since feline appetite hinges on sense of smell, cats refuse to eat if a stuffy nose interferes with scent.

Good nutrition fights disease and keeps pets healthy, and a sudden refusal to eat, or a gradual decline in appetite over days or weeks, causes loss of weight and depression and can make the pet even sicker. In severe cases, the veterinarian may recommend drugs to help stimulate your pet's appetite. The tranquilizer diazepam (Valium) is particularly helpful in cats because it has a side effect of increasing hunger. Other times, force feeding may be recommended; a paste of the regular diet is made and syringe-fed to the cat or dog.

"One of the biggest problems we have with hospitalized chronic-care and critical-care patients is nutrition," says Dr. Andrew Mackin, an associate professor in small animal internal medicine at Mississippi State University. "Trying to tempt or force them to eat is not an effective way of getting calories into them." Only two or three days' refusal to eat significantly impairs a sick pet's ability to recover from disease.

In people, a feeding tube for liquid nutrition inserted down the nose works fine for a day or two. These tubes can even be placed without anesthesia, an important concern for patients who are already in precarious shape from their illness. A nasal feeding tube for cats and dogs must be even smaller than for people, and works only with expensive liquid diets. Pets rarely tolerate the tube for more than a few days before they dislodge it, or develop problems with sneezing or nosebleeds. "That's fine if you have a patient you want to get over the hump for a day or two," says Dr. Mackin. "But you need a much bigger tube for significant nutritional support. And a much bigger tube can't go down the nose."

For the past ten to fifteen years, the traditional approach has been to place a large-bore feeding tube into the stomach. A flexible endoscope sent down the throat to view the stomach aids the veterinarian in positioning one end of the feeding tube in the stomach. The other end exits through the abdominal wall through the pet's side. This gastrotomy tube allows the pet to be fed for days, weeks, or even months.

Doctors employ the same technique in people, and for them only a mild sedative is required. Dog and cat patients must be anesthetized to place the feeding tube. Although anesthesia entails increased risk for the patient, an awake pet would bite and destroy the $10,000 scope.

A New Twist on Feeding

About the same time Dr. Mackin was brainstorming a way to improve feeding tube placement, the Cook Introducer became available. With a slight modification, Dr. Mackin developed a protocol using the Cook Introducer to place large-bore feeding tubes in awake dogs and avoid the problems associated with general anesthesia.

Sedation calms the dog just enough for her to accept the metal tube of the Introducer into her mouth. It's threaded down the throat, where it's used to tent up a small area of the esophagus. You can actually see the movement of the instrument on the outside of the throat as the Introducer manipulates the tissue so that it protrudes a bit to give the veterinarian the needed target. The corresponding area on the outside of the dog's throat receives a local anesthetic. Then a special instrument pierces the tissue of the numbed throat and the feeding tube threads through the opening into the esophagus. The metal Cook Introducer is removed from the back of the dog's throat, leaving the tube exiting from the neck, where it is then fed down the throat into the dog's stomach. A neck bandage covers the tube opening to keep it clean, and twice a day the bandage comes off for the dog to be fed.

For a month, the dogs in the study lived entirely on what could be fed down the tube—and remained healthy, happy, and active, says Dr. Mackin. He predicts the final results will prove the technique a success.

Evaluation of the study dogs' swallow reflex and esophageal well-being will be judged by an impartial clinician to ensure the dogs are as healthy at the end of the trial as when they started. Success would mean that veterinarians—and pets—would gain a new and safer technique for maintaining nutrition even in the sickest patients.

Diagnosis by Breath Tests

Many conditions can interfere with the passage of food from the stomach or intestines and cause vomiting in cats and dogs. Signs may include anorexia, weight loss, chronic and intermittent vomiting, and even gastric dilation, in which the stomach rotates on its axis, as in bloat. Standard methods used to evaluate gastric emptying in cats and dogs include feeding barium or other contrast mediums to the pet, and then taking X-rays or CT scans. Sometimes a tube is inserted through the mouth and down the throat to the stomach to take samples of the stomach contents. The techniques are rather invasive and take a relatively long time to run, since the barium takes from four to seventeen hours to move through the digestive system. Also the barium mixed with food can complicate readings.

Recently, breath test technology has been used in dogs to detect and measure gas produced in response to eating test material. The test meal, or substrate, is readily digested and absorbed, and the appearance of the gas in breath indicates how the substrate travels in the gastrointestinal tract. In studies performed by Dr. Philippa S. Yam, of Glasgow, Scotland, the stable isotope of carbon is used. The results of this study indicate that the test, C octanoic acid breath test (C-OBT), is a simple, reproducible, and safe method to assess gastric emptying of solids in the dog.

ARTHRITIS

Degenerative joint disease is the most common form of arthritis, accounting for 40 percent of all orthopedic diagnoses in dogs. "Roughly 20 percent of the dogs going into a veterinary hospital have pain because of arthritis," says Dr. James H. Sokolowski, a veterinarian at Waltham USA. Dogs, especially large breeds, can suffer severe pain and disability from arthritis. Cats suffer from degenerative joint disease, too, but because of their lighter weight, they seem better able to cope and show fewer signs of pain or stiffness. Rather than limping or holding up a leg the way arthritic dogs do, the arthritic cat typically stops moving around. Feline arthritis often isn't diagnosed until further in its progression, when the cat begins showing signs that the owner notices.

A healthy joint contains several key parts: two or more bones that come together; tendons that hold the bones in place; muscles that move the joint; and a specialized connective tissue called cartilage that lets the bones move freely against each other. Smooth articular cartilage is designed like a spring mattress that cushions the ends of the bones where they meet (articulate) at the joint. Encasing this joint is a smooth, flexible joint capsule lined on the inside by the synovial membrane, which produces fluid similar to plasma that coats and lubricates the somewhat spongy cartilage. The sponge action of healthy cartilage can squeeze fluid and waste into the joint space or absorb nutrient-rich synovial fluid that maintains cartilage health, helps repair damage, and washes away toxins that cause cartilage to erode. The fluid also protects the joint capsule from inflammation, which can cause joint pain. Motion of the flexing joint pumps the fluid where it's needed. Natural cartilage and synovial fluid offers one-tenth the friction than any man-made ball-bearing system.

What causes arthritis? The most common culprits are misaligned or malformed bones that don't fit well together; loose or torn tendons that cause joints to become unstable; and trauma that damages the cartilage. When the bone-to-bone fit isn't perfect, friction wears down the cartilage and eventually the bone. Usually, it's the weight-bearing joints—hip, knee (stifle), shoulder, and elbow—that are affected. Less commonly, dogs and cats suffer from rhumatoid arthritis, in which the immune system mistakenly attacks the joints and causes arthritis.

When injured, cartilage releases excess enzymes that attack its own elastic properties. As the cartilage loses its elasticity, it's less able to get rid of waste products and absorb nourishment. It also loses the ability to repair itself. The first signs of pain appear when the waste products and attacking enzymes reach the synovial membrane and cause inflammation, or when cartilage erodes until bones rub together. The increasing pain restricts movement, which causes further damage, since the joint must move to distribute the protecting fluid.

Diagnosing Arthritis

Arthritis diagnoses are based on X-rays that show what's going on with the bones and joint. Surgical repair can restore function and prevent further damage, if it's done before the cartilage has been injured, but changes in cartilage aren't easily seen on X-rays until the damage is severe.

Signs of joint pain also help pinpoint the problem, and a computerized test identifies not only which legs hurt but also how sensitive each is. Dogs are led across a platform called a force plate with a computer hookup. "We can see exactly how much weight they put on each leg," says Dr. Darryl Millis, a surgeon at University of Tennessee. The force plate test also offers a way to evaluate improvement.

Chewable Aspirin for Dogs

Human-dose aspirin can offer dogs effective pain relief, but giving them the pills can be a problem. Pain-relief medicine designed for dogs adjusts the dosage and adds a tasty flavor to help the medicine go down. Pala-Tech Laboratories has introduced Pala-Tech Canine Aspirin Chewable Tablets in beef and liver flavors the dog takes as a treat. The buffered aspirin is also microencapsulated to minimize any gastric irritation. Pills are available for twenty-pound dogs (150 mg) or sixty-pound dogs (450 mg), and are scored for easy pill splitting to get more accurate doses.

Traditional Treatment

Once arthritis develops, it can't be cured, but early treatment can keep most pets more comfortable. Traditional therapy for arthritis includes weight management, exercise to maintain muscle tone and prevent stiffness, and pain relief.

Arthritic pets tend to gain weight because of their reluctance to move. Lack of exercise also causes a loss of muscle mass and tone. Losing weight removes some strain from painful joints. Generally a veterinary-supervised weight loss diet works best. Exercise preserves the joint's range of motion, helps with weight, and maintains muscle mass. Sound muscles help support arthritic joints, but once lost, muscle mass will almost never be completely regained. Generally, treatment includes as much low-impact movement such as walking or swimming as the pet can stand on Monday, Wednesday, and Friday. Rest the pet on alternate days, and treat him every other day with a recommended pain medication.

Nonsteroidal antiinflammatory drugs (NSAIDs) like aspirin have been the gold standard for treating arthritic dogs. Unfortunately, aspirin-type drugs have the same potential side effects as in people, and a daily dose over the long term may cause digestive problems, ulcers, kidney damage, or even further cartilage damage. Cats are even more at risk because the most common pain-relieving drugs are toxic to them.

Antiinflammatory steroid drugs have uncomfortable side effects and potentially great health risks when used long-term.

New Therapy Options

Innovative arthritis therapies operate on the premise that no one size fits all. Veterinarians are quick to point out that the best treatment offers a combination of therapies, designed for the individual patient. Some work better in certain animals, while others seem to offer benefits across the board.

Physical Therapy Whether arthritis is involved or not, everyone gets stiff and loses range of motion in their joints as they get older. "That's the number one reason pets lose their ability to walk and get around," says Dr. Robert Taylor, a surgeon in Denver. "If we can improve their range of motion with physical therapy, then their quality of life improves." More and more orthopedic specialists include physical therapy programs for postsurgical patients. But Dr. Taylor says physical therapy benefits a wide range of pets, particularly creaky older pets and those suffering from arthritis.

New physical therapy techniques include, on the one hand, the ancient art of massage, and on the other, whirlpool soaks, jet-water swimming pools, and even treadmills. Water therapy uses buoyancy to relieve weight strain on joints, and offers a nearly painless way to exercise and build muscles, and loosen up stiff joints. The newest innovation, borrowed directly from human athletes, is the underwater treadmill, which has shown dramatic results in pets and other animals. For instance, when two polar bear cubs from the Denver zoo, Klondike and Snow, were orphaned, they stopped eating right and failed to develop normally. "They could only scoot or crawl around on the floor," says Dr. Taylor. "We used the underwater treadmill to literally teach them how to walk."

Pain Medicine One of the newest pain relievers for dogs is Rimadyl (carprofen), an NSAID (nonsteroidal antiinflammatory drug) similar to aspirin but without its side effects. Studies suggest that nearly 80 percent of dogs showed up to an 80 percent drop in pain, with side effects of less than 1 percent. For many dogs, pain relief means they can return to the active life they've been missing. Since its introduction, countless pet dog owners have praised Rimadyl as a blessing that gave them back their active companion.

However, increasing concern about side effects reported by some dog owners prompted the manufacturer, Pfizer Animal Health, to release warnings regarding signs of drug intolerance. Arthritic dogs tend to be older animals and may have preexisting problems with their liver, kidneys, or digestion that make them more likely to develop appetite loss, vomiting, and diarrhea when using Rimadyl. In some cases these complications have led to death. All drugs have potential side effects, of course. Veterinarians recommend that all pets undergo proper screening to reduce the risk before beginning any drug therapy.

Feeding the Joint From the world of natural medicine come oral nutraceuticals, nutritional supplements used like a drug to treat a health condition. Nutraceuticals such as glucosamine and chondroitin sulfate products are touted for supporting joint health. These products are recommended for cats as well as dogs, and help protect and regenerate connective tissues within cartilage by providing the raw materials for building new cartilage. They also have natural antiinflammatory properties. Few of these products have undergone tests for safety and effectiveness, though, and so results are hard to predict. Currently, Cosequin is the most common of these medications recommended by veterinarians, based on trials conducted at Cornell College of Veterinary Medicine and elsewhere.

Along the same lines, a number of pet foods now incorporate a variety of nutraceuticals to benefit joint health, and this trend will likely continue. For example, Canine Joint Support Veterinary Diet (by prescription only) contains New Zealand green-lipped mussel (perna mussel). "We've designed it to be a complete and balanced maintenance diet, and we put it through double-blind controlled clinical studies," says Dr. James H. Sokolowski, a veterinarian with Waltham USA. Double-blind studies means neither the researchers nor the subjects know who gets the "real" test and who gets the placebo. "The studies demonstrated that in a period of three to six weeks a majority of animals fed the diet will show significant improvement in their motion, and their demeanor." Eicosatetranoic Acid (ETA), a unique omega-3 fatty acid found only in the green-lipped mussel, has a strong antiinflammatory action. It's also a rich source of chondroitin sulfate, a component of cartilage and synovial fluid that helps lubricate the joint.

Adequan (polysulfated glycosaminoglycan, or PSGAG), made by Luitpold Pharmaceuticals, is one of the newest classes of antiarthritis drugs for dogs. "We've used this [drug] since 1986 in race horses for cartilage injuries, and it's been used off-label in dogs for quite some time," says Dr. LeeAnn McGill, a veterinarian in Alabama. Basically, this drug, now FDA-approved, is similar to the oral glucosamine-type drugs. Controlled studies have shown that a concentrated dose, given by injection, delivers the drug to the synovial fluid within two hours, where it's maintained for seventy-two hours. The latest recommendation suggests a dose of 2 milligrams per pound of body weight by intramuscular injection, twice a week for up to eight injections. Adequan, described as a disease-modifying osteoarthritis drug (DMOAD), reduces joint inflammation, relieves pain, inactivates damaging enzymes, and restricts their release, stimulates the repair of damaged cartilage, and promotes joint lubrication.

"Dogs show a dramatic change after the second or third injection," says Dr. McGill. "I've seen relatively no side effects, and 85 to 90 percent of dogs I've treated have responded very favorably." Controlled studies indicate 78.5 percent of dogs that respond to the drug continue to show benefits for more than six months. After the initial four-week treatment, a follow-up injection is needed every six to eight weeks. "Dogs run through the door to get their shot—they seem to know it makes them feel good," says Dr. McGill. Like other arthritis-control options, the sooner treatment begins, the better the response. "We counsel people to use Adequan early in the disease, not as a last resort," says Dr. McGill. "If you can stop or slow the progression of degeneration of the joint, that will enhance quality of life down the road."

Modern Miracles:
Melody's Fountain of Youth

Melody loved her life with Frances Bush of Alberta, Alabama, but by the time the dog turned three years old, the joy had been replaced with constant, frightening pain. The 160-pound Mastiff moved like an old dog, and often stumbled and fell when she tried to walk. "Mastiffs are gentle giants, that's their nature," says Frances. So it was heartbreaking to see the happy face turned haggard. Melody became grumpy with the other dogs, and even stopped greeting Frances at the door because it hurt too much to move.

"We took the dog to an orthopedic specialist, but surgery wasn't an option for her," says Frances. Melody had dysplasia (an abnormality of the fit of the joints) in both elbows and both hips, and compensating for the pain had damaged both her knees as well. Even if they fixed one knee, it would take two or three months before Melody would have recovered enough for the Bushes to even think about doing the second knee. And by the time they did the other one, the first one would probably be gone.

For four weeks Frances gave the dog Rimadyl at the high doses recommended by the orthopedic specialist, but Melody just got worse and worse. "Melody was hurting so much, she had tears in her eyes, and we still had to help her walk. I couldn't stand to have her in such pain," she says. "You have to think quality of life—and she didn't have it. So I made up my mind to put her to sleep—and I called Dr. McGill."

Dr. McGill had used Adequan in a number of arthritic dogs with good results and offered the drug as a last-chance hope for Melody. Frances eagerly embraced the idea. At $60 a shot, the treatment was expensive because of Melody's size—she needed two full vials for each shot, twice a week for several weeks—but the dog's life was at stake.

Dr. McGill explained that Melody would probably need at least four shots before any improvement could be expected. Frances spent her lunch break each day with Melody, lying on the floor talking with her since it hurt for her to move.

The day after the fourth shot, Frances came home to a miracle. Melody met her at the door, danced around like a different dog, and wanted to play! "She regained her puppyhood just like that," says Frances. "I had not seen her like that for a year—she was really happy, and I was absolutely thrilled.

"Adequan was the miracle drug for her," says Frances. They finished the eight-shot treatment nine months ago, and Melody has shown no relapse—except for when she overdoes play sessions with a fourteen-month-old puppy friend.

"When you have Mastiffs, you learn that everything you do is doubled or tripled," says Frances about the cost of the treatment. But she has no doubt the miracle was worth it. "Melody is double or triple the love, too."

BACK INJURIES

Dogs suffer back problems much more frequently than cats, especially long-bodied and short-legged conformation breeds like Dachshunds and Basset Hounds. The spine can be injured from trauma—jumping and landing wrong. Other times, back problems develop over time due to degenerative disk disease.

The spine, composed of short bones strung together by ligaments, has built-in shock absorbers called intervertebral disks. These fluid- and collagen-filled disks located between each vertebra cushion the bones and allow for flexibility. The spinal cord travels through a bony canal inside each vertebra. Any damage to this canal potentially can encroach on the spinal cord and result in pain or neurologic problems. For instance, if the disk leaks fluid, it turns bony and loses resiliency until the disk ruptures and compresses the spinal cord. In the degenerative form, disk disease typically begins as early as seven months of age and progresses over the dog's life.

Ruptured disks in the lower back cause a weak, wobbly gait in the rear legs. Ruptured disks in the neck result in a hunched, painful posture and possibly front leg weakness. More severe damage can result in complete or partial paralysis below the point of the injury.

Confinement and enforced rest for four to six weeks has been the standard treatment for many years, and this may return the dog to mobility. Modern therapies tend to be much more aggressive. Rather than the "wait-and-see" recommendations of the past, advocates promote treatment as soon as possible—and in some cases, suggest therapies that prevent further injury. Surgery is offered as a last chance to dogs that are not helped by rest. Surgery creates a "window" in the vertebrae by removing the encroaching disk material from the spinal canal, to decompress the spinal cord. Uncomfortable rehabilitation after the surgery returns most dogs to at least partial mobility, but recovery often takes as long as six months.

Holistic Therapy Options

Veterinary acupuncture treatments have proved quite helpful for pain relief in pets suffering disk disease. The centuries-old technique places therapeutic needles at specific points on the body to stimulate positive reactions. Although the exact mechanism still remains a mystery, studies have shown that needle stimulation of certain acupuncture points release neurochemicals like endorphins that relieve pain naturally. Acupuncture can also trigger the release of cortisol, a natural hormone that fights inflammation.

A much newer unconventional therapy is Veterinary Orthopedic

Manipulation, or VOM, developed by Dr. William Inman of Seattle. It offers a nonsurgical technique to relieve pain and return pets to mobility. "A chiropractic mallet device triggers reflexes down the neck and spine all the way down to the pelvis," says Dr. Matthew Fricke, a veterinarian in Oregon. The spring-loaded reflex hammer has a powerful, rapid but tiny (1- to 2-millimeter) range of motion. Theoretically, the device triggers a reflex similar to the knee-jerk reaction.

By triggering spinal reflexes, Dr. Fricke says VOM not only pinpoints problem areas, but also helps relax areas of muscle spasm or pinched nerves. Pain causes muscles to tense or spasm, and that pressure on the spine causes more pain, creating a vicious cycle. "VOM breaks the loop," says Dr. Fricke. "The device triggers a reflex that tells the muscles to relax. There's no reaction in the normal back."

Most pets feel better immediately after the first treatment, but it takes a while for the muscles to "relearn" to relax. Dr. Fricke says the first treatment usually lasts a week, the second two weeks, the third relieves the pet for up to three weeks, and so on until the pain is permanently gone after five to six treatments.

The VOM technique is available through independent practitioners who have taken Inman's seminars to learn the technique. However, VOM continues to be regarded with skepticism by many veterinarians. People tend to remain suspicious of new therapies until they are scientifically proven safe and effective. Manipulative therapies like VOM are still so new that no definitive research has been done on their potential benefits, says Dr. David H. Jaggar, a veterinary chiropractor in Boulder, Colorado. But after two and a half years of using VOM, Dr. Fricke is convinced his cat and dog patients have benefited from it. "It's simple, noninvasive, nondamaging, and effective," he says.

Modern Miracles:
Jenny Takes a Stand

When Jenny the Dachshund stopped climbing the stairs, her owner, Connie Mallory of Redmon, Washington, knew something was wrong. "I put some ice on her back and she got better," says Connie, "but it didn't last." Within a few days the thirteen-year-old dog couldn't walk and had to drag her back legs. Her rear end was totally paralyzed.

Connie tearfully called her sister, who urged her to attend a lecture held that same day by Dr. William Inman, a veterinary chiropractor from

Seattle. He had a new therapy called VOM that was supposed to offer new hope to pets that suffered from back and other orthopedic problems. Connie was skeptical.

She didn't want Jenny to suffer, and she was reluctant to put her through the trauma of surgery. Feeling she didn't have much choice, she made an appointment to have Jenny put to sleep. But that Sunday, on the way to the vet's office, Connie stopped on an impulse to listen to what Dr. Inman had to say. She arrived in time for the last half hour of the lecture.

Connie sat with the paralyzed Dachshund on her lap in the back of the room, petting Jenny and trying to stop her tears. Jenny wasn't the only dog in the room—Dr. Inman was conducting demonstrations during the lecture—but before Connie knew it, her dog was being examined by the veterinarian.

Dr. Inman used the activator to examine and treat Jenny. The paralyzed little dog lay quietly on the table without moving throughout the treatment. Then the doctor stood her up on the table. "She took three or four steps—and everyone in the room started crying!" says Connie. "She's sixteen years old now, and still walking and even running. Jenny moves a little sideways, but she keeps on ticking."

Water Therapy

Swim therapy has been used for decades to rehabilitate horses recovering from injury or surgery, says Dr. A. D. Elkins, a surgeon in Indianapolis. The buoyancy of the warm water relieves pressure on recuperating muscles, soothes the pain, and speeds the healing process. "It allows us to push our animals a little harder in rehab and get them back to normal sooner," he says.

Water therapy rehabilitation benefits orthopedic and muscle injuries, and especially back surgery patients, says Dr. Darryl Millis, a surgeon at University of Tennessee. Some swim therapy proponents claim up to a 92 percent success rate in dogs that have fairly severe spinal cord problems.

As effective as it is, water therapy for canine patients is enjoying a significant advance, again following in the footsteps of equine medicine. The underwater treadmill at University of Tennessee, one of the first built specifically for small animals, typically benefits postsurgical patients within the first two weeks after the surgery. "The patients are still pretty sore and getting over the pain and discomfort from surgery," says Dr. Millis, "and a lot of those animals refuse to swim because it hurts."

The underwater treadmill provides them with exercise that has a lower impact than swimming.

Dogs are able to walk while relieved of most of their weight. The 90-degree water also keeps muscles loose and soothes pain. "It's less work for them than trying to keep themselves afloat with swimming," says Dr. Millis. "They just walk very slowly and build up pretty rapidly to recovery."

Laser Disk Ablations

One of the newest therapies, used more as a preventative than cure, uses lasers to address back pain and paralysis. "We've done over two hundred cases here at Oklahoma State University as a prophylactic [preventative] procedure in dogs like Dachshunds that have come in with histories of having back pain and paralysis," says Dr. Kenneth E. Bartels, a professor of laser surgery at OSU. In the past, surgeons made a long incision down the back to expose the spine and then removed the seven disks that could prolapse, or fall out of place, in the future. Instead, in the new procedure seven spinal needles are inserted through the skin directly into the disks, and a laser vaporizes the center of each of those disks via the needles. Vaporizing this material means there's nothing left to prolapse. "It takes about twenty minutes, we pull out the needles, and they go home the next day," says Dr. Bartels.

Modern Miracles:
Double the Trouble

For thirty-five years Bill and Roberta Armstrong had shared their lives with a long line of pet Dachshunds. The Stillwater, Oklahoma, couple knew the long-bodied dogs were prone to back problems but luckily they had never experienced difficulties. Their luck ran out several years ago when first Oscar and then Schnitzel, their current miniature wirehaired Dachshunds, developed back trouble.

During Thanksgiving week they noticed that the normally playful eight-year-old Oscar was acting subdued, and moped around the house. "He turned overnight into an old-man dog," says Bill. When they noticed Oscar refused to jump the one step up onto the deck to come into the house, they feared the worst.

The Armstrongs scheduled an exam, and the veterinarian recommended conventional surgery to relieve Oscar's back pain—it would cost about $1,000. The steroids he was given in the meantime didn't seem to help much, and they decided to seek a second opinion at the nearby Oklahoma State University veterinary hospital. "I knew about the new surgery from our neighbor, Dr. Ken Bartels," says Bill. "We made an appointment, and they said Oscar was a prime candidate for the surgery."

Oscar went into the hospital one day, had the surgery the next, and went home the day after that. The laser disk ablation surgery cost about $400, and was a huge success. "He's a new dog!" says Bill. "He came home in excellent shape and didn't need any rehab." He says Oscar did look like a Teletubby dog with half of his back shaved. "You could see the little pinpricks where they had put the needles in and done the laser procedure."

A year later, Schnitzel exhibited the same symptoms as Oscar. "We took him to the OSU veterinary emergency room that Saturday because his little back feet were toeing under," says Bill. The hospital kept Schnitzel for observation and scheduled a thorough exam for Monday. "But instead we got a one A.M. call Sunday that he was paralyzed and needed immediate surgery. We said of course!"

The preventative laser surgery wasn't an option at that point, so Schnitzel underwent conventional surgery at two o'clock that morning. Unlike Oscar, Schnitzel needed extensive rehabilitation following his surgery and was hospitalized for a week. It took two to three months before he could use his back legs. "At first he had limited control of his bladder, but that pretty quickly went away. But he didn't recover fully," says Bill. "His back end would fishtail when he'd run."

Schnitzel finally stopped improving, and the Armstrongs talked to the surgeons at OSU about the laser surgery for him to prevent a relapse. "I don't want to put him through it ever again," says Bill. "After his laser surgery, he's still not perfect, but we can see an improvement. He's doing fine. Oscar and Schnitzel are both fine."

Degenerative Myelopathy

Dr. Roger Clemmons, an associate professor of neurology and neurosurgery in the Department of Small Animal Clinical Sciences at the University of Florida's College of Veterinary Medicine, specializes in research on degenerative myelopathy (DM). DM is thought to be an autoimmune disease, in which the immune system mistakenly attacks the spinal cord, resulting in progressive paralysis. It most commonly affects German Shepherds. Although no cure has been found, Dr. Clemmons's combination of drug and natural treatments appears to prevent progression of the disease or bring about remissions in up to 80 percent of patients.

The therapy includes aminocaproic acid, an oral liquid amino acid that addresses inflammation caused by blood clots and their breakdown; and N-acetylcysteine, a type of amino acid found in protein that acts as a potent antiinflammatory antioxidant that helps protect the nerves. He also incorporates a combination of holistic therapies that include vitamins, herbs, a natural diet, and gentle exercise to keep muscles toned.

BLOAT

Gastric dilation-volvulus (GDV), also known as "bloat," is a leading cause of death among large and giant breeds, affecting up to 60,000 dogs each year. GDV develops from air that rapidly accumulates in the stomach until the stomach twists and traps stomach contents that can't be expelled either by vomiting, burping, or traveling into the intestines. Bloat can also refer to the stomach distention with or without the stomach twist, but the twist causes the most serious problems. The twist cuts off blood circulation to the stomach and spleen, and compresses a vein that returns blood to the heart, severely restricting normal blood circulation and leading to shock. That can cause death within hours.

Dogs become restless from the discomfort within a few hours of eating. Typically they whine, lie down then get up, and pace in an effort to get comfortable. The dog may try to vomit or defecate without success. The stomach becomes swollen and painful, and signs of shock—pale gums, irregular or shallow breathing, rapid heartbeat—are soon followed by collapse.

Any dog can suffer bloat, but purebred dogs of large and giant breeds have a threefold greater risk than mixed breeds. "Nobody really knows for sure why the stomach ultimately rotates," say Dr. Dale E. Bjorling, an internist at the University of Wisconsin. "But Great Danes have the highest incidence, with about a 40 percent chance they'll have an episode before they reach age seven." A recent survey estimated the lifetime risk of bloat at 24 percent for large breed (50 to 99 pounds) and 22 percent for giant breed dogs (over 99 pounds). The chances of bloat in large breed dogs increases dramatically at three years of age, compared to six months of age in giant breeds. Dogs that are underweight also have an increased risk, which may be an indication they already have problems with their gastrointestinal tract.

Research from Europe suggests many affected dogs may have subtle swallowing abnormalities that interfere with their esophagus so they swallow more air or are less able to burp to rid themselves of trapped stomach gas. In this country, Dr. Larry Glickman of Purdue University has done the most thorough research into GDV. He conducted a five-year study of nearly 2,000 show dogs (Akita, Bloodhound, Collie, Great Dane, Irish Setter, Irish Wolfhound, Newfoundland, Rottweiler, St. Bernard, Standard Poodle, and Weimaraner) to determine how often they suffered from GDV and to identify both breed and individual risk factors. The study was funded by a grant from the AKC Canine Health Foundation, the Morris Animal Foundation, and by the eleven breed clubs included in the study.

Some of the study results seem to correspond with the European findings. "Dr. Glickman's work suggests that the deep, narrow-chest conformation of certain breeds may create a more acute angle at the junction of the esophagus with the stomach, and predispose them to accumulate gas in their stomach," says Dr. Bjorling. But that alone doesn't cause the problem. "There's a constellation of things that all converge to result in GDV," he says. "Anxious, irritable, nervous, and aggressive characteristics seem to make the dog predisposed." Some research indicates nervous dogs have a twelve times higher risk than calm, happy dogs.

"The survival skyrockets if you get them early on and get them decompressed," says Dr. Bjorling. Simply passing a stomach tube down the throat and into the stomach will manage the distension problem, but a twisted stomach requires surgical correction—and an X-ray doesn't always offer a clear picture of the problem, he says. "I'd perform surgery early, after they've had an episode, because I think you can decrease the incidence of reccurrence."

In corrective surgery, the abdomen is opened and the surgeon massages the juncture of esophagus and stomach so the tube can pass into and decompress the gas. Then the surgeon returns the stomach to its normal position, and addresses any damage to the stomach, spleen, or other organs from blood loss. The bill for emergency surgery and after-care treatment ranges from $1,000 to $1,500, and it's not unusual for dogs with complications to go home with a bill of more than $10,000, says Dr. Bjorling.

Even when the stomach decompresses by stomach tube without surgery, Dr. Bjorling recommends gastropexy surgery, which fixes the stomach to the body wall so it can't twist again. That prevents a recurrence of the condition in more than 90 percent of cases. "I recommend it as preventative, particularly in the Great Danes," he says. It can be done at the same time as spay or neuter surgery, and laproscopic surgery techniques can make the procedure much less invasive and reduce recovery time. "You intentionally create a scar that fixes the stomach to the body wall," he says. This elective surgery costs about $800 to $1,000 when done by a specialist, or a bit less when performed by a general practitioner, says Dr. Bjorling. "If you have a strong emotional bond and are concerned about the possibility, it's probably a good investment."

Although bloat can't be completely prevented, predisposing factors can be reduced, particularly with large and giant dog breeds. Dr. Glickman's study confirmed that bloat risk increases with advancing age, larger breed size, greater chest depth/width ratio, and having a sibling, offspring, or parent with a history of bloat.

"I think multiple feedings of smaller quantities is a good idea," says Dr. Bjorling. "Don't give them a bucket of water they can bury their head in and suck down five gallons at one go." Eating too fast also increases risk. To slow the rate of gulping, researchers recommend placing a heavy chain with large links in the bowl with the food. That forces the dog to slow down to eat around the chain.

Dr. Glickman's study showed that limiting water and exercise before and after meals, commonly recommended in the past, in fact does not reduce the incidence of bloat. Another recommendation—raising the food bowl—actually increases the risk of bloat by about 200 percent! High-fiber diets have been suspected to exacerbate the problem, so the next step in the analysis of Dr. Glickman's Purdue University data will be to assess risk factors in a dog's diet.

Modern Miracles:
Wookie's Tummy Ache

Of the nine Malamute pups in the litter, Wookie impressed Patricia "PJ" Kendrick from the beginning. "Wookie was hell on wheels!" says the Nolensville, Tennessee, breeder, and easily pushed the other puppies out of his way to find his mother. By the time he was six weeks old, he weighed a healthy eleven pounds.

But shortly after, PJ found him bloated and lethargic. "He cried in pain when I moved him," she says, "so I rushed him to the veterinarian." Dr. Barry Fly of the Nolensville Animal Hospital admitted the puppy. After an hour of tests, Wookie was close to death and they still had no idea what was wrong. The only alternative, they told PJ, was exploratory surgery. "I told them to do whatever they had to do to save his life," she says.

The emergency surgery opened the puppy the length of his abdomen, and revealed a defect in Wookie's pylorus. "That's the outflow valve that controls the flow of food from the stomach to the small intestine," says PJ. It was thickened and had spasmed shut. In most animals, the problem causes vomiting when the gastric emptying time takes too long.

Dr. Fly performed a pylorimyotemy, which restructured the valve to prevent future spasms. "I don't think gastric torsion has ever been seen in a puppy," he says, "but Wookie's gastric dilation is the early form." He told PJ that Wookie had the worst case of bloat he had ever seen in a puppy his age.

Two days later when he was to be released, Wookie developed a complication. The abdomen needed reinforcement with sterile mesh before the sutures would hold enough for healing to begin. Two days after the second surgery, Wookie finally came home.

"Despite all he had been through, Wookie always mustered up kisses, and greeted me with a soft woo-woo and a tail wag," says PJ. He needed constant care when he came home, and was allowed to eat only two tablespoons of gruel four times a day. "But we survived the two weeks until he was allowed to eat larger and more solid food," she says. Today, he's a healthy adolescent Malamute happy in a new home. Dr. Fly says the corrective surgery should ensure Wookie never has another problem with bloat.

Altogether, the cost ran about $600. "I never question cost when there's something they can do to save a dog's life, and ensure quality of life," says PJ. "Wookie survived against the odds, and he is smart, loving, and full of life. I would do it again in a heartbeat."

BONE GRAFTS

Nowadays, bone grafts are used widely. Broken bones that heal slowly or not at all can be stimulated to heal by applying bone grafts. Cysts or tumors on bone that are removed and leave weak places can be "patched" with donor bone in the form of a powdered composite that is packed into the open spaces.

The body doesn't reject bone grafts as it would a kidney transplant or liver transplant, because the bone marrow is first removed. That means there's no need to cross-match between the donor and host. The body will build a new blood supply and generate new marrow in the donor bone.

The graft provides not just a scaffold for building new bone. "It also has growth factors in it that stimulate bone formation," says Dr. Helen Newman-Gage, a donor specialist located near Seattle. A fracture turns on certain cells that remove calcium from the bone, which exposes growth factors that cause the body to lay down new bone. "A transplanted bone graft tells the host bone, hey, there's been a trauma here, send in some cells to rebuild this bone," says Dr. Newman-Gage. Eventually the patient incorporates the graft as its own bone.

Bone grafts have greatly reduced the need for amputation. Limb-sparing surgery was devised mainly for dogs that had arthritis or neurological conditions or other problems that would prevent them from being able to function without a front leg, says Dr. Maura O'Brien, a surgeon in Los Angeles. Limb-sparing surgery especially benefits pets diagnosed with bone cancer (osteosarcoma). Traditional treatment for the disease has been to amputate the affected leg, which is where the cancer usually starts.

Amputation can often cure the feline patient because bone cancer in cats doesn't tend to spread, says Dr. William G. Brewer, Jr., an internist at Auburn University. But with dogs, very often by the time of diagnosis the cancer has already spread beyond the leg, so amputation alone won't significantly benefit the dog. Owners of these pets are often reluctant to have amputation done since it likely won't increase survival, and they are concerned about the quality of the dog's remaining life.

"We adapted our limb-sparing procedure from techniques used in people," says Dr. O'Brien. Osteosarcoma occurs most commonly in teenagers, and doctors replace diseased bone with either bone grafts or prosthetic devices made of metal that can be lengthened as the young patient grows. Most canine bone cancers or traumatic bone injuries affect adult dogs, so the metal rods aren't necessary. As long as the surrounding muscle, nerves, and tissue remain intact, surgeons can use a bone graft to replace what is removed, avoid amputation, and save the leg.

Bone tumors usually occur near a joint. "We remove the affected portion of bone, along with a three- to four-inch margin, and preserve all the blood supply, muscle, and tendon tissue," says Dr. O'Brien. "Then we place a size-matched graft back into the segment, and attach it to the remaining bone with a bone plate and screws." The radius—the bone right above the wrist in the foreleg—offers the best chance of success. "The plate usually spans across the joint, and that works well because dogs function fine with a fused wrist joint," she says. "They can walk and even run and be fairly comfortable with only a minimal limp." Another common area targeted by bone cancer is the humorus by the shoulder joint, which on occasion can also be spared. Tumors in this area tend to be bigger, though, and a fused shoulder joint may not allow the dog as much mobility. "We're also working on different ways to do limb sparing in the back leg and up in the pelvic region, too," says Dr. O'Brien.

The recovery for limb-sparing surgery is similar to that for broken bones, but usually less painful, because a surgical break causes less trauma than one from being hit by a car. Also, osteosarcoma is extremely painful, and removal of the tumor offers a lot of relief all by itself, says Dr. O'Brien. Dogs typically get narcotic drugs for pain control while in the hospital and aspirin-type medications once they go home. "They're usually up and walking within the first few days of the surgery," she says. It takes about twelve to sixteen weeks for the graft to fuse to the dog's existing bone and heal.

Cost of the procedure, including the surgery, graft, anesthesia, and medications, runs about $3,000, but may be lower when performed as part of a funded study. "The implants that we get, the plates and screws, cost the same as they do for a person, and the surgical equipment is the same," says Dr. O'Brien, "so our costs are very similar in that respect." Bone grafts can provide a permanent cure for the dog that has no other complications, and he'll be set for life.

However, for 90 percent of all dogs with osteosarcoma, limb sparing offers only one part of a cure, because the cancer has already spread to other areas of the body by the time the tumor appears on the leg. "If you simply amputate the leg, only ten percent are alive at the end of the year, and average survival is four months," says Dr. Brewer. "With chemotherapy, average survival is about three hundred days, with forty percent alive at the end of the year and twenty percent alive at the end of two years," he says. The newest work with immunotherapy and innovative chemotherapy techniques extends average survival time to about five hundred days—50 percent do better, and 50 percent do worse. For a ten-year-old dog, a therapy that extends quality of life by an additional year or two is eagerly embraced by many pet owners.

Dr. O'Brien, who is in private practice, does cooperative studies with other researchers in order to offer some of these innovative treatments to her patients. A biodegradable implant that contains chemotherapy, developed by Colorado State researcher Dr. Steve Withrow, offers one of the most promising treatments. "You implant at the surgery site with the bone graft," says Dr. O'Brien, "and it releases high doses of drug there to kill any tumor cells left behind in the wound bed that could spread." The implant also has fewer potential side effects than traditional whole-body chemotherapy. The cooperative studies give researchers additional information on how the therapies work. "The implants aren't readily available yet—only through surgeons or clinicians who participate in these studies."

Modern Miracles:
Rhys Rises to the Challenge

Kim Pitts fell in love with Ri-dzong's Drakyi Rhys Merak—"Rhys"—the moment she saw him. Born October 1991, Rhys was a three-month-old stubborn, independent black puppy when he arrived at her Lakewood, California, home. Tibetan Mastiffs, herd dogs from Nepal, are known to be independent thinkers, devoted and loyal, and Rhys didn't disappoint. "He considers the house, the cats, and my husband and me to be his property," says Kim, "and he takes his protection duties very seriously." Rhys quickly became part of the family. But Kim didn't realize just how much the big 132-pound dog meant to her until February 2000.

That's when she noticed Rhys limping after their daily walk. "I thought he'd strained or sprained something," she says, "but the next day it wasn't any better, so we took him to the vet." Rhys went home after his X-ray with a steroid shot to reduce pain and swelling, and a pain patch. "The X-ray showed a tumor," says Kim. "I knew that wasn't good."

Kim had worked for the past twenty years with cancer patients as a critical-care respiratory therapist. She'd also had another pet dog die of a bone tumor, and she knew what to expect. "Osteosarcoma is one of the most rapid, insidious cancers known to man or beast, and spreads to lungs," Kim says. "Rhys is my son," she says. "He's been part of the family for eight years. I thought I was going to die."

A chest X-ray showing that the lungs were still clear offered some hope. Kim made an appointment with Dr. O'Brien to discuss treatment options. "The first option was to do nothing," says Kim. They'd give him pain medicine only to keep him comfortable as long as possible. But Dr. O'Brien expected the cancer to quickly erode the bone to the breaking point, and spread throughout the body, and that Rhys would die or be put to sleep within three months. The second option was to amputate his leg and follow up with standard chemotherapy. The third option was limb sparing, a bone transplant that replaced the diseased tumor with donor bone. Kim was told Rhys's otherwise excellent health, the placement of the tumor, and the early diagnosis made him a perfect candidate for this option. They would also implant an experimental biodegradable sponge impregnated with chemotherapy drugs to reduce the chance of the tumor coming back.

"There is no cure," says Kim. "We know osteosarcoma comes back, maybe tomorrow, next year, or three years from now." Their decision wasn't about curing Rhys, but about buying him additional quality of life. After twenty-four hours of total hysteria and tears, Kim's husband, Jerry, said, "You can't go on like this. I don't care how much it costs. We'll do everything to preserve his life."

The limb-sparing surgery took place on March 5, 2000, which also happened to be Kim and Jerry's twelfth wedding anniversary. The couple considered it a wonderful anniversary present for the whole family.

The hospital didn't have a cage or kennel large enough for Rhys, so they created a private critical-care recovery area just for him. He went home the day after the surgery, with pain pills, a transdermal pain patch pasted on his skin, antibiotic pills, and a bandage that covered him from toenails to shoulder. To Rhys, the worst part of the treatment was the Elizabethan collar restraint that he had to wear to prevent him from worrying the bandage. He returned for a bandage check each week—it came off April 30—and he began monthly chemotherapy. His last chemo was Sunday, June 25, and that same day an X-ray of his chest showed his lungs were still clear.

Rhys and his family continue to enjoy each day as it comes. He plays with the cats, does his Mastiff five-minute stutter-step romp, eats normally, and moves from room to room, staying close to Kim and Jerry. The couple has spent more than $10,000 on his treatment, and they wouldn't hesitate to make the same decision again.

"If you have animals, you take responsibility for taking care of them," says Kim. "I know Rhys is going to die. If I could give him more time, I would do it. But it has to be best for him." She doesn't understand people who look at animals as "just pets." "They are my family," says Kim. "You take care of your family."

Prosthetic Limbs Offer a Leg Up

Dogs that lose legs due to trauma or therapeutic amputation typically adjust quickly and do extremely well with only three legs. Prosthetic limbs, though commonplace in human medicine, are not widely available for pets. However, they can work well for front-leg amputees when the elbow joint remains intact. "Dr. David Knapp here at Angell has had very good results with the front leg," says Dr. Paul Gambardella, a surgeon at Angell Memorial Animal Hospital. But the back leg can be trickier to fit. He says Dr. Knapp works with a Boston area human orthotics specialist from one of the Veteran Administration hospitals. "We give him the measurements and he comes over, designs, and makes the prosthesis for the specific dog."

But according to Dr. O'Brien no one has developed canine prosthetics on a consistent basis. "Dogs vary so much in size and shape that nothing can be standardized," she says. Also, teaching the dog how to use the prosthetic can be a huge challenge. "In most cases, the dogs do better without it."

Fascinating Facts! Bone Regeneration

University of Illinois veterinary cancer surgeon Dr. Nicole Erhart often performs limb-sparing procedures, but she has taken her current research to a new level. Her experimental procedure, distraction osteogenesis, removes the diseased bone, then stimulates the remaining sections to grow the new bone needed to fill in the gap.

Availability of Tissue for Transplant

Veterinary Transplant Services, started in mid-1999, serves as a tissue bank for veterinary patients. Dr. Helen Newman-Gage, who worked in the field of human tissue banks for nearly twelve years, recognized the need and used her background to establish the first-of-its-kind company just outside Seattle.

People are familiar with human organ transplants, but tend to be less familiar with other types of donor tissues. In dogs and cats, these donor tissues are equally beneficial but can be hard to find in the proper form, or in a timely fashion. That's where Veterinary Transplant Services comes in.

"We recover tissues that can be transplanted, then screen, process and store them, and provide them to veterinarians," says Dr. Newman-Gage. The service routinely provides bone, tendon, and corneal grafts for dogs and cats and occasionally for horses. Other tissues may also be provided as requested. Although donor bone can be harvested from the same patient—for instance, a bit of bone can be taken from a hip and used for a spinal fusion—using an outside donor eliminates the pain and recovery from the second surgery site.

Bone and tendon offer the fewest complications for transplanting and are easiest to store because they don't need to be cross-matched to the recipient. They contain no living cell membrane markers that stimulate the immune system to reject foreign tissue. "The corneas are a little bit different in that we absolutely need to have viable living cells in the corneal graft, at least on the inside," says Dr. Newman-Gage. The patient will cover over the graft with its own corneal surface cells, but the inner ones need to function to help keep the cornea clear. "But the cornea is kind of a privileged site that doesn't have a lot of blood vessels, so the body's immune system basically doesn't find the foreign cells to reject them."

Some veterinary schools, such as Colorado State University, bank whole bone grafts for their own use in limb-sparing procedures. But Veterinary Transplant Services ships requested tissue anywhere and is currently the only tissue bank that provides processed bone grafts and other hard-to-find tissues. Cancellous bone, the spongy bone inside the harder outer surface, can be packed into sites to form a scaffolding for new bone to grow. Demineralized bone powder, made from the cortical, hard-surface bone, has had the calcium removed to expose the growth factors that stimulate new bone to grow. Large segments of donor bones, such as an entire radius, are also available.

BRAIN TUMORS

A variety of brain tumors occur in cats, dogs—and people. Although they are common in people, brain tumors develop with even greater frequency in dogs, says University of California-Davis neurologist Dr. Richard A. LeCouteur, and most occur in dogs that are more than five years old. "Brain tumors affect any and all breeds of dog and cat," he says, but Boxers and Golden Retrievers have an unusually high incidence. Reported cases of primary brain tumors are 14 to 15 in 100,000 for dogs, and 3 to 5 in 100,000 for cats. "So here at UC Davis, surgeries for removal of brain tumors are now literally a weekly occurrence," says Dr. LeCouteur. "I think we do more than anybody anywhere in the world."

Most brain tumors in dogs and cats are difficult to treat because pet owners don't recognize the signs early enough. In many dogs and cats the symptoms may be as subtle as hiding during the day, reduced frequency of purring, or less activity. The fact that such behavior is naturally common in many pets, and can be caused by a host of problems, can further confuse the issue. The location of the tumor determines the type of signs you see. A tumor of the forebrain typically prompts seizures or changes in behavior, while brain stem tumors, depending on location, can result in a head tilt, weakness, circling, or muscle atrophy on one side of the face.

Because tumors arise most often in aging pets, owners may attribute the behavior change to simple aging. The pet might have trouble recognizing familiar people or places, or lose house training. Seizures, problems with balance, or any change in behavior could stem from a tumor. Some pets become aggressive or hyperexcited. By the time symptoms become noticeable, the tumor may be too advanced for treatment to be effective.

Improving the Diagnosis

The ability to diagnose brain tumors has undergone a revolution in the past twenty years. Computed tomography (CT) and magnetic resonance imaging (MRI) offer more accurate determinations of the location and extent of brain tumors than ever before. These advances in imaging also make it possible for precise CT-guided needle biopsies that aid diagnosis and help deliver drugs to the tumor.

In conjunction with Ohio Medical Instruments and Dr. Philip Koblik of the Radiology Service, Dr. LeCouteur and Dr. Robert Higgins of the Pathology Service have developed a "stereotactic" frame that positions the head of a dog or a cat so that, using CT imaging, a fine-needle biopsy of the animal's brain tumor can be taken.

Traditional Therapy

The major goals of treatment are to eliminate the tumor or reduce its size, and to control the secondary effects of the tumor. Steroid therapy can help reduce the swelling, and in some types of tumors (such as lymphoma), it can reduce the size. That can help reduce the symptoms. In some cases seizures can be controlled for a time with drugs like phenobarbital. Researchers report that using these support therapies alone offer an average survival time of only between six and fifty-six days.

Surgery, radiation therapy, and chemotherapy are the standard ways of treating brain tumors. When the tumors are caught in time, modern surgical techniques alone may offer amazing cures, particularly in cases of benign growths. For instance, meningiomas, tumors of the covering of the brain, may often be completely removed, particularly those in cats. Surgery with follow-up treatment can allow cats to live four to five years after treatment without recurrence.

But even when tumors are benign, they have often infiltrated other areas of the brain, and so are difficult to tell apart from normal brain tissue. The possibility of causing brain damage to normal tissue during surgery often makes complete removal impossible. As a result, pets have historically had less than good results with brain tumor surgery. Average survival varies but tends to run 140 to 150 days, according to Dr. Patrick Gavin, a professor at Washington State University in Pullman. The outcome for humans' and pets' brain tumors has not improved significantly over the past three decades.

For tumors that can't be reached surgically, or in cases where some of the tumor is left behind, radiation can control the growth of the tumor, and in some instances can eradicate it completely. But radiation affects normal brain tissue as well as cancerous tissue. Also, brain tumors don't seem to react in the same way to chemotherapy as other types of tumors. Even with aggressive therapy, brain tumor patients usually have a poor prognosis.

Researchers are addressing the problem by developing new strategies.

Targeting Tumors

Dr. Gavin and his team have developed Boron Neutron Capture Therapy (BNCT). This new form of radiation treatment destroys cancer cells without injuring nearby healthy tissue. The concept was first proposed in 1932, but only recently has technology advanced to the point where the technique could be developed and used in a meaningful way.

BNCT is a two-step radiation treatment. In the first step, the tumor is saturated with a boron compound. When given intravenously, the nontoxic, nonradioactive boron-carrying drug crosses the blood-brain barrier, and is concentrated in the tumor. Tumor tissue soaks up the drug more quickly than normal tissue, because it grows so quickly. The blood circulating through normal brain tissue washes the boron away.

In the second step, radiation is aimed at the tumor, using neutrons with sufficient energy to penetrate the tissue but insufficient energy to do damage by themselves. These otherwise harmless neutron particles (radiation) interact with boron atoms captured inside the tumor. The process releases large amounts of ionizing energy that is primarily confined to the cells that contain the boron. This kills the cancer cells but with relatively little injury to nearby normal tissue cells. Average survival times of dogs treated with BNCT combined with surgery are about double that of conventionally treated dogs.

Gene Therapy

Dr. LeCouteur is also investigating gene therapy, a very new area. "A lot of people think it makes great sense to use the genetic makeup of the tumor cells to actually kill those cells. It's a very natural approach," he says. He works with Dr. Higgins, in addition to others, in developing the pilot program.

In order to grow, tumor cells generate an extensive network of blood vessels to feed themselves. Malignant cells manufacture biochemicals that initiate, then maintain, blood vessel growth. In normal adult tissue, an agent called endostatin counteracts the action of the mechanism that stimulates abnormal blood vessel growth. Essentially, endostatin is the off switch for cancer cells.

When Dr. LeCouteur's team introduced the gene for endostatin into malignant brain tumors in mice, tumor growth was significantly inhibited. The success in the mouse studies has allowed Dr. LeCouteur to take the next step. He is applying the therapy to dogs in what he terms a "suicide gene therapy."

When the DNA from canine endostatin is introduced into the nucleus of brain tumor cancer cells, it switches off blood vessel growth and starves the cancer to death. Researchers introduce the kamikaze DNA into cells in a variety of ways, including a piggy-back virus technique. "Viruses are very effective at infecting cells, so we use a harmless virus like a Trojan horse to carry our therapeutic DNA into the target cells," says Dr. LeCouteur.

A specially manufactured fat molecule called a liposome also works as an effective way to deliver the DNA. The carrier liposomes circulate in the bloodstream, reach the tumor, attach to the tumor blood vessel cell, and deliver an army of endostatin genes. "This therapy may be able to slow or stop tumor growth, or stop tumors that have been surgically removed from reforming," says Dr. LeCouteur. After being genetically modified with the viral DNA, the tumor cells may then be killed by drugs that have no harmful effects on normal brain cells.

The current pilot program treats the tumor by injection, and twenty-four to forty-eight hours later, the tumor is surgically removed so it can be analyzed to measure the treatment's effect. Once the treatment proves successful, it is hoped that surgery won't be needed. Everyone involved benefits, since the dogs receive state-of-the-art care at a reduced cost. And the novel therapy has potential applications not only for pets, but for people as well.

Modern Miracles:
Molly Beats the Odds—Twice!

One day last March, Molly began to wobble when she walked. A day later, the seven-pound cream and red-shaded Persian seemed back to normal. Not until the next week when Molly toppled over did her owners, Marlys and Greg Bartling of Iowa City, Iowa, become concerned. The pair spent the next week at the veterinary clinic. Molly had blood drawn and X-rays taken.

"They couldn't find anything wrong," says Marlys, "but Molly started to withdraw." The normally outgoing, loving show cat hid, whimpered, cried, and didn't want to be touched. They returned for more tests, and while they were at the clinic, Molly went into convulsions. She was referred to Dr. Alan Schreiner and Dr. Karen Klein at Iowa State University in Ames.

That Saturday Marlys left Molly at the university clinic in the intensive care unit, where she was given phenobarbital to control her seizures until the neurologist could examine her the following Monday. "Ames didn't have an MRI, so Molly's was done at the local human hospital," says Marlys. The imaging test revealed the cat had a very large brain tumor.

"The news left me numb," says Marlys. Molly was not quite ten, and by rights should have had many more years to live. Marlys was told there was a one in three chance it would be a "good" tumor—a slow-growing meningioma that surgery could cure. These tumors in cats tend to grow in a clump and are fairly easily removed. A decision had to be made quickly about whether or not to take the gamble. "Molly was failing," says Marlys. "We didn't have a choice." So she traveled back to Ames to be with Molly and hold her the night before the surgery, not knowing if she'd see the Persian again.

"The neurologist said the tumor came out in little pieces, and didn't have 'fingers' like bad tumors," says Marlys. Sure enough, three days later the pathology report confirmed it was a meningioma. Molly had her own cheering section at the hospital, says Marlys, and they all jumped up and down with relief and excitement. "They told me they couldn't get all of the tumor," says Marlys, "but that the surgery had bought her probably four more years."

Molly spent a week in the hospital after her brain surgery, and came home with a feeding tube in her neck to help her eat. But she collapsed three days later, and Marlys made another two-and-a-half-hour trip to Ames for more tests. Molly had developed anemia, possibly a complication of the phenobarbital or anesthesia. She'd also developed corneal ulcers on her beautiful copper eyes from all the stress. After two weeks, Molly finally went home, and by the end of a summer filled with taking medications, she had recovered—to a point.

"She wouldn't jump up on anything, she'd lost a third of her body weight, and she was almost blind," says Marlys. Molly had always been the boss of the other cats, but now they seemed to know she wasn't "right" and left her alone.

Eleven months later, they noticed Molly's back legs seemed weak, so they scheduled another MRI. The tumor was back, just as big as before. "It filled her head, and her little brain was smashed back against her skull," says Marlys. "We were devastated. We couldn't believe it." They'd spent eleven months medicating Molly, sometimes seven or eight times a day to heal her eyes and get her well. The news was even harder to take this second time.

Molly began to decline and suffered seizures at home. This time Molly was referred to Dr. David Lipsitz, a clinical assistant professor of neurology and neurosurgery at University of Wisconsin at Madison.

In March 2000, a year after the last surgery, Molly was admitted to the hospital in Madison, a three-and-a-half-hour drive from her home. "They said the tumor was too big for radiation," Marlys says. "Dr. Lipsitz said it was very risky to do a second surgery." Marlys's greatest concern was for Molly. "I wasn't going to put her through it again," she says. "I was ready to take her home to die. But my husband, Greg, said, 'Let's go for it! It's her only chance.' " She says Greg didn't think twice about the first surgery, either. "He loves her. She's his cat, too."

The professionals at both Madison and Ames treated Molly as if she were the most important cat in the world, says Marlys, and that convinced them to try again with the surgery. "They never made us feel silly for being batty over a cat," she says. "They were truly as concerned as we were."

So the couple left Molly that day, hoping they'd made the right decision. The next morning, the surgeon called to tell them the surgery must be now or never. Molly had spiraled downward and wouldn't survive much longer. "Then they called at two that afternoon to say the surgery was done—and they got it all!" says Marlys.

Molly came home three days later, but this time with no feeding tube, no eye ulcers, and no anemia. "They told me that pets with brain tumors won't jump up," says Marlys, "and after the second surgery, Molly pole-vaulted up on the bed.

"Now she rips up and down the hall, races, and jumps up on things, plays with toys, throws them in the air, jumps on them—she's a totally different animal," says Marlys. Molly's back with the other cats, too, bossing them around. "I'm sure they think she's used up two of her nine lives by now."

All told, Molly's two surgeries, MRIs, and hospitalizations ran about $8,000. "We laugh and watch her go down the hall and say, there goes the siding for our house!" says Marlys. "Molly is just a treasure to us, and she was worth every penny."

CANCER

Dogs and cats suffer from the same kinds of cancer as people—from lymph gland and skin cancers to breast and bone cancers. Considered a disease primarily of old age, the Veterinary Cancer Society says cancer is the leading cause of death in dogs (47 percent) and cats (32 percent), particularly in pets over the age of ten.

In the normal course of a dog or cat's life, old cells throughout the body die and are replaced by new ones in a process called mitosis, in which one cell splits into two new ones that are identical to the parent cell. Sometimes something goes wrong in this process, and the new cells aren't identical—they mutate to something different from the parent cell. For reasons that aren't clear, mutation sometimes creates abnormal, fast-growing cancer cells. Like parasites, they invade and replace healthy tissue with abnormal growth.

In most cases, a healthy immune system recognizes and eliminates foreign or mutated cells. But when the system breaks down, the abnormal cells proliferate and form tumors. Benign tumors are localized and relatively harmless, while malignant tumors are dangerous and life-threatening. They tend to spread—metastasize—throughout the body and interfere with normal body processes. The degree of malignancy determines the seriousness of the disease. "Low-grade" cancers may grow to enormous proportions but tend not to spread until late in the disease. The most dangerous cancers spread very early, even when the point of origin (the primary tumor) is tiny or nearly undetectable.

The exact mechanism that prompts cancer to form isn't known, but a variety of factors seem to be involved. Some families or breeds of dogs and cats are genetically predisposed. Viruses like feline leukemia virus and feline immunodefiency virus can cause cancer, and vaccines cause injection site tumors in some cats. Cats with white on their face around the nose, eyelids and ear tips, and dogs with white thin-haired abdomens are at risk for tumors caused by sunlight. Hormones also influence the risk of cancer. Spaying dogs and cats at an early age markedly decreases the risk of mammary cancer, says Dr. Dennis Macy, an internist at Colorado State.

Mammary cancer accounts for 52 percent of all tumors in female dogs, and nearly half of the cases are malignant. Investigators at Michigan State University College of Veterinary Medicine are studying the molecular genetics of the disease, using known gene mutations in human breast cancer to offer a roadmap to learning more about the canine disease. Four genes in humans have been identified. BRCA1 and BRCA2 cause 40–45 percent of inherited forms in people, and mutations in TP53 and AT also contribute. Preliminary results from the two-year canine study indicate that a mutation of at least one of these genes plays an important role in canine mammary cancer as well.

Exposure to carcinogens over the pet's lifetime may explain why older pets develop cancer most often. Dogs and cats are at risk for the same carcinogens as the owners, says Dr. Macy. Animals live an accelerated lifespan, so the buildup of carcinogens in their bodies affects them much more quickly than in human beings.

Our pets act as sentinels of disease—an early warning system—for their owners. For instance, Dr. Macy says bladder cancer in cats and dogs develops because of secondhand smoke and chlorine, and pets that belong to asbestos workers get the same asbestos-induced cancers as their owners. A study headed by John S. Reif of the Department of Environmental Health at Colorado State University compared 200 dogs with bladder cancer to 200 dogs without bladder cancer to determine the risk of exposure to certain compounds in chlorinated water. In another study, Dr. Reif and his colleagues reported that when exposed to secondhand tobacco smoke, dogs with short noses have an increased risk of lung cancer, while breeds with long noses have an increased risk of nasal cancer. "Dogs and cats share our environments; they're biological organisms. They respond in a very similar manner as people do," says Dr. Macy.

Diagnosis

"The earlier cancer is diagnosed, the better the chance for control or cure," says Dr. Macy. Not all cancers start with an easily felt lump or bump on the outside of the body. Cancer prompts a wide range of physical and behavioral signs. Ultrasound, X-rays, or other imaging technologies allow the veterinarian to see the extent of internal tumors.

But to diagnose cancer, samples of suspect cells must be removed from the tumor and examined under a microscope, or evaluated in a blood or urine sample. Laboratory tests also document the progression of the cancer—determine how advanced the disease is. Certain types or stages of cancer respond better to specific treatments.

Lymphosyntigraphy offers a new diagnostic technique that helps define how far the cancer has spread, says Dr. Barbara Kitchell, a cancer researcher at University of Illinois. Radioactive tracers are injected into the pet's body. Cancer cells tend to absorb these compounds, making them detectable. Affected lymph nodes, for example, should be revealed using this test.

Some cancers are difficult to identify by looking at the structure of the cells under a microscope. Says Dr. Macy, "We can now use genetic probes to determine if those cells are really abnormal. We can detect gene de-arrangements—genetic markers within the cells that are consistent with malignancies." This technique, developed by laboratories at Colorado State University, makes it possible to diagnose canine cancer far earlier than in the past. The cutting-edge test can be run on samples sent to the laboratory, and often provides a definitive diagnosis when preliminary tests have been inconclusive.

Prediction: Diagnostic Evolution

"With the computer age, we're getting better and better and faster and faster at making diagnoses. In the next five to ten years, we'll see even more sophisticated equipment able to pinpoint exact locations and exact pathologies that are occurring in the patient," says Dr. David Ruslander, a radiologist at Tufts University. "That will allow us to deliver an increased dose of radiation therapy to a much more confined area, while limiting the dose to the surrounding normal tissue. This technology will allow us to improve control rates and cure rates in larger numbers of cancers, both in veterinary medicine as well as in human medicine."

Conventional Treatment and Advances

Treatment attacks cancer from many directions to physically remove, shrink, or otherwise stop the cancer with as little damage to normal tissue as possible. Traditional ways of fighting cancer include one or any combination of surgery, radiation, and chemotherapy—the same options used routinely in human cancer medicine. "Many tumors are readily handled by the general practitioner, and others may require more specialized help in a referral practice," says Dr. William G. Brewer, Jr., an internist at Auburn University.

Surgery Removing tumors has been the mainstay of cancer treatment for dogs and cats. Advances such as lasers used like scalpels and arthroscopic techniques using noninvasive tiny entry incisions allow surgeons to remove some types of tumors completely. However, a complete cure with surgery alone is rare because even a single missed cell opens the possibility that the cancer may return or spread. Surgery is nearly always combined with other treatments that target malignant cells that may have been left behind.

Radiation Cancers of the face and head, or those that surround nerves and vital organs, may be impossible to remove with surgery.

Conventional beam radiation that shoots intense X-rays directly into the cancer works well as an alternative, particularly against cancers of rapidly dividing cells, such as skin or bone marrow.

However, radiation doesn't discriminate between cancerous and healthy tissue. It can damage normal areas of the body, and often spills onto the sensitive tissues of the intestinal tract or lungs, a major cause of the side effects seen in human radiation treatment. "People who receive radiation therapy tend to have centrally located tumors," says Dr. Brewer. "In animals, the tumors we treat with radiation tend to be more peripheral in location, like in the head and neck, so we're not irradiating over sensitive tissues." Dogs and cats tend not to experience the same severe side effects as people. At most, they may lose their whiskers or appetite temporarily. Radiation cures up to 80 percent of some kinds of cancer in dogs and cats, but irradiating tumors on the head may also damage the eyes and can cause blindness or brain damage.

The pet must be anesthetized to target the cancer, which raises the cost as well as risk for older animals that may not tolerate anesthesia well. Radiation therapy machines cost a great deal and also have regulatory concerns because of the potential for radiation exposure and toxicity to therapists. Yet today they can be found in nearly all veterinary universities and in many specialty hospitals across the country.

Some of the newest radiation equipment, technically called linear accelerators, like the one at Washington State University, feature a computerized 40-leaf collimeter similar to the iris on a camera. That allows the radiologist to shape the X-ray beam to fit the tumor, and target it with pinpoint precision. The head of the machine rotates around the pet's body, adjusting the beam as it travels. That spares the surrounding normal tissue from being irradiated. The laser-sighting system built into the linear accelerator means patients can be placed in the exact same position for every treatment.

"We now can diagnose and plan treatments with the spiral CT scanner using a three-dimensional planning computer," says Dr. David Ruslander, a radiologist at Tufts. That allows the dose and delivery of the radiation to be aimed more specifically, while avoiding normal tissue. Instead of a shotgun dose of radiation that can also hurt normal tissue, the computer maps a narrow target that treats only the cancer. "It basically does three-dimensional reconstructions of the entire patient, and then we can visualize the dose that's being delivered to the patient in all dimensions," says Dr. Ruslander.

A CT scan often helps define the location of the tumor so that radiation can be aimed correctly. The next generation of therapy will combine CT scan technology with the linear accelerator, says Dr. E. Gregory MacEwen, an internist at University of Wisconsin. Dr. David Vail and other researchers at the University of Wisconsin have developed a hybrid CT scan machine that delivers radiation when the scan detects the cancer, then stops as it scans normal tissue. "It's all driven by the image of the tumor," says Dr. MacEwen. The innovation allows them to deliver very high doses of radiation to the tumor. "It's like a knife that lets you sort of cut around the corners," he says. A prototype of the machine has been built, and dogs with nasal cancer will be treated with it at the medical school in Madison. Conventional radiation may damage the eyes and can cause blindness or brain damage.

Chemotherapy   Cytotoxic or cell-poisoning drugs, referred to as chemotherapy, are used to fight cancers that have spread throughout the body. The drugs are often used in various combinations, along with surgery or radiation. Nearly all chemotherapy drugs used in pets are adapted from human medicine, e.g., gemcitabine and temazolamide.

Unlike human chemotherapy patients, cats and dogs rarely experience side effects, which are minor when they do occur, says Dr. Ruthanne Chun, a cancer specialist at Kansas State. That's because dogs and cats tolerate the drugs better than people do; also, drugs aren't combined in the same way and doses tend to be lower in pets. In addition, because doses are calculated according to the pet's body weight, the cost for a small pet tends to be relatively low. Of course, the cost mounts with large dogs.

Understanding How Cancer Grows

New compounds don't just kill cancer cells; they are designed to stop continued growth of the tumor. Malignant cells think they're supposed to divide. Says Dr. Kitchell, "It's like they're on autopilot and just go crazy." Clinical trials now under way hope to find compounds that are able to stop that kind of automatic replication, she says.

Some of the most intense research in chemotherapy drugs focuses on a class of compounds called angiogenesis inhibitors. "Tumors need to be able to recruit a blood supply to be able to grow beyond two to three millimeters in diameter," says Dr. Chun. They need angiogenesis—the creation of new blood vessels—to help the tumor grow. Anti-angiogenic therapies are intended to keep the tumor from being able to grow to a significant size, she says. "It may be able to survive at a microscopic level, but hopefully not make the patient sick."

For instance, tumors in mice have been found to produce angiostatin, a naturally occurring protein that seems to suppress the growth of smaller tumors. Dr. Chun says this mechanism may enable the primary tumor to gather all nutrients for itself by stopping the growth of new blood vessels and starving other tumors. "Endostatin is another compound that's been found in animals with tumors, which also stops blood vessels from growing," says Dr. Chun. But angiostatin and endostatin are very difficult to get in bulk quantities. A University of Wisconsin gene therapy study tries to get around that problem by giving dogs and cats the gene needed to produce angiostatin on their own. Researchers hope the animal can make enough angiostatin to stop the tumor from growing and actually make it shrink, says Dr. Chun.

Other angiogenic research looks at endothelial growth factor and prostaglandins that encourage blood vessels to grow in tumors. Tumor blood-vessel inhibition is considered one of the most promising areas of cancer research today. A research team at Colorado State headed by cancer specialist Dr. Greg Ogilvie is part of a national animal trial that involves multiple centers participating in a multimillion-dollar study with Bayer Corporation in Europe. The study looks at how these experimental treatments fight lymphoma and osteosarcoma. Results of the blinded study—nobody knows which patients get the real therapy and which get a placebo—won't be known for another year or two, says Dr. Steve Withrow, an internist at Colorado State, but so far no side effects have been reported.

Delayed Drug Delivery

Dogs and cats can benefit from innovative cancer treatments by participating in preliminary trials, says Dr. Kitchell. Her team conducted the animal studies for a chemotherapy gel product made by Matrix Pharmaceuticals in Fremont, California. "You inject this gel into the tumors, and it releases chemotherapy in a time-release fashion. It was very effective, and shrunk the cancer," she says. The news was so good, in fact, the company gained FDA approval to conduct human trials. "So they closed the veterinary trials," she says. "We're waiting for them to get approval to market the product and make it available again for pets."

Other experimental drug delivery systems use polymers, a type of molecule combination, that are inserted during surgery and slowly degrade over a period of weeks, releasing chemotherapy in massive doses right to the tumor site. A biodegradable spongelike material developed by a Duluth, Minnesota, company in cooperation with the National Cancer Institute has been used in veterinary research trials at Colorado State University. The therapy has worked well with bone cancers and other types of solid, localized tumors that can be surgically removed but may leave behind a few cancer cells. "We've been able to decrease the local recurrence rate by probably 50 percent," says Dr. Withrow. The therapy doesn't eliminate the cancer entirely but dramatically improves the patient's prognosis and may eliminate the need for radiation therapy. "We've also discovered it has some whole-body effects," says Dr. Withrow, "and can do the equivalent to intravenous chemotherapy to stop the whole-body spread of bone cancer."

Dr. Withrow is also working with another company to create a polymer treatment that can be injected. "We've treated forty to fifty patients, but it will take another year to see if it's as good as the previous product."

Unfortunately, only the researchers at Colorado State and a handful of investigators across the country have access to the sponge implant therapy. "Even though both the polymer and the chemo drug have FDA approval, the combination is new," says Dr. Withrow, "and FDA regulations require quite a few million dollars for the different phase studies." That may not happen for years.

Thermal Therapy

Cryosurgery has successfully been used on localized, shallow tumors to freeze and destroy cancerous tissue. A substance that produces intense cold—usually liquid nitrogen—is applied directly to the tumor itself, leaving surrounding healthy tissue intact.

Hyperthermia, or heat therapy, is the opposite of cryosurgery—it heats the cancer cells to kill them. At the proper temperature, the tumor is destroyed without damaging normal tissue. "We've worked with a hyperthermia unit that we're testing in animal tumors," says Dr. Kitchell. The heat-producing frequency can be set to reach different depth and dimensions within the body, thus allowing doctors to pinpoint the tumor and spare the surrounding healthy tissue. Work supported by the American Cancer Society indicates that increasing the temperature of the tumor increases the effectiveness of radiation therapy, doubling the time in which local tumors remained under control. And researchers at North Carolina State University in Raleigh, funded by the National Cancer Institute, currently are studying hyperthermia-radiation treatment in pet dogs with soft tissue sarcoma to help determine the best dose of heat in combination with radiation.

Another innovation is photodynamic therapy (PDT), a kind of light-activated chemotherapy using lasers. "Photosensitizing agents, similar to chlorophyll, are used," says Dr. Brewer. For unknown reasons, the tumor tends to absorb these agents, which respond to different wavelengths of light. "Once the agent has been absorbed, then either the laser light is shined on the area or laser fibers are implanted in the tumor," says Dr. Brewer. The agents release the laser light energy inside the tissue and kill the tumor cells. This therapy is used for some skin cancers, oral tumors, and bladder tumors.

Diet Therapy

Dr. Gregory Ogilvie, a professor at Colorado State University, has investigated the role of diet in cancer patients. Studies have shown that cancer causes changes in the body's metabolism, and results in a syndrome known as cancer cachexia. This causes weight loss even when the pet eats enough food. It leads to hospitalization of up to 87 percent of human cancer patients, and affects an even greater percentage of pets. Patients with subnormal nutrition aren't able to use drugs properly, which interferes with their treatment.

Researchers theorize that certain diets can help overcome nutritional deficiencies caused by cancer. For example, tumors thrive on glucose, or blood sugar, and tend to steal it from the body, thereby depriving the body of this essential energy source. Both human and canine patients are also prone to insulin resistance, which means they aren't able to effectively absorb glucose into their cells, leaving all the more for the tumor. Since simple carbohydrates in the diet tend to increase insulin resistance, diets that avoid simple carbohydrates may be best for dogs afflicted with cancer.

Cancer patients are also known to have trouble metabolizing fat, which is linked in turn to such problems as suppression of the immune system. But the fact that some kinds of tumor cells have trouble using fat for energy suggests that a diet relatively high in fat might benefit canine cancer patients. The type of fat may be important as well. For example, omega-3 fatty acid supplements help wounds to heal and shorten the time of hospitalization. Polyunsaturated fatty acids, especially eicosapentaenoic acid (EPA) and docosahexaenoic acid (DHA), may prevent the growth and spread of tumors, and prevent cachexia.

In Dr. Ogilvie's study, increasing DHA prolonged the remission and survival time for dogs with late-stage lymphoma. A diet relatively high in this type of fatty acid and relatively low in simple carbohydrates not only overcomes alterations in metabolism associated with cancer, but also improves the effectiveness of chemotherapy, and decreases the adverse effects associated with radiation therapy.

The ideal cancer diet isn't known, but any nutritional support is better than none. Dr. Ogilvie's experimental diet not only improved quality of life but extended longevity by as much as three years. The study results formed the basis for Hill's Prescription Diet Canine nd.

Gene Therapy

Dr. Kitchell's PhD is in cancer biology, and at a laboratory at University of Illinois scientists are investigating genes associated with the ability of cancer cells to endlessly replicate themselves. Cancer cells don't die, they just keep reproducing. "We've done a lot of research on telomerase," says Dr. Kitchell. This enzyme causes the ends of chromosomes (telomeres) to grow, and this is part of what allows a cancer cell to continue to divide. Without telomerase to replenish chromosomes, the sausage-shaped bundles would shrink every time a cancer cell divided, causing the cells to fizzle out and die. Finding a way to block the action of telomerase may prevent cancer cells from continuing to replicate.

Yet mice and rats are poor models for this study, says Dr. Kitchell. Telomerase is expressed all the time in rodent tissue, but not in normal human and dog tissue. It starts showing up only when cancer is present. "The dog makes a better model because it expresses [makes] telomerase in virtually the same tissues as people, it brings it up in cancers just the same way people do, and the telomere [chromosome] length in the dog is fairly close to the telomere length in people," says Dr.

Kitchell. Such studies will benefit cats and dogs, as well as human cancer patients.

In another approach, genes are manipulated to create genetically engineered vaccines. "I think we're the only place in the world that's developing tumor vaccines for pets with cancer," says Dr. MacEwen. "We do gene therapy at the same time." With a grant from the National Institute on Dental Research, his team studies melanoma of the mouth and skin in dogs, a very common malignant cancer that often spreads to nearby lymph nodes and lungs even after surgery and chemotherapy. People also get melanoma of the mouth, and the dog is the best model for human melanoma.

Dr. MacEwen grows a large quantity of tumor cells from melanoma that has been surgically removed from a dog. "It takes about a month to get enough cells to make a vaccine from the dog's individual tumor," he says, "and then we do gene therapy on the tumor cells." A device called a gene gun injects the human gene for cytokine—a protein that stimulates the immune system—directly into the cells. The dog tumor cells containing the human gene can then make this cytokine in high quantities. Says Dr. MacEwen, "We irradiate these cells—not enough to kill them, just so they won't proliferate and form new tumors. And then we inject them back into the dog in the form of a vaccination procedure once a week for eight weeks. When animals and humans develop cancer, their immune system becomes tolerant and doesn't see the tumor as foreign. So we re-present the tumor to the dog in the form of a vaccine, to try to trick the immune system into recognizing these as foreign cells. With this procedure we try to harness the immune system, which is very potent, to kill remaining cancer cells."

In January 2000, Dr. MacEwen began a four-year trial in which all the dogs with melanoma receive standard surgical care, but only half get the vaccine and half are given a placebo. "Dogs are referred from many local veterinarians, and we also are able to make vaccines long-distance," he explains.

Experts predict that therapies that target an individual tumor will soon be the norm. Today, we're very good at inducing remissions, but we're not so good at effecting permanent cures, says Dr. Kitchell. New cancer therapies will address the genetic defect in the gene that causes the cancer, employ tumor-specific drugs that inhibit tumor growth, and deploy the immune system. But a silver bullet to cure all cancer is not on the horizon, says Dr. Withrow. Each new weapon simply adds more firepower to the arsenal.

"Bottom line, of the chronic diseases that affect dogs and cats, cancer is the most curable," says Dr. Withrow, "and even when it's not curable, we can alleviate pain and improve quality of life. People should approach it with more optimism than they do."

Prediction: Cancer Tests

In the next decade, cancer researchers will develop "predictive assays" that will determine how each dog or cat—or human—will respond to a particular treatment. "It will be similar to the way we now culture bacteria to find out what antibiotic to give," says Dr. Withrow. Gene analysis, hormone analysis, drug resistant markers, and other as-yet unknown tests on the tumor itself may help doctors customize the perfect treatment for a particular pet's cancer.

Modern Miracles:
Algebra's Legacy

Simon was only four months old when he began what Lynn Miller of Princeton Junction, New Jersey, thought was simply "recreational vomiting." As a championship-quality Oriental Shorthair from Lynn's "Algebra Cattery," which breeds and shows purebred cats, the kitten had a glorious show career ahead of him. But a couple of days later, when Simon began to gulp and make funny noises, Lynn took him to the veterinarian. "They diagnosed pharyngitis and put him on antibiotics," says Lynn, "but a day later he had such trouble breathing we went back." She had a bad feeling that Friday, and she insisted they take an X-ray.

Sure enough, there was a tumor in his chest. "It was so big it obliterated his lungs and heart," she says. Lynn planned to take Simon to a specialist on Monday, but before she could schedule an appointment, the kitten ended up in the University of Pennsylvania veterinary emergency room. "He was beyond hope by then," she says. "The cancer had spread all over."

Lynn was saddened by the kitten's fast-growing lymphosarcoma, but not truly alarmed. All the Siamese and Oriental Shorthair cats at Algebra Cattery tested negative for FeLV. Lynn was a stickler for health checks and proud of the care she gave. The cancer was a one-time strike, she thought.

But a week after Simon died, Lynn got the news that his brother, another four-month-old kitten, with a family in California, also had the cancer. She quickly notified the owner of the kittens' sire, who lived in the next town, and she called a friend in Connecticut who had another of her kittens. Sure enough, Calypso also had lymphosarcoma.

The disease was very different from FeLV-associated cancer, and seemed to affect only young cats, typically before they were two. And the incredibly aggressive and fast-growing disease lurked somewhere in the family tree of Lynn's championship cats.

"At that point we were going a little nutsy," she says. Anytime a cat looked funny, she had it checked. Calypso had begun chemotherapy immediately when diagnosed and was doing well, so Lynn insisted treatment be started immediately when Calypso's little sisters, QT-Pie and later Equal, came back positive for lymphosarcoma.

Chemotherapy lasts about two years as a combination of pills and injections. "It starts off with treatment every week, then the treatments are farther and farther apart. The pills we do at home and the IVs we do at the hospital," says Lynn. Cost varies depending on the type of medication—some drugs are expensive, but less costly substitutes are often available. "My veterinarian really works with me," she says. It shouldn't cost more than a few hundred dollars for a diagnosis—a chest X-ray runs about $50—and then up to $50 for each re-exam and round of chemotherapy.

The chemotherapy shrank the tumors, which went away within a few days, says Lynn, and haven't come back in any of the cats she knows of. Both QT, a blue lynx point, and the seal-point Equal temporarily lost their whiskers from the treatment, but they weren't slowed down at all by the chemotherapy. Their fur was so short the whisker loss didn't even show. "We showed QT most of the time she was on chemo, and she did great," says Lynn. "She was Best Colorpoint Shorthair in that region and made Best Cat eight times—nothing would stop her from getting those rosettes."

QT and Equal have both finished their two-year chemotherapy treatments, have no sign of any tumor, and continue to do well. Their big sister Calypso, also doing well, is now a three-year survivor of lymphosarcoma. "QT is a typical Siamese-type cat," says Lynn. "Active, demanding, she runs, plays, and jumps, and just loves people. She's so cute."

Over the past few years Lynn has shared her experience with other cat fanciers to educate them about the problem. "A lot of veterinarians will say you have to schedule a bunch of tests over a week's time, but the cancer grows too fast, and you'll lose the cat. Do everything quickly," she advises.

Lynn also contacted Heather Lorimar, a feline geneticist who collects and compiles pedigrees in a large database and works with Leslie Lyons at the University of California-Davis, to track the disease and try to pinpoint the family link. "Hopefully, somebody will get to the bottom of this," she says. "On the Cat Fancier's e-mail list, there have been more than 135 people on the support group," says Lynn. "It's out there in all the breeds." By talking about lymphosarcoma openly instead of trying to hide the problem, Lynn Miller and her Algebra Cattery will save the lives of future cats.

CATARACTS

The clear lens directly behind the pupil in the eye works like the lens of a camera. A cataract turns the lens cloudy, and vision loses sharp focus. The pet can even become blind. The severity of the problem varies, from a tiny spot of white to total blockage. Essentially, the lens changes in the same way a clear raw egg white becomes opaque as it cooks.

Cataracts in cats are not common and most often result from chronic inflammation in the eye as a result of diseases like feline infectious peritonitis, feline immunodeficiency virus, or feline leukemia virus. Dogs, on the other hand, suffer from cataracts more than any other species. "People think it's an old-dog problem, and actually more likely it's a young-dog problem because [cataracts are] inherited so often," says Dr. Carmen Colitz, an ophthalmologist at Louisiana State University. Many dog breeds are predisposed for cataracts, and American Cocker Spaniels and Poodles are the two most common. "Cats really don't get an inherited cataract except maybe the Maine Coon breed," she says, "and that's rare."

"A normal dog's visual acuity, as best we can determine, is about 20/50 to 20/80," says Dr. J. Phillip Pickett, an ophthalmologist at Virginia-Maryland College. "A cat's visual acuity is probably a little less than a dog's." Cataracts gradually impede the pet's vision until it becomes blind. But advances in veterinary ophthalmology can return a pet's sight to nearly normal.

Surgical Treatment

The same surgical techniques used in people can restore the vision of cats and dogs. In the past, pets with cataracts often weren't treated until they had suffered a significant amount of vision loss. Waiting too long, though, can allow the cataract to become too mature and reduce the success rate of the surgery to about 85 percent, says Dr. Colitz. "That's still very good, but you have a 95 percent success rate when the cataract is immature, more on the lines of what human surgeons have," she says. "The success rate is so good we want to do them early."

Before the surgery, the pet's eyes are examined to be sure there's no other problem. "We test their retinas with an electraretinogram and with ultrasound to make sure their retinas aren't degenerated or detached," says Dr. Colitz. "If they pass the test, then we set them up for surgery."

"The instrument we use for phakoemulsification [breaking up and removing the cataract] is the same as in human hospitals," says Dr. Paul A. Gerding, Jr., an ophthalmologist at the University of Illinois. "It removes the lens using ultrasonic sound waves." Most veterinary ophthalmologists in private practice or at a university can perform the surgery. "The technique passes a hollow sharp-tipped needle into the eye through a three-millimeter incision where the cornea—the clear part of the eye—and schlera—the white part of the eye—come together," says Dr. Pickett. The needle acts like a tiny jackhammer using ultrasound in thousands of cycles per second. "It vibrates back and forth, and that energy and sharp edge breaks up the lens. Then the pieces are sucked out through the hollow part," says Dr. Pickett.

After the initial surgery, the pet can see again, but he's left severely far-sighted, says Dr. Colitz. Instead of 20/50, he'll see 20/800. "He can see the tree across the way but not the food bowl," says Dr. Colitz. So after the surgery, artificial lenses implanted in the eyes, just as in humans, correct the focus. "We can restore animals' vision to as good or better than it was before they had the cataracts," says Dr. Gerding.

Rigid implants have been used in pet eyes since about 1991 and require a surgical incision of about 8 millimeters. More recently, paralleling advances in human ophthalmology, replacement lenses made of pliable, foldable materials, can be inserted through a smaller surgical wound. That allows the eye to heal more quickly and with less inflammation.

After surgery, the pet stays in the hospital one to two days to make sure the inflammation remains under control. Dog eyes suffer much more inflammation than people's do. The pet must receive eye drops four to six times a day for at least two weeks, and possibly up to six weeks, says Dr. Colitz, but they tend to recover very quickly. The cost, says Dr. Gerding, runs approximately $1,000 per eye. Most often, both eyes are done at the same time.

Modern Miracles:
Razz Sees His Future

When Champion Milki-Way Afpint Razzle Dazzle CD ("Razz" for short) bailed out on an exercise during agility practice, his owner, trainer, and best friend Terry Graham of Tallahassee, Florida, knew something must be wrong. Razz had just reached his second leg on the obedience achievement ladder—the "CD" title at the end of his name stands for "Companion Dog"—and Terry knew he'd easily earn his CDX (Companion Dog Excellent) very soon and shine in agility competition. In fact, Razz was such an enthusiastic performer, he'd been invited to be a featured performer on a television show about canine agility.

Although Affenpinschers can be stubborn, refusing to complete an exercise just wasn't like Razz. "He went up the ramp, then balked at the walk," Terry says. The narrow, high catwalk spanning the two ramps was a standard part of agility he'd flown across before, but now it seemed to frighten the little dog. "He ran and hid under the porch."

The next day at the veterinarian's office, Terry learned that Razz had cataracts in both eyes so severe her veterinarian was surprised he hadn't walked into walls. "It was so sudden!" she says. "I just sat and cried, because I knew it was the end of all our teamwork."

Terry feared the cataracts might be hereditary. Though he had since been neutered, Razz had been bred once and had pups. She wanted to make sure the talented dog had passed on only his good qualities and not cataracts to his offspring. So once she found a veterinary ophthalmologist, she rounded up eleven of Razz's relations and had everybody's eyes checked. To her relief, Razz was the only dog in the bunch with cataracts.

Despite having only peripheral vision left, Razz finished his CDX title even before Terry had him scheduled for cataract surgery. "They pulverized the cataracts and suctioned them out," she says. It gave him useful vision back, she says, but she retired him from competition. "He still likes to feel as if he's working, so we still do exercises," she says. "The cataract surgery gave him vision for these past eight years."

Seeing More Clearly

Dogs live through their noses, and have great hearing, so does it really matter if they're nearsighted? Yes, says Dr. Christopher J. Murphy, a professor of ophthalmology at the school of veterinary medicine at the University of Wisconsin-Madison. If measured against human standards of 20/20 vision being most desirable, the average dog sees about 20/60, he says. Certain breeds see better. Labradors, commonly used as guide dogs for the blind, have been bred for better eyesight and may have vision closer to 20/20.

But Dr. Murphy's research suggests some dogs inherit even worse eyesight. "Our initial survey of German Shepherds showed that almost half were myopic, or nearsighted," he says. "And we found a pretty high frequency in Rottweilers and Miniature Schnauzers." He said surveys also showed that about 10 percent of Labrador Retrievers are nearsighted, and Collies have problems, too.

Slight myopia probably doesn't matter to a pet dog, he says. But for working dogs or performance animals, like field trial retrievers who need to see that bird drop three hundred yards away, better vision could make the difference between a mediocre and a championship performance. "Some of these dogs serve as guide dogs for the blind, or are search and rescue animals," says Dr. Murphy, "and all things being equal, why wouldn't you want a normally sighted dog?"

He says dogs destined for performance careers should be screened for vision prior to breeding. That could help lower the incidence of poor vision in some of these breeds. Dr. Murphy hopes further research will help determine the underlying mechanism that causes the myopia, so that scientists can develop new drugs and therapies that would benefit not just dogs but people as well.

CLAWING

Cats claw objects to mark territory. This natural behavior leaves visual and scent cues that signal "ownership" of the designated property. Scratching also offers aerobic stretch exercise, and keeps claws healthy. Claws are used for everything from grooming to defense, hunting, and climbing. But indoor pet cats scratch whatever objects are available to them, and when claws destroy furniture, cats may lose their homes—or even their lives.

Today, behaviorists recognize that cats have both a physical and a psychological need to scratch and claw. Rather than fight nature, you can train your cat so that this normal behavior takes on a less destructive form. With consistent food, play, and verbal rewards, and the proper choice and placement of claw objects desirable to cats, clawing can be redirected to a "legal" target.

Scent-Training Tool

An innovative product called Feliway, developed by Sanofi Nutrition Animale S.A., is an effective way to fight inappropriate clawing. The liquid spray smells like the chemicals that cats produce in their cheeks, called pheromones. They mark territory by rubbing against furniture or other objects. Cheek pheromones calm cats and reduce stress.

Originally designed to stem urine-marking behavior, the spray also diminishes or eliminates scratching on illegal targets, like furniture. That's probably because calming and reducing stress with the scent eliminates their urge to claw-mark. In a study of twenty-three cats, spraying the scratching target once a day for twenty-one days stopped the scratching completely.

Recent studies have identified two categories of scratching behavior. In the first group, scratching is an inherent part of territorial behavior. Early separation from their mother, at or before six weeks of age, predisposes cats in this group to display claw behavior near their most important areas of activity—hiding places, litter box, hunting areas, sleeping spots. This basically posts a note to other cats saying the area is owned, and warns them away. To train these cats to avoid scratching forbidden objects, you need to provide a legal target near the original one.

In the second group scratching occurs during or after situations that worry the cat or cause stress. In particular, the cats claw in highly visible strategic locations, like the front door or sofa, when their environment is too big for them to keep under control, or the area is shared by other animals, especially other cats. For this group, scratching may be completely eliminated if the stressful events—i.e., a strange cat crossing their lawn—can be controlled.

Behavior Training

Because clawing marks territory, scratch objects must be placed in prominent locations for the cat to use them. Cats want the whole world to see their scratch graffiti, and scratch training most often fails when the commercial post gets hidden away in a back room that the cat ignores. Equally important, the textured surface—wood, sisal, carpet, or fabric—and shape of the object must meet the cat's expectations. Some cats prefer to scratch vertical surfaces, while others want horizontal targets. Cats may be induced to use commercial scratch posts with the help of a bit of catnip.

Training can be done at any age, but earlier works best, when the kitten first begins to experiment with his claws. Behavior modification requires a combination of rewarding good behavior with positive reinforcement and redirecting poor behavior with negatives that discourage the cat.

Innovative deterrents to scratching forbidden objects can also be helpful. The best of these "self-train" the cat by providing a negative reinforcement prompted by the cat's own inappropriate behavior. For instance, double-sided tape products like Sticky Paws applied to furniture repels the cat that is foolish enough to touch the sticky surface. Vinyl nail covers like Soft Paws reduce the potential damage.

Surgical Intervention

Surgery to declaw the cat also remains an option, but in recent years it is more often reserved for "last-chance" cats. Usually only the front claws are removed, since rear claws are not used to scratch furniture. Cats can still climb trees with the remaining rear claws.

Declaw surgeries raise controversial ethical questions, since this elective surgery does not benefit feline health. The cosmetic surgery amputates the last digit of each toe from which the claw grows, and serves only to eliminate a normal behavior the owner has been unable (or unwilling) to modify with kinder, gentler training options. "Using a Resco nail trimmer, a surgical guillotine-type device, and scalpels to remove the claws is a little traumatic to the animals. It's a little painful," says Dr. Kenneth E. Bartels, a professor of laser surgery at Oklahoma State University.

Cats without claws continue scratching behavior but no longer damage furniture. They are also rendered defenseless, and some behaviorists believe certain cats compensate for the loss of claws with an increase in biting behavior. Proponents argue that when the surgery is properly performed, a cat suffers no ill effects, and ensures that he won't lose his home (or life) once his destructive scratching is eliminated.

A more recent procedure, called a flexor tendonectomy, leaves the cat her claws, but prevents her from extending them by cutting the tendon that controls the claws. The claw base tends to thicken and nails tend to become blunter, since sharpening the claw is no longer possible. This makes it even more important for owners to clip the claws as needed.

Advances in surgical techniques have reduced postoperative pain, and current declaw surgeries are more humane than in the past. "The surgical laser allows us to remove those claws, and seal the blood vessels and nerve endings so the animal is much more comfortable after the surgery," says Dr. Bartels. However, laser surgery, which uses heat energy (burns!), takes longer to heal than cuts from a scalpel. So although the cat feels better, he may bounce around on his feet too soon and develop complications if the incisions open. "It's gentler, but you must compensate for slower recovery time," Dr. Bartels adds.

COGNITIVE DISORDERS

As pets age, normal changes such as slower gait, gray hairs, or finicky eating habits often develop. But cognitive dysfunction syndrome (CDS) goes beyond normal aging. It is a medical condition that can cause a variety of behavior signs. The condition is thought to stem from physical and chemical changes in the brain that affect how it functions.

Every dog and cat is different and so signs vary from pet to pet. But typical signs of cognitive disorders include general confusion or lack of recognition of familiar people, pets, and places. The stricken pet may get "lost" in the house. They often bark, howl, or yowl inappropriately in the middle of the night or other times. Their internal time clocks become confused, so sleep and awake cycles become reversed. Housebroken pets "forget" to tell owners they need a bathroom break, or confuse the indoors with the yard or litter box, and soil the house. Most heartbreaking of all, CDS can cause drastic personality changes, turning affectionate pets aggressive or outgoing pets fearful.

More is known about canine CDS than the feline form, but Dr. Gary Landsberg, a veterinary behaviorist at the Doncaster Animal Clinic in Thornhill, Ontario, says 36 percent of cat owners report behavioral problems in the seven- to eleven-year-old age group. By age sixteen, the figure rises to 88 percent. Cats with CDS have deposits of amyloid material in the brain similar to those found in human Alzheimer's patients, but other brain abnormalities seen in human senile dementia are not found in pets.

In a pet owner survey, nearly half the dogs age eight and older showed at least one of the signs associated with the condition. A study conducted at the University of California-Davis showed that 62 percent of eleven- to sixteen-year-old dogs showed signs in at least one category of CDS. Also, previous surveys of veterinarians have indicated that in the United States, up to 500,000 elderly dogs are put to sleep each year with cognitive disorder. "The number of dogs at risk, meaning those ten years of age or older, is greater than seven million," says pathologist Dr. William Ruehl.

Human medicine prescribes selegiline hydrochloride as a treatment for Parkinson's disease, Alzheimer's disease, and Cushing's disease. The veterinary version of the drug called Anipryl (Pfizer) has FDA approval for treatment of Cushing's and CDS in dogs. Dr. Dawn Merton Boothe, an internist at Texas A&M College of Veterinary Medicine, says Anipryl may prevent the formation of chemicals that damage the brain. Also, the drug may boost the immune system to prevent the development of slow brain damage. Anipryl also has been used off-label in cats.

The response to the drug varies among dogs. Some show rapid improvement and others less dramatic results. In one study, owners reported that 69 percent of the dogs improved in at least one symptom after a month of Anipryl therapy compared to 52 percent of placebo-treated dogs. A second clinical study showed that 75 percent of dogs improved after a month of therapy, and the dogs continued to improve up to three months later. Most dogs are prescribed one tablet a day for the rest of their life. Interruption of the therapy can lead to reappearance of the signs. Depending on the size of the dog, Anipryl costs about $1.50 to $2.50 a day.

Prior to receiving any drug therapy, the dog must be thoroughly examined and screened for other possible reasons for his behavior problems. "Many dogs never get their brain tumor diagnosed because people think they're just getting old," cautions Dr. Richard A. LeCouteur, a neurologist at University of California-Davis. Seizures and behavior changes are the most common signs of brain tumors in dogs and cats, and brain tumors are a disease of older pets. "So we see the dog three to six months later when the Anipryl has not worked, and by that time the tumor has grown so much we can no longer help the dog," says Dr. LeCouteur.

Supplementing the Memory

Compounds called phospholipids found in food supplements can perform similarly to the natural chemicals that are manufactured and released by the nerve cells. These chemicals trigger the nerve cells to fire and send messages. Pets can suffer from cognitive disorders because their brain cells can't send or receive the necessary messages.

Researchers have discovered that choline and phosphatidyl-choline, two of the most common of these message-sending compounds, can help reverse the signs of age-related senility in both cats and dogs.

MVP Laboratories in Nebraska (www.mvplabs.com) combines these compounds into a dietary supplement called Cholodin. Some studies have shown that an average of 75 percent of all dogs with CDS have improved with Cholodin, which is a less-expensive alternative to Anipryl. Cholodin-Fel is specially formulated for cats. The products have recently become available through veterinarians, and come in bottles of 50 and 500 tablets, or one-pound bottles of powder for sprinkling on the pet's food.

Canine Fountain of Youth

Deprenyl, also known as selegiline (Anipryl), originally received attention as a longevity drug. "We've known for fifteen or twenty years that deprenyl increases longevity in mammals like rats and mice," says Dr. David S. Bruyette, an internist in Los Angeles. His 1997 study showed dogs that received the drug each day for six months lived longer than dogs in a placebo group.

"We think the drug affects the way that the brain ages," says Dr. Bruyette. By altering the chemical toxins in the brain that contribute to aging, the drug may help slow down the aging process, increase survival, and prolong the time before a dog develops an old-age disease.

Dr. Bruyette also completed a two-year longevity trial of deprenyl in four hundred pet dogs throughout the United States. "Two hundred dogs got a placebo and two hundred got the active ingredient," he says. Once the statisticians have finished crunching the numbers, he expects to see an increase in survival in the dogs taking deprenyl. He says drugs like the commercial product Anipryl will be the first of many. "We're going to see lots of these longevity drugs," he predicts.

How Old Is Old?

Pets become elderly at different ages, and the way they age is determined as much by size and breed as it is by preventative care. Old age in cats is thought to begin around age twelve, and small and medium dogs that weigh fifty pounds or less reach elderly status between age nine to thirteen years of age. Large dogs that weigh between fifty to one hundred pounds tend to become old by age eight. And dogs that weigh over ninety pounds—like Great Danes—can become old as early as six years old.

Modern Miracles:
Chelsea Bounces Back

Nobody knows how Chelsea wound up in an abusive home. But the West Highland White Terrier quickly bounced back when Terry Graham of Tallahassee, Florida, rescued her at five-and-a-half months of age. Chelsea had every reason to grow up shy, defensive, and suspicious, but instead she blossomed, says Terry. Like many rescued pets, the little white dog appreciated living in a happy home. "She's been the most loyal, loving, and protective dog I've had."

From the beginning, Chelsea took her duties as queen dog very seriously. She fit right in with Terry's show dogs, and she ruled the unruly Affenpinscher pack with a firm paw. "She's also always been my self-appointed frog gooser," says Terry. The little white dog patrols the perimeter of the pond and nose-pokes bullfrogs back where they belong. Despite some painful joint problems that plagued her as a young dog, life was sweet for more than a decade.

A year ago, Terry noticed that her aging pet was starting to have trouble hearing. "I had no problem communicating with gestures," she says, "but it was more than hearing loss." Chelsea would stand over her food and look confused, as if she didn't know how to eat. She couldn't find the pet door and began having accidents in the house. She lost her alpha position within the pack, and the younger Affens started to chase her and pick on her.

"I felt so sorry for her, it was really sad. I knew she was senile," says Terry, "So I took her to the vet and asked if Anipryl would help her." Although her veterinarian couldn't guarantee results, they agreed to try Chelsea on the medication.

"I had my old dog back in three weeks!" says Terry. Chelsea once more policed the frog pond, and resumed playing with the other dogs. The hazing from the delinquent youngsters stopped. At fourteen years old, Chelsea was back in charge where she belonged.

Chelsea doesn't stray far from Terry's side these days. "I know my time with her is limited, and I think she knows it, too," she says. "Having this little abused dog for fourteen years has been a gift to me, and it's so nice to have her back. She was a lost soul, and now she has a full life! We've had a whole extra year together so far, because of Anipryl."

CORNEAL TRANSPLANTS

Injuries to the surface of the eye can create a slow-to-heal sore that develops into an ulcer, which can cause progressive tissue damage or loss. Dogs and cats get eye ulcers from being scratched, or from dust or seeds that get into the eyes. "We see lots and lots of corneal disease, scarring, ulcers, perforated eyes, and injuries in those breeds that have really buggy eyes like the Pekingese, Persians, and the Pugs," says Dr. J. Phillip Pickett, an ophthalmologist at Virginia-Maryland College. In many of these instances, a whole cornea transplant or a graft of part of the cornea offers the best chance for recovery.

Like bones and tendons, corneas can be stored in banks and made available for pets that need them. They can be frozen and kept indefinitely. Freezing kills the cells, so the cornea becomes cloudy, but the frozen cornea tissue can still be used for patches in traumatic injuries. Many veterinary ophthalmologists keep frozen corneas on hand for their own use, says Dr. Helen Newman-Gage, owner of Veterinary Transplant Services, but fresh corneas preserved in a special media must be used within about fourteen days of harvest. Veterinary Tissue Bank routinely provides fresh corneas as needed to veterinarians across the country.

A corneal transplant is most often used in the event of acute injury or to treat an ulcer that perforates or almost perforates the eye. The white part of the eye has a membrane called the conjunctiva, and the ophthalmologist moves a small part of the conjunctival tissue, then grafts it onto the damaged area of the cornea. "That brings the direct blood supply to the area," says Dr. Carmen Colitz, an ophthalmologist at Louisiana State University. "The cornea is clear and doesn't have a blood supply, so you have to help it sometimes."

The second most common scenario for a corneal transplant occurs in older dogs when problems of the inside layer of their cornea, called the endothelium, cause the cornea to turn blue. According to Dr. Colitz, since the cornea is otherwise healthy in this case—not infectious or inflamed—it is kept intact except for a small central portion, which is removed and replaced with a fresh corneal graft.

Cats can develop corneal sequestration, in which an area of collagen in the cornea dies and turns brown to black. "It's usually associated with chronic herpes virus infection," says Dr. Colitz, "and can happen in any cat, but brachycephalic cats like the Persians are predisposed." That's because flat-faced cats with large eyes don't blink well, and often sleep with their eyes partially open, so the strip of the cornea not covered by the eyelids tends to get very dry. Dr. Colitz says ophthalmologists used to put conjunctival grafts over the area. That protects the eye, but the graft isn't clear and doesn't improve the cat's vision. "So in our newest innovation we surgically remove the piece of cornea that's dead or mummified, and then just fill in the defect with a partial thickness corneal graft," she says. "You sew it in place, and in about six weeks the eye has healed, the cornea becomes clear, they look beautiful. Cats are excellent eye patients; they're very forgiving." Most ophthalmologists now perform this technique. Corneal graft surgery typically costs around $800 per eye.

Visionary Solution

"I often use contact lenses as a diagnostic aid if dogs come in with ill-defined visual problems," says Dr. Christopher J. Murphy, an ophthalmologist at University of Wisconsin. Contact lenses can correct nearsighted vision in dogs, but aren't particularly practical for dogs. "About half the dogs lose their contacts within two weeks, and that's not inexpensive," says Dr. Murphy. But dogs with poor vision or that are prone to eye damage like hunting dogs may benefit from being fitted with glasses, he says.

A routine eye examination includes a technique called retinoscopy, or refraction, and can be done on dogs by the veterinary ophthalmologist. "It's the same way you fit a child for glasses when he can't tell you what he sees," says Dr. Murphy. The exam determines if the dog's eyes focus in front or behind a given target, and then his focal point is corrected with the appropriate lenses.

Even dogs with perfect vision benefit from the protective aspect of glasses, and products like Doggles (www.doggles.com) or Sun Pups are designed to fit the canine face in all its various shapes and sizes. Clear safety or tinted lenses are standard fare but prescription lenses can, of course, be made for the individual dog. "After I took the third corneal foreign body out of one hunting dog, the guy started making his dog wear hunting goggles," says Dr. Murphy.

CYSTITIS

Bacteria, a virus, or a fungus that irritates the lining of the urinary bladder causes cystitis. Pets that feel discomfort or even pain while urinating typically lose house-training. They feel the need to urinate more frequently. Dogs and cats may cry or appear to strain during urination, and may pass blood.

Urinary tract infections affect more than 10 percent of all dogs—females more often than males—and often lead to the formation of bladder stones. Cystitis may be associated with the formation of urinary crystals in dogs and cats that are typical of lower urinary tract disorders (LUTD). Testing the urine identifies the type of infection, and if infection is present, the appropriate medication, often an antibiotic, is given for two to three weeks to help speed recovery. A therapeutic diet helps prevent the recurrence of some types of crystals or stones.

More than half of all cystitis cases in cats are idiopathic, which means the cause is a mystery. Researchers estimate that this disorder affects nearly half a million cats every year. Researchers believe that such cases parallel interstitial (or idiopathic) cystitis that some women regularly suffer. Stress appears to be the major trigger of inflammation. Something as simple as a change in diet may bring on an episode.

"This is a challenging, major pain in the rear end for pet owners," says Dr. Sarah Stephenson, a veterinarian in Charleston, West Virginia. "Nobody wants their cat peeing all over the place, and nobody wants their cat to be uncomfortable." She says cat owners quickly reach the end of their patience, and they may consider putting the offending cat down unless something can be done.

The newest treatment for feline idiopathic cystitis borrows from the human approach in this area, addressing both the stress and the inflammation with a single medication. Amitriptyline (brand name Elavil) works in people to counter anxiety and depression, and this stress relief helps calm the urinary condition as well. Amitriptyline also inhibits the release of mast cells in the bladder wall. "We believe the inflammation is largely due to the activity of mast cells," says Dr. Stephenson. By stabilizing these cells, inflammation in the bladder wall is reduced.

It may take several weeks for behavior drugs like amitriptyline to make a difference, although Dr. Stephenson has seen some cats improve much sooner than that, even within days. That may be due to the drug's antiinflammatory properties, or the drug might even create a kind of placebo effect. In other words, giving the drug builds confident expectations in the cat owner, and this human confidence reduces the cat's stress over the owner's displeasure—and that helps relieve the symptoms.

Amitriptyline doesn't help in all instances, and some veterinarians consider other brand-new experimental treatments promising. Dr. Dawn Merton Boothe, an internist at Texas A&M, says pentosan polysulfate, derived from beechwood cellulose and approved for use in humans for treatment of interstitial cystitis, may also help the condition in cats. Researchers have also noted the similarity between the chemical structures of amitriptyline and hydroxizine, a common antihistamine. In Dr. Stephenson's experience, hydroxizine works well. That's good news, especially when cost is an issue. "Elavil can be pricey, but the generic amitriptyline and the antihistamine hydroxizine are both dirt cheap," she says.

A Possible Culprit

An ongoing study at Michigan State University by Dr. John M. Kruger and others is investigating the possiblity that a feline upper respiratory agent, calicivirus, plays a role in idiopathic cystitis. In 1998 the team isolated a calicivirus from urine obtained from a cat, and genetic analyses funded by the Winn Feline Foundation concluded that it was different from other caliciviruses. Further research will help determine if these urine caliciviruses cause idiopathic cystitis. Researchers hope to develop specific diagnostic tests, antiviral drugs, or more effective calicivirus vaccines to treat the condition.

Fascinating Facts! Diagnostic Litter

In 1999, Pet Ecology Brands Inc. of Dallas began to market the first "diagnostic cat litter." Total Concentrated Cat Litter and Scientific Brand Concentrated Cat Litter contain a pH detector that turns pink when a cat's urine exceeds the healthy, normal 7.0 pH value, and will help monitor urinary tract health in cats prone to urinary problems. The products are available in pet specialty stores and from veterinarians.

Modern Miracles:
Shady's Relief

Two years ago, Anne McCulloch of Charlestown, West Virginia, acquired a two-year-old grand champion Ocicat show cat named Auxarc's Night Shade of Catiators, or "Shady" for short. When his original family got out of showing, he went back to his breeder first and then on to Anne's house. "He rapidly moved through three catteries, which ought to be enough stress for anybody," says Anne.

Anne noticed that Shady almost immediately began straining in the litter box. "He wasn't blocked," she says. "He'd pass tiny amounts, but just kept trying to go to get some kind of relief. And he'd sit humped over in his bed. He was just miserable."

So Shady paid a visit to Dr. Sarah Stephenson, and she ran tests that ruled out infection. Although they found no crystals in his urine, they decided to feed him Hill's cd, a therapeutic prescription-only diet designed to prevent the formation of struvite crystals, a common type of stone. The diet alone didn't seem to help, and after Dr. Stephenson exhausted all the tests, she diagnosed idiopathic cystitis.

They tried Elavil first. The drug calmed his symptoms but had side effects Anne didn't like. "It just zapped his personality and made him droopy," she says. When Shady suffered a relapse six months later while still taking the Elavil, Anne returned to the veterinarian to ask about other options.

Dr. Stephenson had since learned about the possible benefits of hydroxizine, and she offered it as an alternative. "It worked fine!" says Anne. Shady gets a single tiny 10 milligram pill once a day, which costs Anne about $15 a month. Shady hasn't had a relapse since he began the new treatment over a year and a half ago. And Shady has regained his outgoing Ocicat personality—which is a major relief to everyone.

DIABETES

The pancreas, a gland located near the stomach and liver, produces the hormone insulin, which stimulates the movement of glucose (sugar) from the blood into the cells of the body, where it is used for energy. Diabetes mellitus is a disorder in cats and dogs that results from conditions that either suppress the action of existing insulin (Type II, non-insulin-dependent), or interfere with the production of insulin (Type I, insulin-dependent). In other words, although food eaten by the pet is turned into glucose by digestion, the animal is unable to use that energy to power his body.

The level of glucose in the pet's blood continues to increase because it's not being used, and it ends up in the urine, where it pulls more water out of the pet's system in a process called osmotic diureses. Consequently, signs of the disease include increased consumption of water and food, increased urination, and weight loss. Diabetic dogs can also suffer sudden blindness as a result of cataracts. The increased need to urinate may cause a break in house-training, which may be one of the earliest signs an owner notices. Left untreated, the diabetic pet eventually begins to lose weight rapidly.

Diagnosis is based on the signs of disease, along with an evaluation of the blood and urine. Sugar and sometimes acetone in the urine indicate diabetes mellitus. Pet owners may also notice sticky urine.

An estimated 1 in 400 cats and 1 in 200 dogs develop diabetes. Breeds that are more prone include Beagles, Cairn Terriers, Dachshunds, Miniature Poodles, Miniature Schnauzers, Keeshonds, Golden Retrievers, Labrador Retrievers, and Doberman Pinschers. Diabetes mellitus cannot be cured, but in many pets it can be controlled by replacing the missing insulin that the body can't produce.

Oral Medications

Most diabetic pets are insulin-dependent, Type I diabetics and require insulin injections. But for the rest, particularly cats, oral medication may help control or even reverse signs of the disease.

"In most diabetics there's still some function of the pancreas left to produce insulin," says Dr. Dan Carey, a veterinarian at the Iams Company. Banking on that notion, glipizide (Glucotrol) appears to stimulate the secretion of insulin from the pancreas. Strict diet control coupled with the drug has been shown to help as many as 56 percent of all Type II diabetic cats.

Dr. Mark E. Peterson, from the Animal Medical Center in New York, has launched a study of metformin, a new oral drug. Unlike glipizide, metformin works to lower blood sugar by helping the cat's body respond better to insulin already present in the body. Dr. Peterson's study, funded by the Morris Animal Foundation, hopes to establish a safe, effective dosage of metformin as an alternative to using injectable insulin or other oral drugs.

Mineral supplements also show promise for both dogs and cats. "Chromium helps to time insulin release and effectiveness," says Dr. Carey. "Vanadium has a similar effect but a slightly different mechanism." Both continue to be explored in terms of their potential benefits in managing diabetes.

Diet Therapy

The Iams Company, which started researching diet therapy for diabetic dogs in 1996, has found that certain types of fiber in the intestinal tract slow absorption of blood sugar and help regulate the diabetic pet. "That makes it easier to match the insulin you're giving by injection," says Dr. Carey. Diets high in fiber have been recommended for both cats and dogs. The diets also help slim overweight pets. This is helpful because fat cells tend to become resistant to insulin, and lose the ability to respond to the insulin that the body does produce.

"By minimizing the amount of blood sugar, you minimize the total insulin requirement so the animal may still be able to adapt and compensate," says Dr. Carey. Diabetic cats, more often than dogs, develop "transient diabetes." After giving these cats insulin injections for a time, the cat's total glucose metabolism begins to self-regulate, until eventually some cats wean themselves off the insulin. "That suggests if we can correct some of the imbalances, maybe we can get things back to normal," says Dr. Carey. He says dogs and cats benefit from diets that carefully select the carbohydrate sources in the food.

Dr. Grace Long, a veterinarian at Ralston Purina, agrees that special diets can offer great benefits, but she believes cats need a different approach. "Cats have an extremely high protein requirement across the board compared to dogs," she says, "and cats tend to break down protein at a steady rate whether you feed it to them or not." If they don't get protein in the diet, they break down their own muscle and lose weight and body mass. CNM DM-Formula (diabetes management formula), introduced in July 2000, takes its cue from the cat's natural metabolism and combines extremely high protein with low carbohydrates, says Dr. Long. "Cats can take the protein, process it through the liver, and make their own glucose at a much slower, steadier rate than if you give them carbohydrates." That allows many Type II diabetic cats to live normal lives without insulin injections.

DNA Test: A Simple Solution

An inherited medical condition called glycogen storage disease type IV (GSD IV) has been identified in the Norwegian Forest Cat breed. It is inherited as a simple autosomal recessive trait, which means both parents must be carriers for a kitten to be affected and show signs. Twenty-five percent of the offspring from such a match will be affected, and two-thirds of the unaffected litter mates will be carriers. A single carrier parent will pass carrier status to 50 percent of offspring when mated to a noncarrier cat.

Here's what happens. The body normally stores excess glucose from the diet as glycogen. A special biological catalyst called glycogen branching enzyme (GBE) is necessary for the glucose molecules to be added and removed from glycogen efficiently. But affected Norwegian Forest Cats have a deficiency of GBE that causes the kittens to store abnormal glycogen. The most common type of the disease causes stillbirth or death of the affected kitten within a few hours of birth. Rarely, kittens survive to five months or so before suffering months of severe neuromuscular degeneration and, ultimately, heart failure and death.

The University of Pennsylvania has developed a DNA-based test to help breeders eliminate the problem in Norwegian Forest Cats with selective breeding. The new DNA test detects whether the mutation is present in a cat's DNA in two copies (as in affected kittens); one copy (as in carriers); or not at all (as in normal cats). The blood test is available for $75.

Getting on Their Nerves

Many cats with diabetes develop a nervous system disorder called peripheral neuropathy. This nerve disease leads to weakness and wasting away of muscle, especially of the hind limbs. Neuropathy rates in diabetic cats is reported as 8 percent, but many veterinarians believe the percentage is much higher. What causes the condition and how it works isn't known.

In an ongoing study, Dr. Paul A. Cuddon and his colleagues from the College of Veterinary Medicine and Biomedical Sciences at Colorado State University are determining the incidence of neuropathy in diabetic cats. They also evaluate the severity, type, distribution, and peripheral nerve and associated muscle involvement. This Morris Animal Foundation–funded study may lead to new treatments for diabetic cats to improve their quality of life.

Modern Miracles:
Floppy's Sweet Success

When Floppy urinated outside his box two years ago, his owner Debbie De Louise of Hicksville, New York, knew something was wrong. "Floppy was fastidious, and it was the first time in six years he'd ever had an accident," she says. The gray cat had suffered from asthma since he was twelve weeks old, though. She'd been warned that long-term use of prednisone, which prevented his asthma attacks, could also cause other health problems.

Dr. Mitchell Kornet of Mid-Island Animal Hospital drew blood and took a urine sample to run tests. Sure enough, Floppy came back positive for diabetes. "It was my worst fear," says Debbie. "I blamed myself for giving him too much of the asthma medicine."

Floppy's pudgy physique—he weighted twenty-two pounds—was the likelier culprit, though, because extra fat can interfere with the body's ability to use its own insulin. The doctor prescribed Hill's Prescription w/d, a weight reduction diet, which cost a dollar a can and had to be purchased by the case. He also took Floppy off prednisone. Then he prescribed insulin injections. "I was terrified," says Debbie. "Floppy needed insulin injections every twelve hours and I didn't think I could give a shot. But I had to try." Before long, she discovered that giving shots was much easier than giving the prednisone pills.

Debbie picked up the human insulin, called humulin, and syringes at the drugstore. The doctor had to do repeated tests to figure out the exact amount of insulin Floppy's body needed. "We started on a low dosage, and then increased as needed," says Debbie. She home-monitored the sugar level in the cat's urine with dipstick tests, strips of treated paper that she stuck under Floppy's tail as he urinated in the litter box. The strips changed color when there was too much sugar. "Every couple weeks, I took Floppy to the vet for blood tests every hour for twenty-four hours to see how he was doing."

After two months, Floppy had lost three pounds on the diet, which was great news. He had been regulated to six units of insulin twice a day. But suddenly, Dr. Kornet said the tests showed the diabetes had gone away, possibly because he was off the prednisone. Debbie was ecstatic. "Floppy went on a honeymoon from the diabetes, where he didn't need insulin at all," says Debbie. "Then eight months later, his diabetes came back." They had to start from scratch to regulate Floppy. After two months, he needed higher doses of the insulin than before. "He had another honeymoon, but this time it was only four months before he became diabetic again."

Floppy's honeymoons got shorter, and the periods between them grew longer. Each time, he needed more and more insulin to regulate his blood sugar. By April 2000, "Floppy was getting sixteen units of insulin twice a day and was not responding anymore." The cat was developing insulin resistance and there soon would be nothing else they could do for him. His glossy gray fur and white socks turned dry and brittle, he acted listless, and he started hiding under the bed.

Debbie heard about a new diet said to work miracles in some diabetic cats, by reducing or even eliminating the need for insulin. Floppy was still young—only seven years old—he had been diabetic less than two years, and honeymoons showed that his body could still produce some insulin. That made him an ideal candidate for the diet. Suddenly, Debbie began to hope that her cat could have a normal life.

The diet was still in trial phases and not available for several months. By the time the Purina CNM DM-Formula diet was released and Floppy was well enough to try it, September had come. At that point, the insulin wasn't working anymore. Floppy's resistance to disease was so low he'd get sick and stay sick for weeks. Debbie feared the stress of a change in diet could make him sick again, but she also worried his next illness would kill him without some sort of help. She decided to try the food, thinking it was the last chance Floppy might have to ever be well again.

The eight-week feeding trial would determine if Floppy's insulin dose could be reduced. "Dry foods have very high carbohydrates," says Debbie, and dry, high-fiber diets have traditionally been used to reduce weight and control diabetes. The new diet, a high-protein and low-carbohydrate canned food, was the exact opposite of the weight-loss food Floppy had been eating. Insulin was stopped immediately, and the new food was to be introduced slowly over a month's time.

Meanwhile, Debbie tested his urine every day, and closely monitored his health. She wanted to know the minute Floppy acted sick again, so she could stop the food and get him quick medical attention. "Two days after starting the food, the dipstick test said he was negative for diabetes!" she says. "I couldn't believe it, but my vet said yes, it can happen that quickly."

Floppy hasn't needed insulin at all since he started eating the Purina CNM DM-Formula diet. Debbie says the hardest part was taking him off dry food, because she can't leave the canned food out overnight or it spoils. "Now he wakes me up in the morning to be fed," she says, "but that's fine. He's running around like a crazy cat again, he's muscular, his fur is shiny and healthy. He's got his purr back." She can't quite believe that the answer to all Floppy's problems was the right kind of food. "He's like a kitten again," says Debbie. "He has another nine lives ahead of him."

ELBOW DISORDERS

Large-breed dogs in particular may suffer joint pain in the elbow as they grow, due to elbow dysplasia. "They end up having arthritis of the elbow," says Dr. A. D. Elkins, a surgeon in Indianapolis. "The elbow is an extremely complex hinge joint, with three bones involved," he says. For this reason, it's been difficult to develop a workable artificial joint similar to those used in hip-replacement surgery.

The first choice for elbow treatments has been pain relief with drugs. Currently, Rimadyl offers the best help. Some elbow problems result from "floating" fragments of bone or cartilage, and surgery that removes these fragments can relieve the pain. The newest arthroscopic techniques allow bone fragments to be removed through tiny incisions through the skin and muscle to reach the joint. This eliminates the need to make a long incision that cuts through a large area of muscle. "There's much less pain associated with arthroscopy," says Dr. Paul Gambardella, an orthopedic surgeon at Angell Memorial Hospital in Boston. "The healing is quicker, and the athlete gets back on the field a lot sooner."

The Veterinary Medical Teaching Hospital at UC Davis handles five or more cases of canine elbow dysplasia every week. Kurt S. Schulz, an assistant professor of surgical and radiological sciences, and his colleagues use new treatments to relieve elbow dysplasia. These include debridement—cleaning out the diseased tissue (cartilage and bone) with a tiny grinder like those used by dentists—and microfracture, a technique used to cause cells in the diseased tissue to be replenished with healthy ones. Both of these surgical procedures require intensive postoperative physical therapy and antiarthritic medications for about four weeks.

It used to be that you'd find such advances only in a university setting, but Dr. Gambardella says arthroscopic orthopedic surgery can now be found at most private specialty practices as well. "The public puts enough value on it that they're willing to pay what it costs to be able to provide that service out in the private sector," he says.

As a last resort, Dr. Elkins says athrodesis—freezing the joint—can be an option. "The motion of bone rubbing on bone as cartilage deteriorates causes the pain," he says. "So if we freeze the joint to keep it stationary, even though they lose some function, there's no longer any pain."

Shrugging Off Shoulder Pain

Lameness of the shoulder, called tenosynovitis, usually affects older large-breed dogs. The signs can be similar to arthritis, but are caused from inflammation of the tendon that controls shoulder motion. The tendon can calcify—become brittle and stiff like bone—and no longer flexes the way it should. Some cases respond well to pain medication, but others require surgery. "In the past you had to go in and make a big incision, dissect a lot of muscle, and cut the tendon and reattach it," says Denver surgeon Dr. Robert Taylor. Of course, that left the dog sore from surgery with a prolonged healing, recovery, and rehab period ahead of him.

Instead, his new procedure uses an arthroscopic technique to go into the shoulder and cut the tendon with a laser. "We let the tendon fall away, and then it scars in by itself," he says. There's no need to surgically reattach the tendon because scars that form during healing reattach it naturally. "Instead of a three- to four-day hospitalization and long recovery, these dogs literally walk out of the hospital the same day," he concludes.

Cartilage Transplant

Arthritis, dysplasia, and joint diseases like osteochondrosis dissecans (OCD) of the shoulder result in a loss of cartilage. Cartilage, a specialized connective tissue, grows from the ends of the bones to cushion and lubricate joints as they move. When cartilage wears away, degrades, or breaks off due to disease, the body can't grow new cartilage and the joint becomes so painful the pet becomes crippled. "There is a huge need for some type of cartilage-resurfacing technology in animals," says Dr. Robert Taylor, a surgeon in Denver.

Following in the footsteps of human medical technology, Dr. Taylor has developed a new procedure that his hospital is using on an investigational basis. "We harvest normal cartilage either from a cadaver [deceased pet] or from the patient's own body," he says. For instance, in humans you can get the extra cartilage from the knee. Not all of the cartilage in the knee makes contact with another bone in the joint. Some extends farther up, so from these noncontact areas it's possible to harvest plugs of bone with cartilage attached. "We core plugs from one area and put it into a defective or diseased area, like the heavy-weight-bearing part of the elbow joint, to resurface the joint with healthy cartilage," he the major organs of the body, and stimulation of this nerve has helped human epileptics.

In vagal nerve stimulation (VNS), a device similar to a cardiac pacemaker is surgically implanted in the neck, where it repetitively stimulates the vagus nerve. Studies in cats as early as 1938 showed that VNS changed brain wave activity. A number of animal studies in dogs, rats, and monkeys led to the development of the Neurocybernetic Prosthesis (NCP), an implanted pulse generator for human epileptic patients. The first human patients were implanted with the NCP system in 1988.

In July 1997 the FDA approved use of VNS devices to help treat hard-to-control seizures. The exact mechanism of how VNS affects seizure activity still isn't clear, but the therapy allows some patients to become seizure-free, while others are able to dramatically reduce dosages of anticonvulsant drugs. To date, over 3,500 human patients have been implanted with the device, and the overall results have been positive. Surgical implantation in human patients takes less than two hours.

Now the studies have come full circle, and Dr. Munana hopes to demonstrate benefits for the 30 percent of epileptic dogs that drugs don't help, or that suffer from side effects. The results of the ongoing study are not yet available, but to date, Dr. Munana reports there have been no significant complications. Dogs tolerate the implant quite well, and no side effects have yet been identified.

Acupuncture

Acupuncture treatment for seizures has been used for centuries—documented as early as 770 B.C. by a group of Chinese physicians. Until recently acupuncture was used in Western medicine only as a last resort in seizures that could not be managed by conventional means. No one knows for certain how acupuncture works, but a major advantage is the lack of side effects like depression or drowsiness that are common with drugs. Dr. Munana reports that acupuncture appears to increase the level of inhibitory discharges in the cortex of the brain, which suppresses seizures. Research has documented that acupuncture increased levels of endorphins, natural painkillers produced in the brain that are known to have anticonvulsive effects.

Dr. Munana says the results of several studies indicate that epileptic dogs benefit from acupuncture therapy. Gold beads are often implanted

says. The bone/cartilage plugs are able to grow more cartilage, which spreads and covers the deficit. The first canine patients to undergo this treatment are doing phenomenally well a year later. "We continue to be excited about being able to provide that procedure," says Dr. Taylor.

Modern Miracles:
Puddy Paves the Way

By the time he was four months old, Puddy already had the typical outgoing and demanding personality typical of Labrador Retrievers. Nothing got in the way of play for the yellow pup. So when his owners, Sharon and Anthony Regalado of Denver, noticed Puddy beginning to limp, they took him for an exam right away. "We thought maybe he had a piece of glass in his paw," says Sharon. The case was actually much more serious.

The veterinarian took an X-ray of Puddy, and while they waited for the results, she explained all the problems that could go wrong with elbows, including osteochondrosis dissecans (OCD), a defect in the cells that promote cartilage growth. Another possibility with very active, fast-growing medium- and large-breed dogs is that they injure and crack the cartilage from bouncing around and exercising too much, just as bones can break under a lot of stress. Once cartilage cracks, small pieces can come free in the joint and cause painful limping. Dr. Robert Taylor suggested that arthroscopic surgery to remove any stray pieces of cartilage might fix the problem.

"So in February 1999, Puddy stayed overnight for the surgery and ended up with maybe one or two stitches," says Sharon. The surgery was followed a month later by several weeks of physical therapy that included swimming against the current in a whirlpool and working on an underwater treadmill. "He loves water, and he enjoyed it," says Sharon. The surgery and therapy had Puddy back up and playing in no time.

But five months later, the limp came back, especially when the pup was tired. X-rays showed no improvement, and a follow-up arthroscope of the joint revealed Puddy had no cartilage left. "I felt horrible for him," says Sharon. "He was not even a year old at this time."

That's when Dr. Taylor described the experimental cartilage transplant. The two-part procedure would first surgically remove the diseased bone and cartilage from the end of Puddy's right ulna, the major weight-bearing bone in the foreleg. A month later it would be replaced with healthy plugs of cartilage-generating bone. Sharon scheduled the procedures, and the second of the two surgeries took place in September 1999.

"It was tough because these surgeries were a lot more invasive than the 'scope," she says. "When I got home, I sat on the kitchen floor with him and he fell asleep on my lap. And I just sat there for an hour because I didn't want to move him. It was so horrible."

Puddy was fitted with a splint following the first surgery, and then he wore a sling for three weeks following the cartilage transplant. Puddy was depressed, and the way the leg was folded back made it look as if it had been amputated. But it was important that Puddy should place no weight on the healing joint. "That was really hard because he was still a pup and so playful and energetic," says Sharon. "I remember thinking, I don't know if I can go through this again."

Yet the end result was fantastic. "When I look at him now after he's recovered, I can't even remember which leg it was. I'd do it again in a heartbeat!" Today Puddy plays and acts like any normal two-year-old Labrador.

The first arthroscope procedure cost about $1,300, says Sharon. And although the cartilage transplant normally would have cost around $5,000, because Puddy was one of the first dogs to undergo the procedure, there was no charge for it. "We were extremely fortunate," says Sharon. "I'm so thankful we did it."

EPILEPSY

Dogs and cats can suffer abnormal nerve impulses in the brain that result in seizures. Epilepsy occurs when neurons that carry tiny electrical messages from the brain throughout the nervous system misfire. A seizure can be described as a biological power surge that blows out the breakers of the brain.

Seizures have a variety of causes. Injuries from head trauma can cause scar tissue in the brain that prompt seizures. Plus, nearly any serious systemic illness—from distemper, heat stroke, and antifreeze poisoning to organ failure—can cause seizures. When they happen for the first time in a pet older than six years old, tumors are often the cause.

Seizures can be cured when the cause is treated and eliminated. But epileptic pets often suffer seizures for no apparent reason. Most epileptic pets are between one and five years of age and act normally between episodes.

Pets most commonly suffer major motor seizures, also called a grand mal or tonic/clonic episode. The dog or cat falls, loses control of bodily functions, and may vocalize while the legs paddle, twitch, or jerk. Psychomotor seizures affect behavior; pets seem to hallucinate, become aggressive or fearful, or exhibit obsessive-compulsive behavior. Most seizures last only a few minutes and are more frightening than dangerous.

Conventional Therapy

Anticonvulsant medication given at home by the owner helps control the seizures, but generally isn't needed if seizures are few and far between. Episodes that are frequent and interfere with the pet's quality of life call for medication to reduce the frequency, shorten the duration of each seizure, or reduce the severity of the seizures with the least amount of side effects. In severe cases, reducing episodes to only one or two a month is considered a success.

Some of the same human medications for controlling seizures are also used in veterinary medicine. Phenobarbital and primidone are most often given to dogs. Primidone doesn't seem to help cats, but they benefit from phenobarbital or oral Valium. Dilantin, which works well in people, is metabolized too rapidly in dogs to be particularly helpful, and it is toxic to cats.

Newer drugs are also being investigated. Pets that suffer from psychomotor seizures have been helped with medications that control obsessive-compulsive disorders. Several universities, including Ohio State and Texas A&M, have researched potassium bromide (an easily metabolized salt) alone or in combination with other anticonvulsants like Tranxene or phenobarbital. Potassium bromide has been around for so long it is even mentioned in Charles Dickens's work, and it seems to control canine epilepsy as well as phenobarbital but without side effects. About 20 to 30 percent of epileptic pets don't respond well to drugs, but most dogs and cats with epilepsy can, with treatment, enjoy a good quality of life.

Vagal Nerve Stimulation

Dr. Karen R. Munana, an internist at North Carolina State University at Raleigh, is currently investigating a promising alternative therapy for epilepsy in dogs. The vagus nerve in the neck connects the brain to the major organs of the body, and stimulation of this nerve has helped human epileptics.

In vagal nerve stimulation (VNS), a device similar to a cardiac pacemaker is surgically implanted in the neck, where it repetitively stimulates the vagus nerve. Studies in cats as early as 1938 showed that VNS changed brain wave activity. A number of animal studies in dogs, rats, and monkeys led to the development of the Neurocybernetic Prosthesis (NCP), an implanted pulse generator for human epileptic patients. The first human patients were implanted with the NCP system in 1988.

In July 1997 the FDA approved use of VNS devices to help treat hard-to-control seizures. The exact mechanism of how VNS affects seizure activity still isn't clear, but the therapy allows some patients to become seizure-free, while others are able to dramatically reduce dosages of anticonvulsant drugs. To date, over 3,500 human patients have been implanted with the device, and the overall results have been positive. Surgical implantation in human patients takes less than two hours.

Now the studies have come full circle, and Dr. Munana hopes to demonstrate benefits for the 30 percent of epileptic dogs that drugs don't help, or that suffer from side effects. The results of the ongoing study are not yet available, but to date, Dr. Munana reports there have been no significant complications. Dogs tolerate the implant quite well, and no side effects have yet been identified.

Acupuncture

Acupuncture treatment for seizures has been used for centuries—documented as early as 770 B.C. by a group of Chinese physicians. Until recently acupuncture was used in Western medicine only as a last resort in seizures that could not be managed by conventional means. No one knows for certain how acupuncture works, but a major advantage is the lack of side effects like depression or drowsiness that are common with drugs. Dr. Munana reports that acupuncture appears to increase the level of inhibitory discharges in the cortex of the brain, which suppresses seizures. Research has documented that acupuncture increased levels of endorphins, natural painkillers produced in the brain that are known to have anticonvulsive effects.

Dr. Munana says the results of several studies indicate that epileptic dogs benefit from acupuncture therapy. Gold beads are often implanted at acupuncture points to cause long-term stimulation of these sites. In one study of forty dogs with epilepsy, 50 percent were able to be taken off all anticonvulsant medication after receiving gold bead implants, another 25 percent were able to reduce their medication, and 25 percent had no response to the therapy.

The Seizure Legacy Explained

Some experts estimate that as many as 4 percent of all dogs suffer from epilepsy, a figure that is much higher with some breeds. In fact, seizure disorders that appear in the first or second year tend to be inherited. Beagles, Belgian Tervurens, German Shepherds, Golden Retrievers, Irish Setters, Keeshonds, Labrador Retrievers, Poodles, and St. Bernards suffer more from epilepsy than others.

Many breed clubs, like the American Belgian Tervuren Club (ABTC), recognize the health problem and are working with researchers to identify how the trait is inherited. Once the epilepsy gene is identified, it is hoped a test can be developed to screen dogs and avoid breedings that would pass on the disease in future pups.

Since 1998, Dr. Thomas R. Famula, a professor in the Department of Animal Science at the University of California-Davis, has collected information from participating breeders in an effort to identify a genetic marker linked to epilepsy. To date, the database includes information from more than 425 Belgian Tervurens. The work is supported by a grant funded by the ABTC and the AKC Canine Health Foundation.

Researchers from the University of Missouri, the University of Minnesota, Ohio State University, and the Animal Health Trust in Great Britain have combined resources to figure out what mutations are responsible for inherited epilepsy in many breeds of dogs. Details about this and other canine epilepsy research can be found on the Canine Epilepsy Network website at www.canine-epilepsy.net.

FEAR

Fear is a strong emotional response associated with the close proximity of another object, individual, or social situation that threatens the animal. This common emotion becomes abnormal or inappropriate only within certain contexts. For example, it's perfectly reasonable to fear water if you fall out of the boat and can't swim, but it's unreasonable to fear a glass of water.

Anxiety is the fearful anticipation of a future event, and tends to be an ongoing but less severe response that can turn into full-blown fear. Phobias develop, on the other hand, from immediate, extreme, and severely abnormal responses, like panic attacks or catatonia. Some experts believe that one phobic experience "primes" the individual to fear future events. The mere memory of the first event is enough to trigger subsequent attacks.

Properly socialized dogs and cats tend to be more confident when faced with new experiences, and they are less likely to suffer abnormal anxiety or fearful behavior later in life. Exposing kittens and puppies to a variety of positive new experiences, people, and places early on— about two to seven weeks for kittens, and six to twelve weeks for pups— can help reduce abnormal fear when they become adults. While pups and kittens may be eager to meet strange people and experiences, many dogs become shy at four to five months of age, then grow out of it as they gain confidence and maturity.

However, pets frightened by something during this impressionable period may forever after react with anxiety when faced with a similar situation. For instance, a kitten traumatized by a small child, or a pup abused by a male caretaker, is likely to be fearful as adult pets when exposed to any other toddler or male.

Pets either try to escape the scary situation and run away, or when that's not possible, they may become aggressive to drive off the perceived threat. Some dogs try to defuse the threat with submissive behaviors, such as urinating to "cry uncle." Punishing pets for fearful behavior doesn't help. More likely, punishment makes the behavior worse or turns the fear into aggression toward the owner.

Nature Versus Nurture

Little is known about how fear works, but researchers have determined that a functioning amygdala (a part of the brain) is required to learn fear, and a functioning forebrain (another part of the brain) is required to unlearn fear. The amygdala is a tiny portion of the "primitive brain." It deals with emotions and the fight-or-flight response. The forebrain is the seat of personality, and it also deals with logic. Many human fear disorders seem to result from the inability to inhibit a fear response. It's theorized that fear arises in part from the overreaction of the amygdala, or the failure of the amygdala to switch off once the threat is gone.

PET (positive emission tomography) scans have been used to study regional brain flow as it corresponds to emotion. Some dogs respond more quickly or with more intensity to various stimuli than other dogs. This "hyperreactivity" is probably truly pathological—that is, caused by a physical or chemical abnormality, says Dr. Karen Overall, a behaviorist at University of Pennsylvania. Once the pet has gone beyond this threshold, it can be nearly impossible to interrupt the fear cycle.

Noise Phobias

Some behaviorists estimate that nearly 20 percent of dogs suffer from noise phobias such as a fear of thunder or fireworks. Thunderstorms are particularly problematic because of the multiple elements that may be frightening—the sound of thunder, flash of lightning, and change in barometric pressure. Some dogs are likely born with the tendency to fear loud, unexpected noises and won't outgrow the fear. Instead, noise phobia tends to worsen with age.

Noise phobias, particularly fear of thunderstorms, are among the most difficult behavior problems to resolve. Counterconditioning or desensitization training works with some but not all dogs. This technique exposes the pet to the trigger situation in controlled settings. For example, recordings of thunder set at an extremely low volume begin the therapy, and the volume is gradually increased to build up the pet's tolerance level. This therapy does not duplicate changes in barometric pressure or lightning flashes, however, and many dogs will still be frightened by the real thing. Desensitization training also has its difficulties, since rewarding the pet with attention for acting scared more likely perpetuates the fear response. Improper desensitization can make the fear worse.

Other behaviorists recommend a behavior-modification program that uses training to engage the pet's mind during stressful situations. By getting the dog to "think" about and concentrate on a pleasant game (which also rewards him for playing), some dogs become too busy to worry about the scary noise.

Antianxiety medicines, including tranquilizers like Valium, have been helpful in the past, and Buspirone shows great promise in treating pet anxiety disorders. But drugs alone rarely cure the problem, for a couple of reasons. To be effective, antianxiety drugs must be given up to four hours prior to the onset of the trigger. These drugs tend to be eliminated from the body very quickly, so another dose is necessary every three to six hours. For thunderstorms, you can get a barometer and give the medicine any time the barometric pressure drops, but that won't work for other unexpected noise triggers like a back-firing car. Clorazepate dipotassium, available in a time-release form (Tranxene-SD), may work well with some dogs, but it also tends to interfere with the pet's ability to learn. Most behaviorists and trainers recommend a combination of behavior modification and drugs, when medication is needed.

Separation Anxiety

Separation anxiety is a common problem with dogs, accounting for 20 to 40 percent of the patients seen by veterinarians. These dogs are commonly anxious and distressed when left alone and become extremely vocal, "forget" house training, and destroy property either as a means to escape confinement or a way to relieve tension. Property destruction is one of the common reasons dogs are put to sleep.

Separation anxiety is most commonly seen in dogs that have been abandoned young and then rescued from a shelter, street, or lab setting. Pups that leave their mother earlier than eight weeks of age are also more likely to develop the problem. Older dogs may develop separation anxiety when household circumstances drastically change—such as children leaving for college, or a new work schedule that leaves the dog alone more often.

Usually, the dog follows the owner about the house, can't bear to have the owner out of his sight, and becomes increasingly distraught as the owner prepares to leave. Full-blown panic takes over once the owner is gone. Dr. Overall says the acting out is most intense during the first twenty to thirty minutes after the owner has left, and the length of absence doesn't seem to matter. As with other fearful behaviors, punishment usually makes the problem worse. It gives dogs a reason to fear being left alone. "This is truly a panic response," says Dr. Overall. "The dog isn't acting or thinking rationally and is abnormal during the episodes."

Recent research in human panic attacks indicates it's not the event or circumstances that cause continuing or escalating attacks, but the memory of how awful the person felt during the attacks. "So it appears an antianxiety drug would help control the condition in dogs, and offer a crucial step in breaking the cycle to teach dogs more appropriate ways to react," says Dr. Overall. Clomicalm (clomipramine, manufactured by Novartis Animal Health) has been approved to treat dogs who suffer from separation anxiety. The drug prevents the metabolism of serotonin, a natural hormone produced by the brain that affects behavior. It has not yet been approved for use in cats but has been safely used off-label to treat feline anxiety.

Drug therapy isn't a magic wand, however. It is merely a tool to help dogs learn better ways to deal with fear. Programs for separation anxiety are designed to desensitize the dog to the triggers of departure—like rattling keys, picking up the coat, or opening the garage door. Staged absences of one minute, three minutes, five minutes, and so on in incremental "doses" help build the dog's tolerance. A "puzzle toy" that contains a treat, such as a Kong or Buster Cube, may distract the dog enough during the critical first twenty minutes after the owner's departure to reduce the chance of a full-blown panic attack. Eventually the dog that receives attention and rewards when he remains calm learns to recognize a benefit to conquering fear.

Placebo Effect

A placebo effect is a positive outcome that comes merely from thinking a treatment will help you. That is, if a person believes that a pill will cure her headache, it may go away even if it's only a sugar pill. That works with dogs and cats too, though they themselves have no expectation of a benefit from a particular medicine. Because of the strong bond we feel toward our dogs and cats, they can "read" our emotions. In other words, pets may not have any expectations about a drug, but their owners sure do.

That can cause a very powerful placebo effect in a complicated way, says Dr. Myrna M. Milani, an ethologist in New Hampshire. "There's a lag time between when you put a pet on a psychotropic drug and when [the drug] actually causes results," she says. Typically, it takes four to six weeks on the drug for chemical blood levels to be high enough to change the behavior.

Despite this scientifically measured lag time, Dr. Milani says quite commonly the pet's behavior improves by a hundred percent on the very first day he takes the pill. "The owner has so much faith in this drug, they relax," she says. "And because they relax, the owner communicates leadership rather than fear and submission to the animal." So the placebo effect on the owner changes her attitude, and that change in attitude impacts the way the pet reacts as well.

Fascinating Facts! Scent Power for Cats

Pets live through their noses. Scent can trigger fear and aggression, or it can calm these emotions. New technology from Sanofi Sante Nutrition Animale, S.A. helps veterinarians and owners soothe upset cat feelings.

Special chemicals called pheromones are secreted by the cats' cheek glands. Cats rub objects to make themselves feel comfortable by spreading this calming scent. Certain parts of these pheromones (an analogue of the F-3 fraction) are used in a spray product called Feliway, and help to prevent urine spraying and claw marking behavior. Feliway also helps calm fearful cats.

The F-4 fraction, though, has proven to be even better for calming aggressive or fearful, fractious cats. It is commercially available in a spray product called Felifriend, distributed by Farnam Pet Products. Veterinarians use the spray on their hands, allow the upset cat to sniff, wait one minute, and then proceed to examine the now-calm cat. Felifriend helped more than 70 percent of the cats in a recent study by Dr. Patrick Pijah. It is currently available in Europe and should be released to U.S. markets soon.

Modern Miracles:
Gordon's Renaissance

Gordon hated noise. That was a problem, since his new home with Leslie McDevitt was in the heart of Philadelphia, where ongoing road repairs and construction surrounded the house. Leslie could only guess what the two-year-old Pit Bull saved by a breed rescue group had experienced to make him so noise phobic, but she was determined to help the dog adjust to his new life.

Her other dog, Maggie, was a canine athlete and always wanted to go outside, so it was hard to accept that Gordon preferred the sofa. But when outside, he'd try to run away from any kind of noise and had to stay on the leash at all times. "Then Gordon decided he couldn't go to the bathroom outside, ever again," says Leslie. "And he got stress colitis, with horrible bloody diarrhea everywhere that ruined the house."

A great believer in dog obedience, Leslie consulted with a dog trainer. "I spent a year practicing obedience with Gordon, thirty minutes a day and taking him to class," she says. The trainer told her all problems could be solved with obedience training, and suggested she train near the train tracks at the dog park to get him used to loud noises. "Gordon became a very obedient, attentive dog. But he was still scared," she says. "I felt like I was abusing him, so I stopped."

Leslie didn't believe in drugging dogs to solve behavior problems. She feared that would just make him sleep all the time. "I tried acupressure, I cooked him free-range chicken and organic vegetables, practiced TTouch and gave him Rescue Remedy," but they didn't work any better than obedience training. "I felt like a failure. I'm his mom, and I couldn't fix Gordon's fear." Half of her friends advised her to put Gordon to sleep.

As a last resort, Leslie contacted Dr. Overall. Once enrolled in a behavior course, Leslie immediately felt better. "There were dogs in the class so much more worse than Gordon, and they were being helped," she says. The answer finally came as a combination of behavior modification and drugs.

The first part of the therapy taught Gordon "deference"—he was expected to sit for anything, from food to attention. "That changed the energy in the house," says Leslie. "Within two days he'd sit just to see if I'd give him anything." Deference therapy can be a part of obedience training, but goes beyond obeying commands. It helps the dog change his attitude so he recognizes his actions have consequences. "The second protocol taught Gordon to relax, and deal with noise," says Leslie. But he'd always had a problem with thunderstorms, and Leslie finally agreed that he needed drugs to help.

To begin, Dr. Overall prescribed Valium daily for five days just to give Gordon a "vacation" from worrying. He had always been so nervous, he worried away any calories he ate. Once he began taking Elavil, for the first time he began to gain weight and look like a normal dog. He also got medication an hour before exposure to noise like fireworks. "He's still afraid, but he just lies down instead of going crazy," says Leslie. Lying down also puts his body in a relaxed position, and he's rewarded with a tasty treat. Essentially, the medicine helped Gordon control his fear, and he learned that when he did, he got rewarded. Eventually, staged "noises" like knocks on the door or other cues that frightened Gordon became a part of the therapy until he learned to accept them.

The Elavil costs about $8 a month, and the behavior consultation cost $300 for five hours. "It was about the same as the obedience class," says Leslie. Today, Gordon doesn't jump up on her and cry, or go nuts when he hears a loud noise. "He looks to me first, before he moves or sneezes. I can take him to the park now, and he keeps playing no matter the noise."

The dog who ran away at the slightest sound now behaves whether on or off a leash, and he never fails to come when called. Leslie wanted him to be a normal dog, and he couldn't be that. But with the right help, he can finally enjoy life.

FOOD ALLERGIES

No one knows how often food allergies occur. They are hard to diagnose and they can appear in combination with other allergies such as atopy (i.e., allergy to inhaled dust or pollen) or fleas. Some surveys estimate that up to 10 percent of all dogs, and 15 percent of all cats, are affected by food sensitivity of one kind or another. These animals react to one or more ingredients in their diet. Protein commonly found in commercial pet foods, such as beef, milk, corn, wheat, or eggs, typically causes the problems.

At least three conditions influence whether or not pets develop a food allergy. First, inflammatory bowel disease, which involves damage or malfunction of the gut, can allow the "leakage" of large protein particles that then come in contact with the immune system and produce an allergic reaction. Second, dogs with a malfunctioning pancreas are unable to digest protein completely, with similar results. Finally, food allergies may develop when the immune system overresponds. The size of the protein particles doesn't matter, and the bowel can be perfectly healthy, but the immune system overreacts and mounts an inappropriate negative response to protein.

Most food-allergic dogs suffer intense all-over itchiness that occurs year round. Cats tend to have an itchy face. Less often, the allergy results in vomiting or diarrhea. West Highland White Terriers, Miniature Schnauzers, Golden Retrievers, and Shar-Peis may have an increased risk. However, any pet can develop the condition at any age, even as early as six months old.

As with other allergies, avoiding the allergen—the food ingredient—relieves the symptoms. A ten-to-twelve-week veterinarian-supervised elimination diet can diagnose a food allergy and identify the culprits (usually more than one protein, i.e., beef and corn).

Traditional Treatment

Food allergies tend to develop only after the pet has been exposed to the protein, be that corn or beef or lamb. Therefore, veterinarians identify the problem proteins by feeding the pet unique ingredients he's never eaten before. Diagnostic diets that contain novel ingredients like rabbit and potato, or kangaroo and rice, are available by prescription and must be used under veterinary supervision. Once the symptoms go away, suspect proteins are added back to the diet one by one to see which prompts a relapse. Once identified, the trigger ingredient can be avoided by choosing foods that don't contain it. Such a "hypoallergenic diet" minimizes allergic reactions. Since every pet is different, there is no such thing as a one-size-fits-all hypoallergenic diet. "If the pet reacted to beef, move to lamb, or if allergic to lamb, move to alligator," says Dr. Steven Hannah, a nutritionist in St. Louis. "There's nothing about lamb or alligator or kangaroo that's hypoallergenic—they just are novel."

Unfortunately, the novelty may wear off once the food is fed routinely. "If that pet has any of those predisposing factors like a pancreatic insufficiency, an inflammatory bowel disorder, or an overreactive immune system, it may be only a matter of time before he develops a sensitivity to the new protein," says Dr. Hannah. Complicating matters even further, veterinarians fear running out of novel proteins.

Hydrolyzed Protein

The newest tool in managing adverse food reactions in pets has been borrowed from human infant formulas, which have used hydrolyzed proteins for many years. "More recently, the technology has been employed in AIDS patients, where any challenge to the immune system must be avoided," says Dr. Hannah.

Basically, the proteins are split into tiny pieces and concentrated. The immune system reacts to complete or large pieces of proteins. It doesn't recognize the protein fractions and so has no allergic response.

The Purina CNM-HA diet, based on this idea, was the first of its kind, says Dr. Korinn E. Saker, a nutritionist at Virginia-Maryland College. "They mechanically altered the main protein source in the food," she says. "That really reduces, or sometimes eliminates, any kind of inflammatory reaction that might occur." Purina is now working on a similar diet for cats. Other commercial pet food companies are launching hydrolyzed protein diets. Dr. Saker says that Hill's Pet Nutrition has a hydrolyzed chicken liver diet for both dogs and cats called Prescription Diet z/d.

GLAUCOMA

The inside of the front part of the eye contains a viscous gel-like substance called aqueous humor, which holds the internal structures of the eye in place. The liquid, made by a membrane called the ciliary epithelium, remains constant but not static in the normal eye. It drains out at the point where the cornea and iris meet, while at the same time fresh fluid is supplied to maintain the right amount.

Glaucoma, or increased pressure inside the eyeball, results from an overproduction of fluid, or not enough fluid draining away. The eye overfills like a balloon until the eye swells and causes excruciating pain. Increased pressure pushes parts of the eye out of position. The pet loses her vision unless treatment begins immediately.

Secondary glaucoma develops from an injury, tumor, or disease that interferes with the ability of the fluid to drain out of the eye, says Dr. J. Phillip Pickett, an ophthalmologist at Virginia-Maryland College. While glaucoma progresses relatively slowly in humans, it's very aggressive in dogs. In cats, it usually strikes pets older than seven years old as a result of feline leukemia or feline immunodeficiency virus, which scars the inside of the eye and prevents drainage of the fluid.

Primary glaucoma, by contrast, arises spontaneously. Dr. Pickett says primary glaucoma is rare in cats, but may be inherited in Beagles and commonly affects Cocker Spaniels, Basset Hounds, and Arctic Circle breeds like Siberians and Samoyeds.

The painful eye tears excessively, turns cloudy or bloodshot, and the pet typically squints or paws at the eye. Although signs tend to be very subtle, it only takes a few days for permanent damage to occur. Ultimately the pupil dilates and no longer responds to light. Once that happens, if medication doesn't control the pain, then the pet's eye is removed. Usually, the eyelid is sewn closed over the empty socket.

Difficult Diagnosis

A device called a Schiotz tonometer has historically been used to measure pressure inside the eye. Drops anesthetize the eyeball so the pet feels no discomfort, and then the veterinarian gently balances the instrument on the cornea. A scale on the tonometer measures the pressure. Schiotz tonometers are the most economical choice for the general practitioner and cost about $200.

Today, more and more veterinarians are purchasing a more accurate and convenient instrument that costs about $2,500. The TonoPen, designed for human use, is a hand-held computer microchip device that only requires a tiny tap on the surface of the eye to register a diagnostic reading. "It's not much bigger than a pen, probably 8 inches long and less than an inch thick," says Dr. Pickett. "It allows veterinarians to screen pets with potential problems and get them to a specialist in time for treatment. The earlier you get them in, the better off they are—just like people." The TonoPen also allows the general practitioner to accurately keep track of how the eye responds to therapy, says Dr. Paul A. Gerding, Jr., an ophthalmologist at University of Illinois.

Troublesome Treatment

New advances in helping cats and dogs parallel those in human medicine, says Dr. Dennis Hacker, an ophthalmologist in California. "Prostaglandins such as Xalatan and latanoprost are very useful in dog glaucoma," he says, but these eye drops don't work nearly as well in cats. Beta blockers like timolol and metipranolol, and carbonic anhydrase inhibitors like acetazolamide, are also used, says Dr. Pickett, and combination therapies tend to work better than a single drug alone. Eye drops help relieve the pain, contract the pupil, reduce inflammation, and may even promote water transfer and reduce fluid production in the eye. But Dr. Gerding says drugs don't tend to help pets long-term as much as they do human patients.

"Surgery that implants shunts has also been shown to control the pressure," says Dr. Hacker. This surgery is generally done by a veterinary ophthalmologist. Cryosurgery, which freezes the fluid-producing cells in the eye, has also been used in the past, says Dr. Carmen Colitz, an ophthalmologist at LSU. "We've kind of mooched off of human medicine as far as the drainage systems, different filters, and devices that are used," says Dr. Pickett. Although the devices work really well in humans, in pets they often ultimately lead to the buildup of scar tissue, which undermines their effectiveness.

Laser Therapy

The latest and most successful therapy for glaucoma in dogs and cats uses an ophthalmic-size diode laser (Nd:YAG laser). The technique is rarely used for human glaucoma. "The procedure, called laser ciliary body ablation, selectively destroys the fluid-producing tissue in the eye and decreases the production of the fluid," say Dr. Gerding.

The laser surgery takes place from the outside of the eye. "You place the laser three to five millimeters behind the edge of the cornea, and zap the structure," says Dr. Colitz. If the procedure doesn't work the first time, it can be repeated, and it has shown to be very effective in saving pet vision.

Laser technology can also repair retinal detachments caused by glaucoma, but the procedure is not commonly done in pets. "Dr. Sam Vinicy's practice in Illinois has that available as a new technique," says Dr. Hacker. He says the equipment costs between $70,000 and $100,000 minimum, so not many ophthalmologists can afford to make the service available.

Prosthetic Eyes

In some cases of glaucoma, the eye cannot be saved and must be removed in a process called enucleation. When the outside of the eye has not ruptured and remains intact, the cornea and schlera—the shell of the eye—can be preserved, says Dr. Colitz. "In a cosmetic procedure, the inside structures can be removed and replaced with a silicone sphere," she says. "It just looks like a cloudy eye, but it still moves the same and works very well." Because the muscles are still attached, the blind eye continues to move in concert with the other normal eye. The procedure runs about $650, depending on where you have it done.

In a more dramatic and rarely requested procedure, the eyeball is removed, the muscles preserved, and the eye replaced with a prosthetic hydroxy apatite ball. "It's porous like coral, so muscles and normal structures grow into it so it moves in concert with the other eye," says Dr. Colitz. Then an ocularist, an eyeball artist, creates a shell that matches the normal eye. People who have lost an eye most commonly benefit from the procedure, but Dr. Colitz notes that, though expensive, it can certainly be done in pets as well.

Fascinating Facts! Hope for Canine Glaucoma

Dr. Kirk N. Gelatt, a professor of comparative ophthalmology in the College of Veterinary Surgery and Medicine at the University of Florida, continues research to develop genetic tests in an effort to eliminate inherited glaucoma in dogs, especially Beagles. How it is inherited is not yet completely understood. Part of his research includes gene therapy that tries to replace the faulty section of DNA with a healthy section to treat dogs that are already affected by glaucoma. Future drugs may help regenerate and heal portions of the eye that have been damaged by the disease.

HEARING PROBLEMS

Hearing loss is being recognized more and more in many purebred dogs. There are several causes. Conductive hearing loss occurs when there's a problem with sound waves traveling through the inner ear. Pets can be born with conductive hearing loss or can acquire it later in life. The most common cause is chronic ear inflammation and infection (otitis) of the external or middle ear. Ear mites, inhalant and food allergic dermatitis, and the yeast *Mallasezia canis* are the most common causes of ear inflammation and infection. Temporary hearing loss may occur with the rupture of the eardrum but should return as the membrane heals.

A sensory disorder is caused by nerve problems in the inner ear. Sensorineural hearing loss, usually congenital and possibly inherited, is present from birth. The pet can have partial or complete hearing loss. Dog breeds predisposed to congenital deafness include Dalmatians, English Setters, Bull Terriers, and Jack Russell Terriers. In cats, those with white fur and blue eyes are prone to deafness. Chemical or noise-induced damage can also cause irreversible or progressive hearing loss. Nearly two hundred drugs and chemicals can prove toxic to hearing. The most common include certain antibiotics, diuretics, the anticancer drug cisplatin, and some antiseptic preparations.

Age-related hearing loss (presbycusis) is not associated with a specific cause, but is a gradual degeneration of one or more areas of the ear. It is believed to be the most common form of hearing loss in cats and dogs.

Dogs and cats often overcome deficits in one of their senses by compensating with another. That's why it's hard to detect hearing loss in pets, even if it is present from birth. In general, dogs and cats are able to hear sound frequencies within a range that's close to three times larger than that of humans, so pets can often suffer both congenital or acquired hearing loss without the owner ever noticing. That means that hearing loss may not be detected until the loss is permanent or until breeding carrier animals pass the inherited condition to their offspring.

Diagnosing Hearing Loss

Dogs and cats can't tell us they don't hear something, so diagnosis can be tricky. Behavioral audiometry, or a hearing test, presents sounds to the patient, and the resulting behavior indicates if the animal detects the sound. Both conscious and reflexive responses can be monitored, but are still tough to interpret. For instance, did the pet actually "hear" the sound or "feel" the vibration through the floor?

Impedance audiometry measures changes in eardrum mobility as pressure in the external ear changes. In a healthy ear, the air pressure in the external ear canal will be the same as the air pressure in the middle ear. By comparing the two, a hearing impairment can be diagnosed.

Acoustic reflex is the involuntary action of the middle ear in response to a sound. When a loud noise is heard, the muscles of the middle ear in normal pets contract to decrease the movement of the eardrum, protecting the inner ear from damage. The reaction can be measured, and an acoustic reflex less than normal indicates inflammation of the middle ear, or disease of the cochlear nerve, which transmits the sound impulses to the brain.

BAER Test

Evoked potential audiometry is an electrical recording of the brain's reception of and response to external stimulus. This test goes by several different names: brain stem auditory evoked response (BAER) or brain stem auditory evoked potential (BAEP), says Blanche L. Blackington, a clinical audiologist in San Diego. The test allows sensory systems like hearing to be evaluated by recording the brain's activity in response to sound. "We do this test on newborn babies," she says, and it works equally well on pets.

Several types of responses can be recorded, as well as responses within different parts of the ear, so the hearing impairment can be pinpointed to a particular area. The BAER test can be used to measure both conductive and sensorineural deafness. Because this test measures recorded brain waves that can be compared to a "norm," it is often the test of choice for very young children—and pets.

The test detects electrical activity in the cochlea, the spiral-shaped hearing organ of the inner ear, and auditory pathways in the brain in the same way an antenna picks up radio signals. The response is collected with a special computer via fine needle electrodes placed beneath the skin of the scalp, says Blackington. One is placed in front of each ear, one on top of the head, and one between and behind the eyes. The needles are so little, pets are rarely bothered by them.

A "click" produced by the computer directed into each ear via a foam insert earphone—the ears are tested separately—provides the stimulus. A printout of the test results shows the actual recorded waveform with the series of three "peaks" of response. Dr. George M. Strain, a professor of Neuroscience at the School of Veterinary Medicine at Louisiana State University, explains that the first peak in the wave printout reflects the cochlea response to the click, and the last two reflect brain stem response. A flat line response indicates the ear is deaf. Dr. Strain conducts ongoing deafness research and collects information about the prevalence, causes, and management of cat and dog deafness in order to educate pet owners and veterinarians.

Hearing Aids for Pets

Just as in people, some types of hearing loss in pets—particularly age-related loss—may be helped with a hearing aid. In the past, attempts to develop canine hearing aids have not been successful because of the problems involved in fitting the aid into the unique shape of a pet's ear. In humans, the ear canal offers a straight shot to the eardrum, but pet ear canals are shaped like an L with the eardrum located at the foot of the L.

Blanche Blackington became interested in developing a hearing aid for dogs after being asked by her veterinarian to help test the hearing in some of his canine patients. Once the degree and type of hearing loss has been determined, Blackington designs the hearing aid for the specific pet. "We take an impression of the external canal with a silicone-based product that hardens very quickly," she says. An auditory engineer experienced in designing hearing aids for people uses the impression to build the aid to Ms. Blackington's specifications. "We've made two canine hearing aids for two dogs so far," she says, "and both have been successful."

Mollyroot, a tiny Lhasa Apso, was one of the first dogs to benefit from the innovative technology. "The pet becomes more active and social when the device works," Blackington says. Hearing allows the pet to become reconnected with the human family, and improves quality of life.

Dogs are the focus for now, but cats may also benefit once the technology becomes more established. Currently, a hybrid BAER system is used that reduces the testing time by two-thirds; that's a huge benefit when applied to wiggly, impatient pets. Blackington hopes her designs and collaboration with veterinary partners Dr. Richard Johnson, his wife, Dr. Nancy Hampel, and engineer Henry Eisensen will create a system they can make available to veterinary offices all over the country. They have formed the Canine Hearing Company to provide testing equipment, along with the unique hearing aid designs.

Modern Miracles: Peter's Sound Success

Fourteen-year-old Peter's hearing had faded so gradually over the years that his owners, Dr. Richard Johnson and Dr. Nancy Hampel, weren't aware just how much the Boston Terrier was missing. "You never know when they're just ignoring you, or they really can't hear," says Dr. Johnson. "Peter had hearing problems probably for a couple of years."

The husband-wife San Diego veterinary team decided to have Peter's hearing evaluated by Blanche Blackington when they heard her on a local radio program describing how she tested a feline at Sea World. "She ran tests and confirmed Peter was hearing impaired," Dr. Johnson says. "We decided it would be interesting to see if we could develop a hearing aid."

Blackington made a mold of Peter's ear canal. "The dog's ear canal is much deeper than in people, so she wanted the hearing aid to go down as deep as possible," says Dr. Johnson. The custom fit would also ensure Peter would have less chance of losing the aid.

The finished device was easy to put in, says Dr. Johnson, and "seated" itself by working its way down to the proper position in the ear canal. Initially Peter shook his head when the hearing aid was in, but then he got used to it and didn't have any problems at all.

The experimental device was a huge benefit for Peter and his family, and the cost was covered in part by Veterinary Pet Insurance. "Pets kind of go around in a stupor, and lie around and sleep all day when they can't hear," Dr. Johnson says. "With the hearing aid they wake up more frequently and hear and become more connected to life."

Peter wore the hearing aid until his death at sixteen years of age. Dr. Johnson says the aid gave the Boston Terrier two additional years of a quality of life he would have otherwise missed.

"New" Deaf Disorder

Dr. Michael Podell, a neurologist at the College of Veterinary Medicine at Ohio State, reports that a particular line of Cavalier King Charles Spaniels seems to present a new type of deafness. Instead of the more typical complete hearing loss in one or both ears from birth, puppies have normal hearing at birth and develop a progressive hearing loss over the first few years of life, even to the point of becoming deaf. Dr. Podell suspects this type of hearing loss is caused by degeneration of the hearing nerve. The new condition poses a complication in screening such dogs to keep potential breeders from passing on the tendency to their offspring. Further studies are underway to identify tests that may be useful in predicting which dogs may develop such a hearing problem.

HEART DISEASE—CANINE

Dogs can be affected by a variety of heart problems. They can be congenital—present from birth—or acquired later in life, and some may be inherited. Heart failure results when the damaged muscle is no longer able to pump blood throughout the body properly.

Symptoms can be specific to the types of heart conditions. General signs can include the dog quickly becoming exhausted from exercise or play. They typically act weak or lethargic. They also may have a bluish tinge to the skin from lack of oxygen.

When the left side of the heart fails, fluid collects in the lungs (pulmonary edema) and results in a cough, labored breathing, and panting. Dogs sit with elbows spread and neck extended while straining to breathe, and may even try to sleep in this position to ease breathing. Right heart failure prompts ascites; fluid leaks from the body and collects and swells the abdomen, accumulates beneath the skin, and may fill the chest cavity (pleural effusion). Accumulation of fluid causes congestive heart failure.

Diagnosis of heart disease is made using X-rays, ultrasound, and electrocardiograms that pick up irregular heart rhythms. Advances in cardiac treatment, including open-heart procedures, today give dogs a much greater chance to maintain quality of life, or even become cured.

The first open-heart surgical program in veterinary medicine began in 1993 at the University of Colorado. "The original focus was on congenital heart defects," says surgeon Dr. E. Christopher Orton. "Today we feel confident [in handling] a variety of congenital heart defects, like ventricular septal defect (VSD), or hole in the heart. And we've had good success fixing a complicated defect called Tetrology of Fallot, which is a combination of four different defects." Because Dr. Orton's program is one of only a handful of facilities able to do open-heart procedures, a three- to four-month wait is typical. "We do about one case a month," he says. "There is a tremendous need for the technology. But we must be very selective because there's such a limited availability at this point."

Patent Ductus Arteriosus

The most common congenital heart disease, patent ductus arteriosus (PDA), affects Miniature Poodles and German Shepherds most often, but any pet may have the problem. It may or may not be inherited. Normally, the ductus arteriosus, a short blood vessel, allows blood to bypass the lungs of an unborn puppy. If the duct fails to close after the puppy's birth, blood leaks back into the heart through the opening and leads to left heart failure. Surgery can cure the problem when performed early, and in the past this has been the treatment of choice. "Young animals recover very well from thoracotomy, and for PDA that's still a viable option," says Dr. Orton. In thoracotomy the entire chest wall is opened to offer access to the heart, and then the hole is repaired.

Neomuscular Transplant

In large-breed dogs, dilated cardiomyopathy (DCM) is the leading cause of heart disease. It is a disease of the heart muscle, rather than of the valves, in which the heart muscle loses its ability to contract and pump blood adequately. The heart enlarges and becomes flaccid with thin walls. Doberman Pinschers and Boxers seem to be particularly prone, usually between the age of two and five years.

Dr. Orton leads a Morris Animal Foundation–funded investigation. The study explores the feasibility of growing a layer of skeletal muscle on the outside surface of the heart to slow progressive expansion of the heart. The muscle layer will be grown from regenerative stem cells (i.e., satellite cells) obtained from muscle biopsies.

A new method, interventional catheterization, is one of the most exciting techniques to reach veterinary cardiology, says Dr. Orton. Coronary artery disease is treated in people by going down the coronaries with a catheter, or flexible tube. Coronary artery disease is not a major problem in animals, but catheter techniques have been developed for pets. "There are a lot of people like Dr. Jan Bright at Colorado State and Dr. Matthew Miller at Texas A&M University who perform closure of PDA with catheters now," Dr. Orton says. Pets recover more quickly from this procedure than from thoracotomy and other more invasive surgeries. "The more you can do with catheters, the less stress for the patient," Dr. Orton concludes.

Dr. Mark D. Kittleson, a cardiologist at University of California-Davis, also uses catheters in an innovative technique called "coiling," to repair PDA or other abnormal holes in the heart. He uses the catheter to lodge little stainless steel fiber-embedded coils into the holes. The fibers stimulate clotting, so that a clot actually shuts off the hole, he says. In effect, the coil induces the body to patch itself. The Amplatzer duct occluder, a space-age-looking mushroom-shaped plug filled with fibers to promote clotting, is another new PDA option for dogs. It is also placed by a catheter and is currently available only at the University of Illinois, says cardiologist Dr. David Sisson.

A handful of centers across the United States are performing the coiling procedure, primarily at universities. "But there are more and more veterinary cardiologists in private practice, too," says Dr. Kittleson, and before long the procedure will be available in every major city. Dr. Orton and other surgeons see only better things to come for veterinary cardiology. "In the future there may be more and more procedures that can be done in people and animals with catheter techniques," he says, citing a septal defect as an example. That currently requires a heart-lung bypass machine, which is available only at a couple of veterinary university teaching hospitals.

Pulmonic Stenosis

Another problem is pulmonic stenosis, a narrowing of the connection between the right ventricle, or lower heart chamber, and the pulmonary artery that leads to the lungs. Affecting small-breed dogs most often, this congenital defect makes the heart work harder to push blood through the narrow opening. Heart muscles sometimes compensate by growing stronger, but many times the heart defect becomes life-threatening.

New catheter techniques can also treat pulmonic stenosis, says Dr. Kittleson. Performed under anesthesia, the procedure requires a small incision into a blood vessel. A catheter is passed through the vessel to reach the heart. A large balloon on the catheter is positioned across this region of narrowing, and inflated with some saline. That opens the passage to its normal size. The procedure is identical to that performed on children with pulmonic stenosis. Heart catheterizations are specialized procedures, and only a few centers across the country do them. They tend to cost $1,000, says Dr. Kittleson.

Open-heart surgery offers a brand-new option for treating stenosis of the pulmonic valve. The technique can very successfully treat this congenital defect by widening the valve to allow more blood to flow from the heart into the lungs. The surgery is currently limited to only two veterinary centers—the University of Pennsylvania and Colorado State University. Patients must also meet stringent requirements to be considered as candidates.

"We use the cardiopulmonary bypass in an open-heart procedure," says Dr. Daniel Brockman, a surgeon at University of Pennsylvania. "A perfusionist [specialist who runs the machine] comes from St. Luke's Hospital in Bethlehem, Pennsylvania, to run the heart-lung machine," he says, "and one of their cardiac surgeons also comes to help with the procedures." The open-heart team consists of four main groups: the preoperative team (medical cardiologists and surgeons), the operative team (anesthesiologists, a perfusionist, two surgeons, and two surgical assistants), the postoperative team (critical care staff and intensive care unit), and ongoing care (attending surgical clinicians). The endeavor is both labor- and facility-intensive and possible only because of all the specialty groups available within the hospital.

Typically patients stay in the hospital for at least seven to ten days after the surgery. Dr. Brockman says he has the resources to perform one or two such procedures a month and that customary fees for an open-heart procedure will run between $6,000 and $10,000 once the program and techniques have been more firmly established. "But right now we're running a clinical investigation—kind of a step up from experimental," he says, "to investigate the feasibility for a mainstream clinical program." His program subsidizes the actual cost and offers pet owners a flat fee at a substantial discount. "The discount is something like a third of the actual fee, somewhere in the vicinity of $2,500 to $3,500," says Dr. Brockman, "but that's still a lot of money."

Large-breed dogs like Golden Retrievers are prone to aortic stenosis, a narrowing of the connection between the left ventricle and the aorta, the large artery that carries blood out of the heart. Surgery is the treatment of choice, but it is risky, expensive, and available only at veterinary schools or from specialists that have access to heart-lung bypass machines.

Heart-Lung Bypass Machine Heart surgery that requires a bypass entails setting up a circuit of blood outside the dog's body. Just as with people, the heart-lung bypass machine takes the place of the heart, pumping the dog's blood and putting oxygen in it.

While the machine can save the dog's life, it also causes damage and can complicate the recovery of the patient, especially very small pets. Rather than the intermittent blood flow created by the heart, a bypass pump creates continuous flow. The constant pressure stresses the peripheral blood vessels and can burst the cell walls so that fluid leaks into the tissues, says Dr. Brockman. Red cells and platelets are often damaged or completely destroyed. "That's very commonly seen in human patients, too," says Dr. Brockman, "but because they're so much bigger, they tolerate it a little bit better." That's why small dogs and cats are not yet considered good candidates for bypass procedures.

Valvular Disease

Acquired valvular heart disease is the leading cause of heart disease in dogs. It is considered a disease of old age and a third of all dogs over the age of twelve are affected. The heart valves simply start to wear out. It's most common in smaller breeds.

When heart valves wear out, they leak blood backward into the heart, instead of pumping it forward. That causes extra strain on the heart muscle. The body retains fluid to compensate for reduced heart efficiency. When the left side of the heart fails, the fluid collects in the lungs and interferes with breathing. When right side fails, fluid collects in the abdomen, chest, or under the skin, so the belly and legs swell, or fluid around the heart interferes with the heart's beating (congestive heart failure).

Dogs with this disease can often be helped with drugs that improve the heart's performance, control lung function and relieve congestion, and rid the body of excess fluid. Therapeutic diets support the damaged heart and compensate for the potassium, chloride, and magnesium lost from increased fluid excretion.

"Our newest frontier in open-heart is valve surgery," says Dr. Orton. His team has had success with repairing a congenital defect of the valve called tricuspid dysplasia. Yet another procedure has not done as well. "One of the most common acquired defects in older dogs is mitral valve disease or mitral regurgitation," he says. "We have performed mitral valve replacement in several dogs, but I'm discouraged about this option for dogs because we've lost about half the dogs within a few months because the valve clotted." Dr. Orton now focuses his efforts on repair of the original natural valve of the dog's heart.

Typically, open-heart procedures last about five hours and involve a team of surgical experts. Similar procedures in human medicine would easily cost $25,000 to $50,000 but generally cost under $6,000 for dogs treated at Colorado State.

"In the next five to ten years, I expect there will be at least three or four centers in North America where open-heart procedures are done frequently," says Dr. Brockman. There are many heart defects common in dogs and cats that don't respond well to current treatments. Perfecting open-heart bypass procedures will offer new hope for these patients.

Pacemakers and Veterinary Medicine

Pacemakers for pets were used for the first time in 1981, and for twenty years they have helped pets lead normal lives, just as they do humans. "They are considered almost standard care these days," says Dr. Kittleson from the University of California-Davis. "We put in twenty to twenty-five of them here each year."

Pacemakers are primarily used when pets have abnormal (slow or irregular) heart rhythms called arrhythmias that cannot be controlled with medication. "Certainly, you shouldn't have any trouble finding someone to implant a pacemaker these days," says Dr. Kittleson. Once implanted, the pacemaker regulates the heartbeat to eliminate fainting spells prompted by the heart condition. It also helps improve heart efficiency, which in turn reduces the chance for heart failure, low blood pressure (hypotension), or sudden death.

Lead wires are placed on the heart and are connected to the pulse generator (battery pack) that's usually positioned either beneath the skin or within the pet's abdomen. Most pacemakers used today are "demand" pacemakers, which sense the patient's heart action. That means that as long as the dog or cat's heart rate exceeds the setting of the pulse generator, the pacemaker will not fire.

Traditional pulse generators can be set at a rate between 70 to 100 beats per minute (cats are set at 120 bpm). Some of the newer programmable ones increase their rate of firing when movement or exercise is sensed.

Complications, from minor to severe, develop in up to 40 percent of animals with pacemakers. Pet owners must be familiar with the pulse rate setting on the pacemaker generator and check the pet's heart rate weekly to monitor the system. Newer pacemaker systems are not sensitive to microwave interference, but older models may require special considerations around such devices.

Modern Miracles:
Zoey Makes History

As a birthday present to herself, Lisa Cioffi of Denver flew to Missouri to pick Zoey out of a litter of six-week-old Weimaraner puppies. "She's very affectionate and lovable, always wanting to cuddle, and extremely bright," says Lisa. "She's the sweetest dog I've ever met." Zoey fit right into Lisa's routine and even joined her for a one- or two-mile run every other day.

During Zoey's four-month-old visit for routine vaccinations, the veterinarian heard something wrong with the pup's heart. Further tests were done, and a CT scan confirmed valve dysplasia. "Her heart was huge—it was pressed up against and filled her chest cavity," says Lisa. She was told heart medicine might help, but Zoey probably wouldn't live beyond a year. "I was devastated," says Lisa. "Zoey had already become my heart and soul."

Frantic to find help for her dog, Lisa was referred to the advanced cardiology program at Colorado State University. Dr. Orton agreed to look at Zoey.

Lisa learned that Dr. Orton's team had performed experimental surgery that transplanted pig heart valves. "He said if he tried it again, he'd use a mechanical valve, but the odds were not great for success," says Lisa. "I didn't want to watch her suffer and die. I wanted to give her a chance."

Zoey's six-hour surgery took place on December 4, 1997, on her five-month birthday. Dr. Orton periodically returned to the waiting room to update Lisa on Zoey's progress. Once the surgery was complete, she was told the first hurdle would be getting off the bypass machine. "Dr. Orton personally kept a vigil for those first seventy-two hours. They took extremely good care of her," says Lisa. She had a minor setback and needed a respirator for about twenty-four hours, but Zoey quickly bounced back.

Lisa picked her up a week after the surgery. "Zoey looked like she'd been hit by a truck!" The fourteen-inch surgery incision ran north-south on the pup's left side, she had a gaping hole in her neck from the tracheal tube, and most of her beautiful silver fur had been shaved. But all the tests showed that her new mechanical valve was doing the job, and Zoey's enlarged heart began to shrink down to a more normal size.

Follow-up tests, including X-rays, CT scans, and sonograms, continued every month for a while, then every three months, and finally at six-month intervals. Zoey continued to improve; on the two-year anniversary of the surgery, Lisa was told a yearly exam at Colorado State would be enough. Zoey continues to make the hour and a half trip to see Dr. Holly Knor at Alameda East Veterinary Hospital every three months for a routine checkup and blood tests to monitor the effects of Coumadin, an anticoagulant medication that Zoey must take for the rest of her life. The drug prevents blood clots from forming in the valve, which could potentially break free and kill her. The artificial valve has given Lisa back a canine friend who doesn't know how to slow down. "Zoey climbed a 14,000-foot mountain with us last summer!" she says.

The operation alone cost well over $4,000, but Lisa says it was worth much more than that. "She's not just my baby. She was the first dog in the world to have a mechanical heart valve—she made history! And paved the way for a lot of animals."

Fascinating Facts! Artificial Pet Heart?

Dr. Michael DeBakey, a famous cardiovascular surgeon in human medicine, continues to research innovations that might benefit heart patients. He is currently working with NASA to develop a self-contained, miniaturized artificial heart. Such an organ might have applications not only for human infants, but also for pets.

HEART DISEASE—FELINE

Heart disease takes many forms in cats and affects as many as 11 percent of the feline population. The most common condition, cardiomyopathy, affects the heart muscles in various ways. Fifteen years ago, dilated cardiomyopathy was the leading heart disease in cats. It causes systolic dysfunction, in which the heart muscle isn't able to adequately contract and has trouble pumping blood out of the heart. The heart becomes enlarged like a balloon, and the muscle walls become thin.

"Back in 1987 we identified a deficiency of taurine [an essential amino acid for cats] as the major cause of dilated cardiomyopathy in cats," says Dr. Mark D. Kittleson, a cardiologist at University of California-Davis. "The vast majority of that disease has subsequently disappeared since cat food manufacturers increased taurine in their cat foods. But it still pops up on us every once in a while." All breeds can be affected, but Siamese, Abyssinian, and Burmese seem to be predisposed to dilated cardiomyopathy. The disease has been reported in cats anywhere from five months to sixteen years of age.

Today, hypertrophic cardiomyopathy is the most common cardiac condition seen in cats, says Dr. E. Christopher Orton, a surgeon at Colorado State University. It is a disease of diastolic function—which means the muscle wall of the heart thickens and reduces the size of the heart chambers until they cannot fill adequately with blood. Any cat may be affected, but most often the condition strikes young to middle-aged male cats.

It is also a genetic disease in humans and in some breeds of cats, says Dr. Kittleson. "The cause is known in humans," he says. "There are certain genetic mutations that cause it." Researchers are using the human benchmarks to help with the feline disease. "We're in the process of trying to identify that gene mutation in the Maine Coon breed," says Dr. Kittleson. "Hopefully once we identify that mutation, then we can test breeding cats and wipe it out of that breed." Future studies may address the condition in other cats as well.

Signs of the disease vary, from cats that appear totally unaffected to those who suffer sudden death. About 50 percent of all cats that show signs die within three months of diagnosis, while cats with minor to no outward signs usually survive more than five years with medical help.

Most affected cats have labored breathing from fluid-filled lungs (pulmonary edema) or from fluid in the chest cavity (plural effusion). Cats act lethargic, depressed, and weak, and may also lose their appetite and refuse to eat. The most dramatic sign, hind limb pain or paralysis, results from blood clots that form in the heart chamber, then break free and travel in the bloodstream to lodge in the hind legs where the artery splits. Called a "saddle thrombus," the clot cuts off the blood supply and causes pain and/or paralysis in one or both rear limbs.

Diagnostic tests include electrocardiograms, which may pick up abnormal heart rhythms, and X-rays, which show fluid in the lungs and chest cavity and the silhouette of the heart itself. The hypertrophic heart looks like a valentine. A third type of test, an echocardiogram, shows the thickness of the wall of the heart and how well the heart muscle pumps.

Treatment won't cure heart disease, but it may prolong or at least improve the quality of the cat's life. Fluid congestion is commonly controlled with a diuretic drug such as Lasix (furosemide) that forces the kidneys to get rid of excess salt and water. Vasodilator drugs open up the constricted blood vessels and help control congestion, which makes it easier for the cat to breathe. Calcium channel blockers and beta blockers may be used to slow the heart rate in hypertrophic cardiomyopathy to give the heart more time to fill. Digoxin may help strengthen heart muscles and regulate blood pressure. About 40 percent of all cats with blood clots regain use of their rear limb within a week without treatment. Clot-reducing drugs help reduce the "stickiness" of blood platelets and so decrease the chances of clots from forming.

Prediction: Breeding for a Cure

How Maine Coon cats inherit hypertrophic cardiomyopathy, and Doberman Pinschers inherit dilated cardiomyopathy, is currently being studied at the University of California-Davis and Michigan State University. Cats and dogs as a whole should benefit from current and future research. "In the next ten years, we'll reap some of the benefits of the human genome project," says Dr. Kittleson. "As they identify specific mutations that cause heart disease in humans, we'll likely find the exact same or similar mutations causing the same diseases in dogs and cats. And in pets, we'll be able to breed to avoid these diseases, so they never occur."

Modern Miracles:
Blue's Murmur

Blue traveled partway around the world to reach Kathy Keely's home in Blackwood, New Jersey. The blue tabby and white Maine Coon kitten arrived from England in March 1999, but his seven-hour flight and hour-and-a-half car ride didn't faze him in the least. He just wanted to get out and meet the rest of the cats, and he immediately fit in. And he quickly purred his way into Kathy's heart. "He's always the first cat to greet me when I walk in the door," she says. "He talks to me, tells me about his day as he follows me around."

A month later, a couple of weeks before Blue was neutered, Kathy noticed the five-month-old kitten panted when he played. "That kind of scared me," says Kathy. She knew panting was normal for dogs but could be a danger sign in cats. Felines typically don't pant unless they overheat, become severely stressed, or have trouble breathing. An X-ray showed his heart to be on the large size, but the veterinarian thought that might be because Maine Coon hearts tend to be bigger than other breeds. "At that point Blue's heart sounded fine," says Kathy. The veterinarian took extra precautions with the cat's anesthesia, and Blue came through the neuter with no problems.

But six months later, Blue developed upper respiratory problems. "We X-rayed him again because it sounded like something stuck in his throat when he coughed and gagged," Kathy says. His heart size was the same, but he'd also developed a heart murmur. The veterinarian thought the murmur was nothing, but they could set up further tests to make sure.

Kathy knew heart problems ran in some Maine Coon lines. She decided to take advantage of the mobile veterinary cardiology practice that could consult right in her general practitioner's office. "First I enrolled Blue in Premier Pet Insurance for $6 a month, just because I'm paranoid," she says, "and then made the appointment with the heart specialist."

The consultation and echocardiogram cost $245, and was covered in part by the insurance. "I've had an echo done on myself," says Kathy, "and that cost $900 for five minutes. This was a deal." She was able to watch Blue's echocardiogram test. "It showed the turbulence of the blood flow through the heart valves," she says, "and you could see the difference between the two sides of Blue's heart." The wall of his left ventricle was clearly thicker than the opposite wall—a sign of hypertrophic cardiomyopathy. "The cardiologist said I'd caught the problem early, and it was still a really mild case," says Kathy, "so my paranoia paid off."

She immediately contacted her friend, Blue's breeder, to let him know the news. "He was just devastated," she says, not only because of Blue, but because he knew the disease could be inherited and there might be a problem in his line of championship Maine Coon cats. So he alerted the owners of Blue's siblings, had both parents screened for hypertrophic cardiomyopathy—and had Blue's mother spayed. "They all checked out fine," says Kathy. "It turns out, Blue was the only cat that had the problem."

Kathy learned that, when diagnosed early, some heart damage can be reversed with proper medication. A daily dose of the human drug Atenolol was prescribed. Atenolol blocks specialized nerve receptors on the heart and blood vessels, to slow and stabilize the heart rate. "I shake the pill bottle, and Blue jumps up on the counter for his quarter of a tiny pill," says Kathy. She says the medicine costs about $8 and lasts two months—and insurance reimburses for the prescription.

After six months on the drug, a second echo test showed the damage to Blue's heart was nearly completely reversed, and his EKG was nearly normal. They reduced his dose to every other day.

"I'm told Blue should live a normal life as long as we medicate him," says Kathy. "Blue is only a year and a half old—and I'm not willing to lose him for a long, long time."

Modern Miracles:
A Valentine for Thurston

It was love at first sight when Cecilia Barrington of West Bloomfield, Michigan, adopted two kittens—brother and sister—from a friend as a Christmas gift to herself. A week later, the little black kitten she named Lovey got a clean bill of health from the veterinarian. But Lovey's tiger-striped brother, Thurston Howl III, prompted a surprised gasp when the veterinarian listened to his heart.

"He had a severe heart murmur," says Christine Cannon, DVM, of Exclusively Cats in Waterford, Michigan. Mild to severe abnormal heart sounds can be caused by a variety of defects in the heart structure or in the way the muscle works. Thurston's murmur was rated a grade 6.

"It was so severe, we were worried he would die," says Cecilia. He wasn't expected to reach his first birthday. Cecilia was devastated. Dr. Cannon recommended an ultrasound to pinpoint the cause. An appointment with mobile cardiologist Dr. William Brown was scheduled for January 5, when the kittens were due to receive their next vaccinations.

The news was grim. "Thurston had two heart defects," says Cecilia. Ventricular septal defect (VSD) is a hole in the heart wall between the right and left sides of the heart. Blood leaks back and forth across the hole, and depending on the size of the opening, may be serious or not. Thurston's hole was rather small, and not serious. "It was the second problem—patent ductus arteriosis (PDA)—that threatened his life," says Dr. Cannon.

Before birth, there's no reason to have blood flow to the lungs because unborn kittens don't breathe, so this blood vessel shunts blood around the lungs. "When they're born, the change in pressure within the chest cavity causes the blood vessel to close, so blood can flow to the lungs," explains Dr. Cannon. Usually the vessel closes within three to five days after birth. "In Thurston's case, it just never closed."

PDA is quite common in dogs and people, but rare in cats. Surgery could fix the defect. Otherwise the kitten was certain to die of heart disease. "The operation costs $2,000 to $3,000. I love my cats, but I'm on a fixed income," says Cecilia. It broke her heart that she couldn't afford to save Thurston's life.

"Sometimes a university has lower prices or programs that help lower-income families," says Dr. Cannon. She contacted Michigan State University in East Lansing to see what might be available. The timing couldn't have been better.

Animal Planet had been filming at the university all week for a veterinary special featuring cardiac surgeon pioneer George Eyster, VMD. Because Thurston's case was so rare, and because of interest from the television producers, Dr. Eyster offered to perform the surgery at a drastically reduced cost of $350. Thurston's miracle surgery was scheduled for Valentine's Day.

Meanwhile, Cecilia's friends took up Thurston's cause. "Lori Cash planned a kitty shower and ten people came to my 'save the kitty' party," says Cecilia. More that twenty people donated money to help with the surgery, and other friends provided transportation for the two-and-a-half-hour car ride to and from the university.

Lovey caused more worries when she went into heat at less than five months old. Cecilia says, "All I could think was, I'm gonna bring Thurston home from heart surgery, she'll be in the loving mood—and I'm not letting him die with a smile on his face!" She scheduled Lovey's spay with Dr. Cannon on the day before Thurston's operation. Thurston would be neutered at the same time his heart was repaired.

When the day arrived, Thurston's left side was cut open from top to bottom, and his ribs spread apart so the surgeons could reach his heart. It took awhile to locate the open vessel—it was in an odd location underneath the heart. The surgery to repair the PDA took about an hour. "The doctors were so sweet to me, I hugged them after they came out of surgery and told me he was okay," says Cecilia.

Recovery usually takes about two hours, but the kitten surprised Dr. Eyster by trying to walk within fifteen minutes. "He wished all his cat patients were like Thurston, and said he was exceptionally well behaved," says Cecilia. The surgery and recovery went so well, Thurston returned home the same day with a pink liquid antibiotic, called amoxicillin, to be give to him twice a day.

"Thurston was shaved naked from his chin to a bit below his middle, with a four-inch incision," says Cecilia. "They said it would take about six months for fur to grow back. I wouldn't laugh at him, but he looked so silly."

Funny looks were the least of his worries. The first night home, he shivered and shook with pain, moaned at the gentlest touch, and refused to eat. At the clinic the next day, Dr. Cannon shaved his other side and put a pain patch on him. The patch stuck to the skin and transferred a pain-relieving drug called fentanyl through the skin for about five days. "What a difference the pain patch made!" says Cecilia. "He ate like he'd never seen food, and I had to be careful he didn't overdo playing. Thurston always lagged behind Lovey. After the surgery, Dr. Eyster said he'll grow by leaps and bounds because the oxygen will get to his tissues more and he'll thrive," says Cecilia.

Dr. Cannon agrees, saying, "Now that we've got the problem fixed, we expect his heart will say, 'Oh, thank you!' and relax and be a normal heart." Thurston's prognosis is for a full and healthy life, without limitations.

Cecilia can't say enough about Dr. Eyster, Dr. Cannon, and all the others involved in fixing Thurston's broken heart. "They saved my kitten's life!" she says. "What a blessing this has been. These kittens have brought me such joy."

Animal Planet ultimately chose to feature a different pet on its program, but Cecilia says that doesn't really matter. "Thurston will always be famous to me—he's already a hero in my eyes."

HIP DYSPLASIA

The pelvis cradles the head of the femur (thigh bone) in a cuplike socket of bone that forms the hip. As a young pet grows, if the alignment isn't just right, a progressive, degenerative abnormality of the fit of these bones, or hip dysplasia, can develop. The misalignment causes wear and tear on the joint that promotes osteoarthritis. Hip dysplasia is the most common cause of rear-end lameness in dogs, especially large-breed animals.

The disease is also frequently seen in a number of purebred as well as mixed-breed cats. The number has likely been underreported due to the stoic nature of felines, and feline hip dysplasia has gained attention only recently.

"Hip dysplasia is very common," says Dr. Gail Smith, an orthopedic surgeon at the University of Pennsylvania, but fortunately only a relatively small percentage of pets suffer the severest, crippling form of the disease. "In our study, 70 percent of the Golden Retrievers at age two have signs of HD, but very few will let the owners know that their hips are anything but normal," he says. Medical treatment can lessen the symptoms, but can't cure the disease.

Genetics accounts for about 25 percent of a dog's chance for developing hip dysplasia, and even dogs with normal parents can develop the condition. Hip dysplasia is considered "polygenetic" by veterinarians, which means a genetic predisposition to HD can be influenced by lifestyle, nutrition, weight, and activity level. Severe disease may be seen as early as four months of age, but usually develops in nine- to twelve-month-old pets. Animals tend to have trouble getting up, have difficulty jumping, limp after exercise, or display a classic wavery or bunny-hop gait, says Dr. A. D. Elkins, a veterinary orthopedic specialist in Indianapolis.

Pets with HD are not bred in an effort to avoid passing on the trait to offspring, but new diagnostic tests have the potential to make great strides in reducing the frequency and severity of HD.

Diagnosis

Outward signs may point to a problem, but for a conclusive diagnosis, X-rays are performed while the pet is under anesthesia. The pet is placed on his back and the veterinarian looks for the typical arthritic changes and subluxation (laxness) of the bone fit. Some changes may not be evident until the pet reaches two years old. "HD is a developmental problem and changes dynamically as the animal grows," says Dr. Elkins. "There can be tremendous changes from six to nine months to a year."

The Orthopedic Foundation for Animals (OFA) provides a consulting service for purebred dog owners and breeders. OFA reviews hip X-rays provided by an owner to evaluate the dog's conformation and, when normal, certifies that fact. OFA certification cannot be done prior to age two in dogs.

"With the newer PennHip technique, we can pick up the degree of joint looseness even before arthritic changes take place," says Dr. Elkins. "Whatever laxity or looseness they have at four months, they'll have for the rest of their life." The PennHip method, developed by Dr. Gail Smith, also positions the pet on his back, but then fits a metal and acrylic form, called a "distracter," between the animal's hips. "It brings their knees up kind of like a frog," says Dr. Elkins, "so their legs mimic what happens when they stand." That X-ray view plus others are used to gauge the pet's laxity score or "distraction index." It takes training to take correct OFA or PennHip X-rays, but can be done by experienced general practitioners.

Dogs can be certified free of hip dysplasia by sending appropriate X-rays to either the OFA registry or the PennHip registry. OFA costs less because there's only one X-ray taken. This is evaluated by three radiologists who score the hips fair, good, or excellent, says Dr. Elkins. PennHip evaluation uses computer analysis to compare the X-rays to all the other dogs of that breed in the registry. It costs about $200, plus $25 for registration in the database.

Medical Management

There are typically three levels of treatment for hip dysplasia. The vast majority of pets do well with medical management to control discomfort. Says Dr. Smith, "They may be real painful in that first year of life, but they get over that, and 76 percent of them do well with conservative management." Weight control and moderate exercise can help keep pets flexible. Dr. Smith considers Rimadyl the best option now available for control of discomfort of the dog that has severe or moderate osteoarthritis.

Limited studies have shown that cartilage-enhancing medications like chondroitin sulfate and glucosamineglycan, used at a very high dose early on, and for the rest of the pet's life, can slow the development of hip dysplasia. "Cartilage never heals itself once it's damaged; the cells do not replicate," says Dr. Elkins. "These agents just help the body keep existing cartilage as healthy as possible."

Studies have also shown that restricting the growth rate of pups during the first four months delays the development and severity of the condition. Foods that promote a moderate growth rate are particularly important in the high-risk large breeds.

TPO and FHO

When hip dysplasia can be diagnosed early before arthritis develops, Dr. Elkins says the state-of-the-art treatment is a triple pelvic osteotomy (TPO). Osteotomy means cutting the bone. "This is a team approach where the general veterinarian is key to recognize these signs early," he says. "We have this window of opportunity only when they're seven to twelve months of age."

A TPO cuts the pelvis in three places with a surgical saw in order to rotate the socket to any angle. Wire and a plate hold the reconfigured pelvis in position with the pelvis socket over the head of the femur, and the plate allows the pet to bear weight during the six weeks needed for the fractures to heal. "The surgery kind of fools Mother Nature," says Dr. Elkins, "so the hip won't develop arthritis." The pet remains hospitalized for twenty-four to forty-eight hours and can then walk out the door.

Most surgeons perform TPO on one hip at a time, with a four- to five-week period between procedures to allow for healing and rehab. "It really takes intensive care to manage these patients afterward," says Dr. Elkins. TPO costs about $2,000 per hip.

Once arthritis has developed, other surgical options offer better results. In a femoral head ostectomy (FHO), the femoral head, or "ball" of the joint is removed, and the pet's body is prompted to create a new "false" joint from fibrous scar tissue. This procedure works best for pets that weigh less than forty pounds, and is the treatment of choice for cats when medical management fails. Total hip replacement surgery, long an option for dogs, has not yet become available for cats because prosthetic joints have not been scaled down to the cat's small size.

Modern Miracles:
Kazie and the FHO

When four-month-old Kazie came to live in Houston with Kathy Joiner in 1993, she knew nothing about Maine Coon cats. She only knew he was an incredibly lovable kitten who acted like a human. "He sleeps with his head on the pillow, all nestled up against me," she says. Love for her pet prompted her to learn as much as she could about the breed. She participated in cat shows, and he won his Grand Champion title in the Cat Fanciers Association.

"After a few years of showing, I got to know about some of the big Maine Coon health issues," says Kathy. She'd heard whispers about hip dysplasia, and so during Kazie's checkup she asked that he be X-rayed to set her mind at ease. "There was really nothing to make me suspect anything, I just had a hunch."

As an MRI/radiologic technologist, Kathy had no trouble seeing that

Kazie's X-ray showed hip dysplasia. Kathy was told to watch for gait changes or difficulty in running or jumping that might require medication—or possibly surgery.

Kazie was fine for another year and a half when a new Maine Coon kitten joined the household. Suddenly, he didn't want to climb, and he refused to jump on the bed to share Kathy's pillow. "I just attributed the change to the new kitten," says Kathy, until she started to hear his hips "pop" as he walked. The stairs he'd once bounded up were taken at a limping, step-by-step hobble. The sight left Kathy crying with worry.

So she made an appointment with Dr. Wayne Whitney, an orthopedic specialist at Gulf Coast Veterinary Specialists in Houston. Kathy was told that Kazie would benefit from total hip replacement, but that the smallest prosthetics available fit twenty-five-pound dogs. Instead, Kazie would have a femoral head ostectomy, or FHO, on each hip. Dr. Whitney explained that cats with great muscle tone and flexibility tend to do extremely well with the procedure.

Surgery took place the following Thursday, and Kathy brought Kazie home on Saturday. "They shaved his whole backside and only left [fur on] his tail and a little bit on his feet, like a lion cut." But the loss of his glorious long fur was nothing compared to rehab, she says. Practicing tough love to help rehabilitate the cat was awful. "When Dr. Whitney made him stand on the floor, Kazie screamed and his back legs wobbled," says Kathy. "It was like putting ice skates on him and pushing him out on the ice." She was told he'd have to relearn to use his legs, and that she'd need to push him to stand and walk. "Kazie wouldn't try for them, but he'd do it for me," says Kathy.

Kazie came home with pain medication including a Band-Aid-like fentynol patch that allowed the drug to be absorbed through the skin. For the first week he remained reluctant to move—or to eat. Finally, a shot of antibiotics and medicine that reduced the swelling at the suture line seemed to do the trick. "An hour later when we got home from the vet, Kazie ran up the steps to the second story," Kathy says, "and by the next day he'd lift his leg in the air to groom himself." From that day on, he showed phenomenal recovery every day, although his fur took a full year to regrow.

The surgery itself cost $1,800, with preliminary X-rays and follow-up care an additional $2,500. But Kathy says she couldn't put a price on Kazie's recovery. "He's wonderful today," she says. "He walks, runs, plays, and jumps on the bed as well as any cats who do have their hips."

Total Hip Replacement

Hip replacement for dogs has been performed for fifteen years, and today it mirrors the procedure done in people. The dog prosthetics are based on prototypes for human hip replacement. "There's now a company called Biometric in New Jersey that does nothing but make hip replacements for dogs—for forty-pound dogs to one-hundred-and-fifty-pounders," says Dr. Elkins. Human artificial hips, of course, are all nearly the same size.

The orthopedic surgeon removes the socket portion of the pelvis and replaces it with a plastic cup fixed in place with screws or cement. The ball portion of the femur is removed, and the end of the bone is hollowed to accept the titanium stem-and-ball inserted into the opening. The prosthetic is usually cemented in place. Other surgeons use press fits with no cements. A recent ten-year study by Dr. Denis Marcellin-Little, assistant professor of orthopedic surgery at North Carolina State, clearly demonstrates that this option also provides long-term success.

When finished, the dog has a new hip with no cartilage, no pain, and no chance of arthritis. "They'll bear weight very quickly, often the very next day, because they're suddenly free of pain," says Dr. Elkins. Rehab for two months following surgery brings the new hip to full function, at which time surgery on the second hip may be done. But for 90 percent of all patients, only one hip replacement provides all they need, because the dog learns to transfer weight to the artificial hip and compensate. The cost varies across the country from $2,000 to $3,000 per hip.

Modern Miracles: Jordan's New Hips

Jordan was only six months old when her owner, Laura Estes of Louisville, Kentucky, noticed that the German Shepherd had trouble getting up. "X-rays showed she had severe hip dysplasia," says Laura. They were referred to Dr. Elkins. "He told me if I didn't do the surgery on her, she would be crippled by the time she was two years old."

Jordan needed to finish growing first before new hip joints could replace her sore, arthritic ones. The surgery on the first hip was scheduled right after Jordan's first birthday. Afterward, Laura was told to keep her caged and walked her always using a leash for about four weeks. That was so the new prosthetic hip would meld to the healing bone, and the staples wouldn't be prematurely removed. "But she has a mind of her own, and keeping her in the cage was a nightmare for her and us," says Laura. "I slept by her cage for three nights to keep her calm, and we kept her mildly sedated." They managed to keep Jordan confined only two weeks, and under leash control for three weeks. "I was a nervous wreck, I was so afraid to do something wrong. But she did remarkably well," says Laura. Six weeks later, Jordan returned to Dr. Elkins for the second hip replacement.

"She is our $3,000 dog now," says Laura. But the bottom line is that Jordan can outrun her three-year-old German Shepherd friend Bugsy, who has perfect hips. She plays, and for the first time she can scratch with her back legs, and even jump.

"Without the surgery, we would have put her to sleep by now because she was in so much pain," says Laura. "Instead, she's like a newborn puppy. It was like God wanted us to have her because He knew we'd be able to take care of her financially and love her just the way she was."

Thermal Protection

At eight weeks of age, even pets destined to suffer hip dysplasia have normal cartilage. It's the laxity of the joint that causes the progressive wear and tear on the cartilage. A new procedure attempts to eliminate the laxity in eight- to twelve-week-old puppies by shrinking the capsule around the joint using thermal techniques. "By shrinking the capsule to provide normal motion in the joint, we hope the cartilage will then continue to develop normally," says Dr. Mark Markel, an orthopedic surgeon at the University of Wisconsin.

The new therapy stems from seven years of research into using thermal energy—first with lasers and now radio frequency energy—to shrink collagenous, or connective, tissues. "Our research helped develop Electrothermal Assisted Capsulorphy (ETAC), initially used by human orthopedic surgeons at Stanford to treat San Francisco 49ers players' unstable shoulders," says Dr. Markel. "There are a whole slew of major league baseball, football, and other athletes who helped develop that, and today it's used heavily in the shoulder, but also in the knee, ankle, and wrist."

Dr. Markel believed the technique could be applied in veterinary medicine as well. Current studies include helping dogs with intact but unstable cruciate ligaments in the knee, and about three years ago, the hip dysplasia pilot study was launched. "We have fourteen dogs which are now about seventeen months old that have had their hip laxity monitored since they were born," says Dr. Markel. The thermal technique is performed on one hip of each animal, and early results offer strong evidence that the heat therapy helps. If the therapy proves successful, it will have an advantage over the invasiveness of TPO. "This surgery can be done with an arthroscope with a very small incision," Dr. Markel says.

Juvenile Pubic Symphysidesis

Dr. Kyle Mathews, an assistant professor of small animal surgery at North Carolina State University's College of Veterinary Medicine, has developed another prevention option that shows great promise. Juvenile pubic symphysidesis (JPS) is less invasive than standard TPO or hip replacement treatments. Dr. Mathews's research is in collaboration with Dr. R. Tass Dueland at the University of Wisconsin.

In JPS an area near the center of the pelvis is heated to kill cells responsible for pelvic development. This alters the "growth plates" to force the bones of the pelvis to grow at different rates. As a result, the pelvis grows at an angle that provides a better fit for the hip. By the time the animal is mature, the hip socket has rotated to a more horizontal angle, thus making it less likely that the ball on the end of the femur will pop out.

The procedure must be performed on dogs between sixteen to twenty weeks of age. After that, the pelvis is probably too developed for a JPS to have any effect on growth. Dr. Mathews says the best time is when the dog is spayed or neutered so the animal only needs to be anesthesized once. The incision for the JPS is about three inches long. So far there appear to be no side effects to the new procedure.

Dogs in the study are showing significant improvement. "After two years their hips are tight. They don't seem to have signs of hip dysplasia, even though they were at risk of developing it," says Dr. Mathews. He's even performed the procedure on his own Labrador Retriever.

Modern Miracles:
Whitney's Wobble

Mark and Holly Hogan of Palo Alto, California, contacted the Golden Retriever Club of America to help find the pup of their dreams, and they chose eight-week-old Whitney from a litter of a dozen fuzzy pups. "Every day I'd take Whitney to the park or beach, and we'd play and have a great time," says Mark. "She lived for retrieving tennis balls."

Whitney had an endearing habit of walking with a swing to her step like a runway model. "We called it the Whitney Wobble," says Mark. "We thought her crazy wagging tail just threw her off balance." But by six months of age Whitney's problems grew worse, and she began to act like an old dog. "She had to position herself just right to get up, and she tired out quickly and wanted to rest all the time." Mark thought she might have a virus and took her for a checkup.

The veterinarian suggested hip X-rays, and later that evening the verdict came in. Whitney had hip dysplasia in both hips. "Holly and I were just crushed," says Mark. The couple had recently moved to the area, and they had a limited income. They didn't see how they could afford hip surgery for Whitney.

But Mark had never forgotten two German Shepherds from his childhood that had both been put to sleep because of hip dysplasia. "I just couldn't do that with Whitney," he says. "She was only six months old, and she wasn't just a dog, not to me."

As a physicist, Mark knew how to conduct research, and he quickly learned that a number of surgical options were available. Whitney was too young for total hip replacement, and he learned about TPO from other Golden owners. But after Dr. S. Gary Brown, an orthopedic surgeon in Fremont, examined Whitney, he said her right hip had too much damage, while the left hip was too small for the necessary plate, so TPO couldn't help. However, she was a prime candidate for a less well known option.

Dr. Barclay Slocum, of the Slocum Clinic in Eugene, Oregon, teaches and licenses veterinary surgeons to use his technique, DARthroplasty (bone graft shelf arthroplasty), which grafts new bone to restructure the hip socket. The procedure provides an option for hips that still have intact cartilage, but are too shallow to be good candidates for TPO. In other words, if the "cup" part of the hip is too shallow, it won't hold the "ball" portion in place even with TPO.

A bone graft from the wing of the ilium bone is placed over the joint capsule at the rim of the "cup" portion of the same bone. If enough bone isn't available from the ilium, a portion of a rib may be used, or a bone bank graft. Strips of cancellous bone (the spongy, inner part of bone) are sutured in place to form a sort of basket in an extended rim over the head of the femur. As the grafts heal, that provides support for the joint capsule rather than the cartilage, and becomes the weight-bearing surface for the hip.

Mark and Holly left their seven-month-old dog with Dr. Brown for the surgery on both hips. The next day, when they arrived to take Whitney home, they expected to see a sedated pup in a lot of pain. "She looked like a Poodle where her back end had been shaved," says Mark, "and she had long incisions in both hips. But her tail wouldn't stop beating, and she was ready to go. She walked out by herself."

The toughest part of Whitney's recovery was the confinement so she wouldn't damage the new bone as it formed. The first two months, spent in Mark's office, seemed to go on forever. She was only allowed to walk to use the bathroom outside, and she was his constant companion as he worked on his dissertation. The next two months she could take walks on a leash, says Mark, but no running or jumping was allowed until after X-rays confirmed that the grafts were healed.

Today at three years old, Whitney has no limits, and she routinely accompanies the Hogans on twelve-mile backpacking trips into the Sierras. "She loves jumping and swimming, and lives for retrieving," says Mark. "She'll play all day with the neighbor dog."

Curing Whitney's wobble didn't come cheap. Mark says that the surgery and all the X-rays totaled $4,000. But he has no regrets. "Whitney is a member of the family. The surgery has been a blessing—thank you, Barclay Slocum!"

HYPERTHYROIDISM

Hyperthyroidism, overactivity of the thyroid gland, has become more and more common in middle-aged cats, although it is rare in dogs. In some urban areas the disease is diagnosed in 1 of every 300 cats, according to internist Dr. Joseph Taboada, a professor in the department of veterinary clinical sciences at Louisiana State University.

The double-lobed thyroid gland, located in the neck, secretes thyroxine and triiodothyronine, hormones that regulate the pet's metabolism, or the rate at which the body absorbs nutrients. Dogs develop hyperthyroidism from a tumor on the gland that often is malignant and spreads to the lungs or lymph nodes throughout the body. In cats, one or both lobes of the gland simply enlarge. In both dogs and cats, the abnormal condition causes an overproduction of hormones, which shifts the metabolism into overdrive.

Pets with hyperthyroidism typically have a ravenous appetite, hyperactivity, and a behavior change such as a short temper or increased aggression. Blood tests and a biopsy of thyroid tissue may be required to diagnose the condition.

In dogs, surgically removing benign tumors can cure the condition, while for cats, removing part or all of the affected thyroid may be the best choice. Daily thyroid supplements take the place of the missing gland after removal. Methimazole (Tapazole) is the drug of choice. This antithyroid drug doesn't cure, but does control, feline hyperthyroidism.

Injecting radioactive iodine that selectively destroys thyroid tissue is another option, and it has a 98 percent cure rate for cats. Only specialized referral hospitals such as university teaching hospitals offer this treatment, though. The government regulates the use of radioactive iodine, and a treated cat must be quarantined for one to four weeks, and his urine and feces monitored for radioactivity before he is released. All material removed from the cage must be handled as radioactive waste. Dr. Taboada says this treatment may be the first choice when effectiveness and few side effects are desired. The drawbacks are availability and expense. In most referral centers this is the most expensive therapy option.

In a brand-new option, often used in humans, ethanol is injected into the thyroid gland. This procedure was first experimentally used to treat cats in 1999. It successfully treated the condition but caused laryngeal (vocal cord) paralysis from inflammation caused by the ethanol. Since that time, ultrasound-guided needles to inject the ethanol have proven more successful with fewer side effects. Complications from the procedure include temporary laryngeal paralysis, mild gagging, minor voice changes, or nerve changes to one or both eyes (Horner's syndrome), which usually go away within two weeks of treatment.

KIDNEY DISEASE

A wide variety of conditions can impair the functioning of the kidneys. These organs screen organic waste and toxins or infectious agents from the blood, and excrete them in the urine. Normal kidneys also govern the fluids in the body, nutrient content of the blood, and manufacture hormones such as ethrytopoien, which controls red blood cell production and blood pressure.

Acute kidney disease comes on suddenly, usually as a result of an injury, infections like canine leptospirosis, or ingesting a poison like antifreeze. The acute disease affects pets of any age. "We also see congenital abnormalities in some cats that can lead to kidney failure at a young age," says Dr. Lillian Aronson, a surgeon at University of Pennsylvania. Some inherited tendencies can also lead to the disease later in life. For instance, a condition called polycystic kidney disease is caused by a problem gene, and has been estimated to affect over 30 percent of all Persian cats. It's now possible to screen for the condition prior to breeding to eliminate the chance of passing the disease on to offspring.

Chronic kidney disease mostly occurs in old age, possibly due to normal wear and tear from a lifetime of use. About 10 percent of all dogs over the age of fifteen, and 15 to 30 percent of cats over that age, have some degree of kidney disease.

Signs of kidney failure are the same whether chronic or acute. In the chronic form they are so gradual that the pet's body tends to compensate. Owners may not notice signs until up to 70 percent of organ function is gone. Earliest signs include increased thirst and urination—and loss of house-training as a result—when the damaged kidneys lose the ability to concentrate waste. Eventually, the pet becomes weak and depressed, loses weight, and may develop constipation or diarrhea. The disease in its advanced stage can cause mouth sores and foul ammonia breath, or even collapse, coma, and ultimately death.

A diagnosis is based on symptoms, along with blood and urine tests. Special examination of the kidneys with X-rays or ultrasound may be necessary. Most blood tests register abnormal function only once it falls to 25 percent or less, but researchers at Michigan State University's College of Veterinary Medicine have developed a test that gives a precise grading of kidney dysfunction. It determines even subtle changes in kidney function, and is called glomerular filtration rate (GFR). An instrument called an inductively coupled plasma-atomic emission spectrometer (ICP-AES) can detect elements in a variety of materials, including solutions that can be injected into the pet's bloodstream to measure kidney function. The ICP-AES costs about $150,000, but is cost effective because diagnostic labs can use the equipment for a wide range of tests.

Medical Treatment

Damage from the acute form of kidney disease may in some instances be reversed, but chronic kidney disease cannot be cured. Treatment tries to stop or slow the disease from getting worse, and relieve symptoms to keep the cat or dog comfortable. "Pets can do well sometimes for months to years," says Dr. Aronson. Fluid therapy injected beneath the skin will keep the cat from becoming dehydrated, and medication can lower phosphorus levels, she says. Phosphorus is a mineral required for many functions in the body, including energy metabolism, but the amount that healthy pets need can make their sick kidneys fail even faster.

Therapeutic diets that help relieve stress on the kidneys are a great boon to pets with chronic kidney disease. Special diets reduce the amount of waste products the kidneys must eliminate, which means the kidneys don't have to work as hard. Reduced phosphorus also helps lessen the strain on the kidneys, and reducing salt helps manage high arterial blood pressure (hypertension) associated with canine kidney disease. "Most renal-failure diets have a lower total quantity of a very good quality protein," says Dr. Grace Long, a veterinarian at Ralston Purina. That means the protein can be more completely digested, and there's less work for the kidneys to do.

Hemodialysis

Dialysis has long been available for human patients, but machines that cleanse the blood have not been available for use in cats and dogs until the last few years. In the past, peritoneal dialysis offered an interim solution for pets with acute kidney failure. The procedure pumps fluid into the pet's abdominal cavity, where it absorbs waste products, then is drawn back out mechanically via a large needle inserted through the abdominal wall. The dialysis allows the kidneys time to heal and keeps the body from being poisoned, while the underlying cause for the problem can be treated and hopefully cured.

In 1998, Dr. Larry Cowgill, an associate professor at the University of California-Davis, developed the world's first companion animal hemodialysis program. This was finally possible when the technology used in human dialysis became sophisticated enough to be adapted to cats and dogs. The pet's blood passes over one side of a "dialyzer"—something like a filter—while the other side contains a solution that approximates blood. The toxic molecules concentrated in the pet's blood are filtered out into the solution, and the cleansed blood returns to the pet's body.

Dr. Cowgill's research includes testing new materials that can be used to remove harmful molecules from the blood. The study also examines nutritional requirements of dogs with kidney failure. His program has served as a model for several other veterinary dialysis programs. The University of Maryland in Gaithersberg has started a program, and Dr. Kathy Langston runs a program at the Animal Medical Center in New York.

Dialysis is used primarily to treat dogs and cats suffering from antifreeze poisoning, kidney infections, and systemic illnesses that secondarily affect the kidneys, like canine leptospirosis. Less frequently, pets are placed on dialysis until a kidney transplant operation can be done. Animals that are not able to maintain their body weight or become anemic despite treatment may be helped by getting a new kidney.

Kidney Transplant

Kidney transplants have become a reality for cats—and sometimes dogs—that meet specific requirements. For these fortunate pets, the donated organ provides a new lease on life. However, it is not a "last-ditch" option performed on an emergency basis.

Kidney transplants date back to the early 1900s, and they have been done for dogs since the early 1950s. The first feline kidney transplant was done at UC Davis in 1984, and the cat, a Persian named Queenie, lived with normal kidney function for two years until passing away due to heart failure.

Dogs must leap an extra hurdle because their body will reject a donated kidney that doesn't match their own tissue. The canine immune system does not tolerate foreign proteins, be they viruses or transplanted organs. "The immune suppression drugs that work well in cats and people, which prevent organ rejection, don't work so well in dogs," says Dr. Aronson. The canine immune system attacks transplanted organs.

The most successful canine kidney transplants have resulted when the donated kidney comes from a litter mate or offspring so the tissues match very closely. Dr. Clare Gregory, director of the Comparative

Transplantation Laboratory at the University of California-Davis, leads research to improve the odds.

Cats are a different story. "As long as they're blood-cross-match compatible, a cat can accept a kidney from an unrelated donor," says Dr. Aronson. That's fortunate because there's a lot more renal failure in cats than in dogs. The best candidates are cats in the earliest stages of the disease that don't have other health problems.

The ideal candidate is negative for feline leukemia, feline immuno-suppressive virus, heart disease, diabetes, or inflammatory bowel conditions. Blood work and urine tests are done, along with an EKG, X-rays, and ultrasound. If it's suspected that the antirejection drugs required after the surgery could bring on dormant health problems like a urinary tract infection, a two-week trial of the drugs may be given prior to the surgery. Age doesn't matter—successful transplants have been done for cats as young as two or as old as sixteen.

Once the cat has been approved for transplantation, a blood cross match pairs the cat to the best donor. The donor cat must be a young, healthy adult. Ideally, this cat is the same size or slightly larger than the recipient cat. An animal needs only one working kidney to remain healthy; part of the "deal" includes adopting the cat that donates the kidney. "The owners love the idea that they are saving the life of the cat that saved their cat's life," says Dr. Aronson. The donors usually go home two days after the surgery.

Recipient cats remain hospitalized for a week before the surgery for preoperative tests, and a week after, to ensure the new kidney works. The recipient cat is fed a protein-restricted diet, and anemia is addressed either with a whole-blood transfusion or erythroipoietin, a hormone that stimulates red blood cell production.

Donating a kidney guarantees the donor cat a home for life, says Dr. Aronson. "We try to get cats for the program that would otherwise not have a long life, and would be euthanized," she says. The University of Pennsylvania has an arrangement with the state SPCA. People who bring in healthy young cats to the shelter are told about the program. "We explain that the cat will be guaranteed a home, he will undergo a surgery but will live a normal life afterward—and would you like this animal to become part of the program?" she says. "We've also had cats come from various research colonies that would otherwise be euthanized. I have a bunch of cats that stay here at the hospital and get pampered."

The procedure requires two surgical teams working on both cats at the same time. The left kidney is usually donated because it has a slightly longer vein. Then the recipient cat is surgically opened and prepared to receive the new kidney. The old organs are left in place as a backup in case the donated kidney fails. The transplanted kidney is sutured to the nearby abdominal wall, and the ureter sutured to the bladder, in order to prevent any future twisting of the organ. Most transplanted kidneys are functioning well within seventy-two hours of the transplant.

The donor cat tends to recover very quickly. The recipient cat typically receives intravenous fluids, and is fed and medicated through a tube.

"After the transplant, the cat must be on antirejection medicine and be pilled twice a day for the rest of his life," says Dr. Aronson. The same medicines used in human transplant patients, cyclosporine and prednisone, work for feline patients. Many cat owners have become accustomed to giving fluid therapy and other medicines and have no problem with a lifelong program. "But for cats that hate pills, that can be a quality-of-life issue," says Dr. Aronson. The average cost for the antirejection medicine runs between 30 cents to $2.40 a day, depending on the cat's size. Follow-up blood work at the cat's local veterinarian monitors the level of cyclosporine and kidney function weekly until the cat is stable, and then every two to three months thereafter—each test costs about $35.

Statistics in 1996 indicated that during the first ten years of transplantation, the average survival rate was twenty-six months following the surgery. But Dr. Aronson believes recent statistics are much more promising. "We've learned how to better deal with complications," she says. "My experience has been that if cats don't have other underlying diseases and are medicated properly by their owners, they can do well for years and years. It's not for every cat, but for the right cat it can be an excellent treatment option." Currently, OJ has survived the longest of all feline kidney transplant recipients—ten years and going strong. The eleven-year-old orange and white tabby is a happy, healthy fourteen-pounder who lives with Nancy and Paul Norris of San Antonio, Texas.

Only a handful of private practices and universities are performing kidney transplants. Some, like Angell Memorial Animal Hospital in Boston, performed transplantation for a while and may do so again in the future should a transplantation surgeon rejoin the staff. The University of Florida, University of North Carolina, University of Wisconsin, and University of Michigan have also been active in transplantation. Currently the two most active facilities are the University of Pennsylvania and University of California-Davis, where the technique was pioneered.

"We've done thirty-two cases here in the first two years of the Penn program," says Dr. Aronson. The cost of the surgery varies depending on where it's done and how well the patient recovers. The entire cost for the surgery and two weeks' hospitalization at the University of Pennsylvania runs about $6,000, while UC Davis estimates the cost from about $3,500 to $4,500 if there are no complications.

Modern Miracles:
Saving Leo

In 1987, Katherine and Peter Karamolengos of Springfield, Pennsylvania, happened across a cinnamon-colored kitten named Leo at a cat show. With copper-colored eyes, a constant purr, and a sweet disposition, the Persian baby was irresistible. "It was love at first sight," she says. "We were just absolutely infatuated with him."

But then in May 1996, when Leo was nine years old, he left a puddle of urine in the bathroom that looked like coffee grounds. Katherine took him to the local veterinarian, who thought he had a kidney infection. But an ultrasound at a specialist diagnosed polycystic kidney disease, an inherited condition most common to Persians later in life. "The specialist told us Leo might have only two months to live," says Katherine. The only hope, they were told, was a kidney transplant, but that wasn't an option because the surgery was available only in California.

Katherine and Peter worked with their local veterinarian to keep Leo as healthy and comfortable as long as possible. "But we knew his condition would only get worse," says Katherine.

After a year and a half of supportive care, the local veterinarian had helped as much as she could, so they took Leo to a feline specialist in November 1997. In addition to regular beneath-the-skin fluid therapy, Leo was given the hormone erythropoietin to stimulate his marrow to make new red blood cells, to fight his anemia. "It's expensive," says Katherine. "A tiny vial smaller than a thimble costs $100." The treatment helped Leo hold his own through the end of the year, but his blood test showed his kidneys were continuing to fail.

A transplant seemed to be Leo's only hope, but by this time he was too sick to travel to California even if they'd been able to afford the trip. "Prospects were dim," says Katherine. Then she heard a radio program mention that the University of Pennsylvania planned to launch a transplant program. "I couldn't believe it," says Katherine. "I called them immediately and talked to Dr. Aronson. And Leo was the first cat admitted to their transplant program."

Leo was admitted a week early to take preliminary tests and to find the best donor cat. "The day of the surgery, I remember sitting downstairs in the waiting room crying," says Katherine. "Then Dr. Aronson and one of her assistants came downstairs, and they were both shaking [with relief]. They said everything went well, and the new kidney was already producing urine." Leo remained in the hospital for another week, and Katherine visited every day, sometimes waiting for hours to get the chance to spend time with him. "The staff were so very kind," she says. "They'd let me come upstairs where he was all hooked up to IVs and pet him in his cage. They said it helped him in the healing process because I was the only person he really knew."

While Leo remained hospitalized, his donor, Tiger, had recovered enough to come home with Katherine. She says the beige and cinnamon-striped tabby has the exact opposite personality of the laid-back Leo. "We were happy to give him a good life," she says.

Then Leo recovered enough to come home. "He still had tubes everywhere, so I had to medicate and feed him through the tubes," she says. "I didn't know I had the strength to do stuff like that, but I did it."

Despite the success of the surgery, Leo developed rare complications involving his thyroid that required further surgery. He also developed diabetes and anemia as a result of antirejection medications and stress. They cut back on the medication dose, but nothing seemed to help. "Even the wound from the catheter wouldn't heal," says Katherine, "and I had long conferences with Dr. Aronson." The specialists wanted to run a bone marrow test and perform exploratory surgery to find out what was wrong. "But I refused," says Katherine. "I didn't want him to go through any more surgery. So we took Leo home to die."

Katherine learned to give Leo shots of insulin for the diabetes, and every week she returned to the hospital for blood tests to monitor his progress. "Three weeks later the tests said everything was close to normal—I stopped breathing!" she says. Three weeks later, his diabetes went away.

Leo still goes for a checkup every few months. "But it's been two and a half years since his transplant—that was February 19, 1998," says

Katherine. "Today he's happy, he purrs a lot, and he's just a pleasure to have around. He's a wonderful cat."

KNEE INJURY

The knee, also known as the stifle joint, contains two crossed ligaments called cruciates that stabilize the joint. All joints are composed of two or more bones that are positioned end to end. Smooth cartilage covers the bones where they meet to provide easy movement, while the ligaments—tough bands of tissue—hold the bones of the joint together. Muscles, specialized tissue able to expand and contract to move the joint, are attached to the bones above and below the joint with other tough bands of tissue called tendons.

Dogs, especially toy breeds, often tear one or both cruciate ligaments as a result of injury or even routine exercise. The dog suddenly starts limping from pain. "It's a major problem in canine athletes, as it is in humans," says Dr. Helen Newman-Gage, the owner of Veterinary Transplant Services outside Seattle. "There are a couple of different kinds of procedures used in animals, but there isn't a very good way to manage the treatment."

For years doctors repaired torn cruciate ligaments by creating a prosthetic ligament, says Dr. Paul Gambardella, an orthopedic surgeon at Angell Memorial Animal Hospital in Boston. Surgeons have used a variety of natural and synthetic materials placed around or near the joint to replace the ruptured ligament and stabilize the joint. For instance, artificial ligaments made from a synthetic called Gortex were used for some time, but were found to cause excessive inflammation in the knee and were pulled from the market, says Dr. Newman-Gage. "Sometimes they use a fishing line to sort of hold the knee together on the outside just underneath the skin," she says. "Although they don't have a replacement tendon, they at least have something that will keep their femur from slipping off the tibia [the two bones that meet at the knee]." These procedures help a great deal, and the persistent lameness is often eliminated, says Dr. Gambardella, but dogs typically end up with lameness that comes and goes and is associated with arthritis.

Emerging technology for cruciate ligament repair includes tendon transplants, used as a substitute for the ligament. These surgeries are performed arthroscopically. "Wayne Whitney, of the Gulf Coast Veterinary Specialists in Houston, has probably done more tendons than any-body," says Dr. Newman-Gage. Dr. Whitney; Dr. Robert Taylor, the codirector of Alameda East Veterinary Hospital in Denver; and others continue to refine the technique. A major difficulty in using donor ten-dons, says Dr. Newman-Gage, occurs during rehab, because dogs are not as sensitive to pain in the joints and tend to overdo too quickly. "Alo-graph [donor] tendons for dogs processed the same as for humans tend to stretch or fray," says Dr. Newman-Gage. "They're used too aggres-sively before they are fully healed."

Tibial Plateau Leveling Osteotomy

Dr. Gambardella says the newest treatment for ruptured cruciate ligament, called Tibial Plateau Leveling Osteotomy, or the TPLO, offers a paradigm shift in treatment options. "The technique changes the dynamics of the knee joint," he says.

Veterinary surgeon Barclay Slocum of Oregon patented the tech-nique, and he grants licenses to other veterinarians to perform the pro-cedure once they have completed his course. During surgery the end of the tibia is cut and rotated so the flat part stays level and the femur can't slide off when the dog stands, says Dr. Newman-Gage. Surgery recon-figures the joint so it no longer requires the anterior cruciate ligament for stability. After the surgery, the knee functions normally.

Dr. Gambardella says results seem superior to the standard tech-niques. "The progress of arthritis appears to be slowed greatly as a re-sult," he adds. The procedure is used only for pets—there is nothing like it in human knee surgery repair.

Knee Replacements

Canine hips that suffer crippling pain can be replaced by artificial hips. The knee suffers from arthritis even more often than the hips, but knee replacement surgery is not available. That's because the ball and socket joint of the hip is relatively easy to duplicate and is held together simply by the dog's body weight. But the knee joint (like the elbow) is fashioned more like a hinge, and must be held together by ligaments. Dogs would greatly benefit from an artificial knee, because arthritis in this joint often causes severe pain as the animals age, even after ruptured ligaments are repaired.

Researchers at Iowa State and a surgeon in the Chicago area are trying to develop an artificial knee for dogs, using human knee replacement as a starting point, says Dr. A. D. Elkins, an orthopedic surgeon in Indianapolis. Any human knee prosthetic joint is about the same size. But in veterinary medicine, size must range to fit everything from a 2-pound Chihuahua to a 180-pound Great Dane. "To get that many different replacements is very, very difficult to do," says Dr. Elkins.

LIVER DISEASE

The liver is one of the most complex organs in the body. It processes sugars and fats, produces amino acids, and stores vitamins and minerals. It also makes hormones, enzymes that aid blood clotting, and bile that allows fats to be absorbed. The organ also filters out waste and detoxifies the blood of drugs and poisons that could damage the body. More than any other organ, the liver is at risk from injury or disease from outside influences. Birth defects, parasites, and cancer of the liver can also cause serious or life-threatening illnesses.

Liver problems tend to produce the same vague signs, no matter what the cause. These include anorexia, vomiting, diarrhea, weight loss, and lethargy. When bile backs up in the blood circulation, light-colored areas of the body such as the whites of the eyes, gums, or inside of the ears turn pale yellow or tea-colored (jaundiced). Increased pressure on the veins that drain into the liver causes ascites, an accumulation of fluid in the abdomen, so that it swells. Advanced liver disease can result in bleeding into the stomach, intestines, and urinary tract; blood in the stool or urine is the sign.

Blood tests look for changes in liver enzymes, and ultrasound also helps diagnose liver disease, but a definitive diagnosis requires a microscopic examination or culture of the liver tissue. Cells for examination may be collected with a fine needle inserted into the liver through the abdominal wall guided by ultrasound imaging.

Treatment consists primarily of supportive care and removal of the cause, if known. For instance, congenital defects like portosytemic shunt most commonly affect toy breeds and require surgical correction. Unfortunately, most cases of canine liver disease have no known cause.

For cats, the most common liver disease is hepatic lipidosis, or fatty liver disease (FHL), which most commonly affects overweight cats.

When obese cats become anorectic—refuse to eat—fat cells move into the liver. The fatty liver makes the cats sicker so they remain anorectic, causing a vicious cycle of liver damage.

When diagnosed and treated very early, liver damage may be reversed in some instances. FHL treatment surgically places a tube into the stomach through the body wall to force-feed nutrition to the anorectic cat. It may take two to eighteen weeks of tube feeding before the cat begins to eat again on her own.

A common treatment in chronic progressive liver disease in dogs involves administering a naturally occurring bile acid that helps protect the liver from further damage. Dogs are given oral ursodeoxycholic acid (UDCA, Actigall, or Ursodiol).

In June 1999, Hill's Pet Nutrition launched the newest tool to manage both feline and canine liver disease. Prescription Diet Canine and Feline l/d are formulated for any type of liver problem. The two innovative diets manage and slow damage by reducing the workload of the liver, supporting liver repair and regeneration, and helping regulate the metabolism of blood sugar.

Preventing Congenital Disease

A study by Dr. Karen M. Tobias of Washington State University is trying to determine if portosystemic shunts in Yorkshire Terriers is inherited. Portosystemic describes the apparatus through which the blood draining from the stomach and intestines (portal circulation) and the blood flowing through the rest of the body (systemic circulation) meet and are directed to the liver.

While still in the mother's womb, the blood of an unborn pup is filtered by the mother's liver. The pup's blood bypasses its own liver through a vessel called a shunt. Once born, the puppy's own liver must take over and the shunt closes. If the shunt fails to close, toxins that the liver normally would remove can affect the brain and cause seizures or other life-threatening problems.

The study hopes to determine common ancestry among affected dogs and to identify how the trait is inherited. It may be possible to devise a DNA test to identify carriers and prevent the births of puppies affected by the condition.

MEGACOLON

For unknown reasons, some cats develop problems with the ability of their colon to move waste material out of the body. The colon is the end portion of the large intestine that connects to the rectum, where waste leaves the body. Affected cats don't pass fecal material for days or even weeks.

An enlarged, flaccid colon, a condition called megacolon, often lacks smooth muscle movement. The condition can be congenital and cause problems from birth, or may develop later in life as a result of tumors, strictures within the tissue that narrow the passageway, or foreign bodies that block the passage or injure the organ. A poor nerve supply to the colon may prevent proper contraction. In most cats, the cause remains a mystery.

The lining of the colon pulls moisture from the waste material. So when feces remain too long in the colon, the dry fecal material becomes harder and even more difficult to move. The colon soon fills up with dry fecal balls, stretching and expanding the colon to gigantic proportions until waste cannot be passed naturally. Fecal balls too large to pass through the cat's pelvis must be mechanically removed by the veterinarian after the cat has been put under anesthesia.

Medical management helps many cats and prevents repeated bouts of fecal impaction. Laxatives, enemas, therapeutic diets, and drugs like cisipride (Propulsid) help the colon to contract, which relieve some cats.

Recently surgery that removes the sick portion of the large intestine has been used to treat megacolon. Dr. Gary W. Ellison, a surgeon at the University of Florida, has performed the innovative procedure. The rectum is left intact and is reattached to the small intestine to create a functional bowel. The surgery, called a subtotal colectomy, is complicated and used mostly as a last resort in severe cases, but it can restore near normal bowel function.

Cats are usually somewhat depressed and refuse to eat for forty-eight hours after the surgery, and sometimes have a mild fever. Recent studies on the aftereffects of the surgery indicate most cats maintain their normal body weight or even gain a little.

For the first three to four days following the surgery, cats typically pass a dark, tarry liquid stool. Feces remain liquid and poorly formed for two to six weeks until the ileum, the last section of the small intestine, increases its ability to absorb liquids. Then the feces usually become soft and poorly formed (cow pie consistency) and remain that way for the rest of the cat's life. Cats usually use the litter box two to three times a day, but the total amount of water loss in the feces equals that of normal cats.

Modern Miracles:
Raja's Last Chance

Skimble's Raja Red, or "Raja" for short, had always yowled in the litter box. "Ever since he's been four months old, he always 'announced' his deposits," says Beverly Caldwell of Tucson, "and both his breeder and I thought that was so cute." The flashy red and white Maine Coon had a number of interesting behavior habits that made him special, and Beverly just assumed that was another of Raja's quirks.

Raja had problems with diarrhea off and on in his youth, but not until age two did Beverly get the first clue he had a major problem with elimination. He began to run around like a crazy cat, search and act anxious, and race back and forth down the hallway, from the tub and shower in each bathroom. Finally he began to "dig" in the bathtub and shower, then ended up in the litter box, where he strained to defecate. "I took him to the veterinarian the day before we left on an RV trip," says Beverly. Because of his history, the veterinarian thought Raja had diarrhea and put him on Imodium to stop him up.

By the time their RV reached Los Angeles, Raja had stopped eating and was in bad shape. At the veterinary emergency room, three enemas couldn't move the blockage. "They sent Raja to a specialist able to do abdominal surgery if he needed it," says Beverly. Thankfully, a drug called cisipride stimulated the colon to move.

Raja was diagnosed with megacolon, and each day he received a teaspoonful of plain Metamucil, a natural fiber laxative, mixed in his food, a dose of a stool softener called Enulose, and 5 milligrams of cisipride three times a day. The medicine worked well for six months before he blocked up again and visited the veterinarian to be cleaned out with enemas. That became the pattern, says Beverly, with episodes of normalcy becoming shorter and shorter. "His X-rays showed the bowel was so distended, it looked like a stomach after three Thanksgiving meals," says Beverly. She knew he would only get worse.

Finally, a decision had to be made. "We had a choice of enemas every five to six weeks, putting him down, or trying the surgery," says Beverly. She knew chronic enemas offered a limited quality of life. "I was a basket case, just in tears," she says, "Raja was so sick I didn't think we could do surgery. I had even decided what prayer I'd say when I held him that last time—I was just going to give him to God." But she says veterinarian Barbara Gores loved Raja too, and didn't want to give up on him. Together they decided to give the special cat a last chance at a healthy life, with the subtotal colectomy procedure. It would cost about $1,800.

The Tuesday surgery opened an eight-inch incision from Raja's rib cage along the length of his abdomen. "Dr. Gores removed all but four or five inches of the colon," says Beverly. Raja came home Friday with a drain along with a wicked-looking incision, and slept all that day. "When he woke up, he felt so good he jumped up on the bed," she says, "and he went up the seven-foot cat tree the third day after the surgery!"

She kept the recuperating cat isolated from the rest of the cats in the house until he felt better. The biggest problem in recovery was getting the big cat to eat. Raja snubbed every canned cat food, baby food treats, and even turkey tidbits Beverly offered, until dry food finally tempted him. "By the end of the first week he was eating fairly well," she says. Raja had been a bit overweight, but lost three pounds after the surgery and kept them off. "Probably a pound of it was the full colon," says Beverly.

Raja's stitches came out on day 9, and by day 21 the fur had grown enough that his scar had disappeared. At first his bowel movements were liquid, but gradually they became normal looking.

Beverly says today Raja is enjoying his second kittenhood, this time without pain. "He's been one uncomfortable cat all his life," she says. Dr. Gores agrees that Raja likely hated to be held or to play with the other cats because he was in such pain. Now all that has changed.

"I'd do it again in a heartbeat," says Beverly. "What's the money? The money's nothing. Now Raja has a chance to live a great life with no limitations." She says Raja's last chance became his second chance—and he's having a ball.

OBESITY

Most pets no longer work for a living. A sedentary lifestyle coupled with highly tasty and nutritious diets have conspired to make obesity the most common nutritional disease, affecting about 25 to 30 percent of dogs and cats. Obesity is commonly defined as exceeding ideal body weight by 20 to 25 percent.

Any pet can become overweight, but most are middle-aged dogs and cats between five and eleven years of age, probably because they are less active as they age. Certain breeds or lines of dogs may also inherit a "fat gene." Obesity tends to be most common in Labrador Retrievers, Cairn Terriers, Shetland Sheepdogs, Basset Hounds, Beagles, Golden Retrievers, Cocker Spaniels, Dachshunds, and Miniature Schnauzers. Neutered pets may not be as active as intact ones that constantly search for romance, so they tend to become overweight unless diet changes match their reduced activity level. There are also metabolic diseases like canine hypothyroidism that can cause weight gain in pets.

A common reason pets get fat is because owners show their affection with treats. "People are killing their animals with kindness," says Dr. Nancy Irlbeck, a nutritionist at Colorado State. "With a tiny dog, a hot dog is worth almost a couple days' calories." Also, when owners themselves are more sedentary, they're less likely to make sure their pet gets exercise. That can create a vicious cycle because the more the pet weighs, the less likely they are to enjoy exercise, and that causes them to gain even more weight, says Dr. James H. Sokolowski, a veterinarian with Waltham USA. A weight gain of a pound or two sounds like nothing, but for a ten-pound pet that is the equivalent of a human gaining twenty-five pounds.

Excess weight puts people at risk for health conditions like atherosclerosis, or hardening of the arteries. Although this isn't a common problem in pets, obesity does increase the risk for diabetes mellitus, cancer, skin problems, cardiovascular problems, and lameness due to arthritis. Fat cats are also at risk for hepatic lipidosis, a liver disease brought on by refusing to eat.

Special "lite" diets that contain fewer calories and/or fat are designed to provide complete and balanced nutrition that also satisfies the pet's need to feel full. "The over-the-counter ones, while somewhat restricted in calories, tend not to be restricted enough for the animal to really lose weight unless they have one whale of an exercise program," says Dr. Sokolowski. Reducing diets rarely work when offered as free choice—dry food left out all day to eat at the pet's leisure—because dogs that are gorgers simply eat more of the reduced-calorie food. Some feline nutritionists believe cats are metabolically programmed to eat a set amount of calories, and eat until this set point is reached. If this is true, special reducing diets may not work when the pet is offered free choice, because the cat simply eats more of the reduced-calorie food to get the same number of calories he'd get from a more concentrated food. Measuring the amount of food given will help pets lose weight and help keep it off.

Therapeutic Diets

Controlling pet obesity usually requires medical supervision and special diets. Slow and steady weight loss maintains the pet's health. Crash diets, especially with cats, run the risk of lethal liver complications, and may also cause a loss of muscle or bone mass rather than fat. For instance, Waltham reducing diets offer a 90-day program for dogs and a 130-day program for cats, designed to lose excess weight in 15 percent increments. "A tailored exercise program for the individual cat or dog is a must," adds Dr. Sokolowski.

"There's a tremendous variation from one animal to the next as to how many calories they actually burn in a day," says Dr. Grace Long, a veterinarian with Ralston Purina. "We give veterinarians a computerized feeding guide that actually calculates the individual animal's metabolic energy requirements so they can tailor the diet just for that individual."

Reducing diets typically replace fat in the food with indigestible fiber, dilute calories with water, or "puff up" the product with air. But not all calories are created equal. "Our studies have shown that the higher you go on protein in reducing diets, the more muscle they'll retain and the more fat they'll lose," says Dr. Long. Today, a number of therapeutic reducing diets have increased the protein levels to reflect that benefit.

Working Within the System

The newest weight-control diets try to use a pet's natural metabolism to control weight. Once digested, the food spills into the bloodstream as blood sugar, and then insulin moves it into the cells to be used. "Insulin is like an usher in the theater," says Dr. Dan Carey, a veterinarian with the Iams Company. "When the movie is over, the usher wants you to leave and he doesn't care where you go." Similarly, when blood sugar goes up, insulin wants the sugar gone. "The insulin doesn't care if the sugar is burned for energy or stored as fat," he says. He considers this concept a fairly significant breakthrough in controlling pet obesity. "The more you keep blood sugar level up and peaking, the more likely you are to deposit it as fat." Therefore, adjusting the diet formulation in reducing diets like the Eukanuba Weight Control foods—and even in over-the-counter "regular" diets—to better fit pet metabolism helps reduce obesity.

Veterinary nutritionists have also discovered that certain nutrients affect the way food is processed and stored. For instance, if you add carnitine to the diet, you can actually increase the rate at which muscles burn fat for energy. L-carnitine, a vitaminlike substance, is a normal component of meat, says Dr. Carey. "At the same time this increases the rate of burning fat, you can maintain the muscle mass," he says. "We've demonstrated that in both cats and dogs."

Other work has examined the effect of vitamin A on the production of a natural body hormone called leptin. "Leptin encourages fat cell production," says Dr. Carey, "and an increase in vitamin A intake results in decreased leptin production and easier weight loss." Two studies conducted at a research facility affiliated with University of Missouri incorporated increased levels of vitamin A, along with adjusting for blood sugar metabolism. "When fed free choice, overweight cats and dogs lost weight," says Dr. Carey.

Testing Nutrition

In human medicine, hospitalized patients are tested in many ways to ensure they get adequate nutrition. Many of the same tests probably apply to pets, too. "We need to establish a way to measure how well we're supporting pet patients nutritionally," says Dr. Andrew Mackin, an internist at Mississippi State University. "We've tried to develop user-friendly tests that veterinarians could run themselves."

Dr. Mackin's study tries to see if nutritional tests that work in humans will apply to dogs. "Blood proteins have a very short circulation time, and if you're malnourished, their production drops and levels of blood protein fall rapidly," he says. Once standard protein levels have been established, veterinarians can use the blood tests to make sure sick pets are fed properly.

PAIN

Pain is designed to be a protective way of helping a pet recognize when something isn't right. For instance, the pain of a flame prompts the paw to retract, rather than linger and receive a more damaging burn. Pain keeps a cat or dog from making an injury worse so, for instance, they'll favor a broken leg, which allows the protected area to heal when rested.

In the past it was believed that dogs and cats don't experience pain to the same degree as people. Current thinking recognizes that pets do suffer similar levels of pain—they just react differently to it. Some pets are so stoic they may feel pain but not show any signs, while others may be critically ill and seem to be in pain but aren't. And excessive pain increases stress, which causes metabolic changes in the body, which interferes with healing. "If pain becomes excessive where the patient can't sleep, doesn't feel like eating, gets depressed, that type of thing, then we're really in a different ball game," says Dr. William Tranquilli, an anesthesiologist at University of Illinois.

Signs of Pain

- Vocalization
- Depression
- Anorexia
- Rapid breathing
- Pale mucous membranes
- Rapid heartbeat
- Missed heartbeats
- Aggression
- Abnormal postures, including lameness
- Restlessness
- Drooling
- Dilation of eyes

When tissue is damaged, it releases chemical substances that make nerve endings extrasensitive. That makes the pain threshold lower than normal. The same thing happens with a bad sunburn, when the gentlest touch is excruciating because the nerves overreact.

Pain management in veterinary medicine has long been complicated by the fact that analgesic drugs, such as aspirin, also interfere with monitoring the condition. Yet in the past ten years great strides have been made in pain management. This has been driven in part by the pet-owner bond. People don't want their furry family members to suffer, and have demanded relief. Today it has become an ethical obligation to address pain in the effort to reduce suffering, says Dr. Steven L. Marks, a surgeon and internist at Louisiana State University.

Treatment for pain is complicated by the fact that, just like with people, pain tolerances vary from pet to pet. "In the human patient there probably is a fivefold variation in pain tolerance for the same surgical procedure," says Dr. Tranquilli, and he expects a similar range in different dogs and cats. Some of that tolerance has to do with experience. For example, a football player at the beginning of the season has a lower pain threshold than he has at the end, when he's used to the pain and the bruises. So you might expect a rough-and-tumble outdoor pet to have a higher pain threshold than a spoiled, couch-potato pet. "With pet pain, we have a moving target," says Dr. Tranquilli.

Response to pain travels through the nervous system, up the spinal cord to the cortex of the brain. Drugs and therapies can be used to control pain at any point along this pathway. A wider variety of medicines today make it possible to take the edge off excruciating pain, but allow the pet to recognize enough discomfort so that they don't overdo it. "It can be tricky trying to get that just right," says Dr. Tranquilli.

Pain Management Therapies

Agents that control pain, called analgesics, are matched to the type of pain. Visceral pain is dull, vague, and achy discomfort located inside the trunk and organs (i.e., intestines, heart, lungs). Visceral pain is caused by the tissue being crushed, torn, or cut; by chemicals like drugs or poisons; or from a lack of blood to the area. Somatic pain is a sharp, localized pain in any tissue other than the viscera, such as the skin, muscle, joints, and bones. Somatic pain is caused by extremes of temperature, or by chemical or mechanical (i.e., crushing, cutting) injury. Neuropathic pain is a sharp, burning discomfort caused by direct damage to the nerves or spinal cord. This kind of pain often cannot be controlled with drug therapy. Acute pain results from a sudden stimulation—hitting your thumb with a hammer—and tends to be the most responsive to pain-relieving medication. Chronic pain is a dull, achy discomfort usually due to old injuries. Cancer pain falls into this category. Chronic pain also tends to be hard to control.

There are many drugs available to manage pain. The most common ones used for pets are over-the-counter NSAIDs, or nonsteroidal anti-inflammatory drugs, which include aspirin. Dogs and cats require different dosages and metabolize drugs differently than people, and so human medicines may be dangerous or even lethal when given to pets. For instance, aspirin works well in dogs but can cause bleeding ulcers, and in cats, it can be dangerous at high doses. Ibuprofen isn't as effective and causes more side effects, and acetominophen (i.e., Tylenol) will kill a cat.

When the pet is critically ill, only a few drugs are safe or can be easily administered. Traditional pain relief comes in the form of pills, liquids, and injections. But oral medicine isn't ideal for pets that are vomiting or refuse to eat. Intravenous medications, though they work quickly, must be given by the veterinarian and don't tend to last very long.

"We're trying to get pain medications that are more user friendly," says Dr. Tranquilli. Instead of a pill, medicines are being formulated in liquids that can be dripped into the pet's mouth or added to the food. Narcotic pain relievers such as morphine, codeine, and Demerol are available by prescription only from the veterinarian. Codeine is preferred for cats and dogs because it's well absorbed in the digestive tract and provides effective relief for all but the severest forms of pain such as cancer pain. Codeine can be compounded into peanut butter or fish paste to help pets accept it. One newer option for pets is Buprenorphine, said to be twenty-five times more potent than morphine. It takes longer to work, but its effects last longer for pets that have severe or chronic pain.

The newest pain-relief drugs are transdermal, meaning they can be absorbed through the skin. Fentanyl (Duragesic) is an opioid drug that comes in a transdermal patch that provides prolonged narcotic relief for both dogs and cats. It comes in a variety of strengths and is particularly helpful for pets that are reluctant to take medicine orally. Today, fentanyl is often used for postoperative pain.

In human medications, the pluronic gel approach—a carrier substance that moves through the skin—allows veterinarians to combine many different analgesic drugs. For instance, DMSO (dimethyl sulfoxide) penetrates the skin within five minutes of application and carries other substances mixed with it into the body. Pain medicine mixed into the gel can be pasted on the skin, the gel carries the drug through the skin into the nerve tissue, and helps lessen the pain at the source. There are many advances on the human side that experts expect to bring to the veterinary world.

The biggest difficulty continues to be the lack of feedback. A person can tell the doctor if a given medicine works or doesn't. With pets, their reactions and the doctor's experience and intuition combine to find the drug that works the best.

Fascinating Facts! Platypus Pain Relief

The male Australian platypus has a spur on its hind legs that excretes venom that has a complex structure similar to a substance found in white blood cells that fights infectious microbes. Many of the proteins and other substances in the venom are unique. One causes muscles to contract; another makes muscles relax and may reduce blood pressure. A nerve growth factor in the venom has been isolated that directly stimulates pain receptor cells. Dr. Allan Torres from the University of Sydney believes platypus venom could be important in designing potent pain control drugs in the future.

Pain Memory and Anesthesia

Veterinary anesthesia has traditionally been conservative because of fears about side effects and respiratory depression. For this reason, pets have been underanesthetized as a rule. In the last five to ten years the profession has become more sophisticated, and uses new techniques for safe anesthesia. "Today we're able to marry pain management into our overall anesthetic techniques," says Dr. Tranquilli.

That's particularly important because of something called "pain memory." Human anesthesiologists routinely administer general anesthesia, followed by a nerve block, which prevents pain in a particular region of the body, such as a leg being set or a joint that's being repaired.

But until recently pets were simply given general anesthesia to keep them immobile and oblivious to any pain during the treatment. Dr. Tranquilli says a percentage of pets, like people, wake up with their nervous system out of kilter if additional pain medicine isn't given. That can also happen if pain continues over many months, without relief. The nervous system wants to keep creating pain, even though the wound has healed or the surgery has stopped. To prevent that possibility, pets can be given a local anesthetic into the spinal cord to act as a regional nerve block that prevents the pain message from ever reaching the brain.

Research has found that pain medication given before the pet undergoes a painful treatment can prevent the problem. Drugs given in advance of pain will reduce the amount of pain after the event. Doing this also decreases the total amount of pain medication needed. After surgery, continued pain control can be accomplished with drains that deliver the medicine into the chest and abdominal cavity, the joint, or even intravenously via a catheter. A much higher percentage of dog and cat patients today are better treated for their pain than just three to four years ago.

PANCREATITIS

Inflammation of the pancreas has recently been shown to be nearly as common in cats as in dogs. But in the past feline pancreatitis was rarely diagnosed. The organ, located near the liver, provides digestive enzymes and insulin. An inflamed pancreas releases digestive enzymes into the bloodstream and abdominal cavity rather than into the small intestine. As a result, the enzymes digest the fat and tissues of the abdomen or even the pancreas itself. Feeding fatty table scraps, obesity, and injury cause many cases of pancreatitis in dogs. The cause isn't clear in cats, but the condition is sometimes associated with diabetes.

Dogs tend to have acute flare-ups more often, while cats suffer chronic disease with vague signs that come and go. Acute pancreatitis can be completely reversed if the cause is identified and removed. However, more than 90 percent of all cases of feline pancreatitis are idiopathic—that is, they have no known cause.

Both acute and chronic forms can be mild or severe, and animals can recuperate from the mild form. The severe form causes extensive death of tissue, involves a number of organs, and means a poor prognosis.

Fascinating Facts! Ear Thermometers

Advanced Monitors Corporation of San Diego has developed the Vet-Temp VT-100 Instant Animal Ear Thermometer. Using infrared technology, the ear thermometer measures core body temperature in one second, and avoids the discomfort of taking rectal readings.

In both humans and dogs, the most common signs are severe pain, vomiting, and a fever. Rather than having too many enzymes, some dogs may suffer from not having enough. Blood tests that measure the level of the circulating pancreatic enzyme, lipase, confirm the disease in dogs.

Cats show vaguer signs. Most are lethargic, anorectic, dehydrated, and have low body temperature. Several new tests for diagnosing the canine disease have been modified for use in cats, according to Dr. David A. Williams, a surgeon and internist at Texas A&M. He notes that some tests, like the feline trypsin-like immunoreactivity (TLI), are even more useful for cats than for dogs. Confirming the diagnosis for both dogs and cats, though, relies on ultrasound. Dr. Williams believes that although it's expensive, a definitive diagnosis of feline pancreatitis should be made by a pancreatic biopsy. That requires exploratory surgery (laparotomy) that can be done noninvasively with a scope (laparscopy).

In most canine cases, support includes intravenous or beneath-the-skin fluid therapy to counteract dehydration, pain-relieving drugs, and medication to control vomiting. Dogs also benefit from fasting—having food withheld—for three to four days until vomiting stops. Low-fat therapeutic diets and dietary enzyme supplements may be prescribed for dogs as well.

Cats typically don't vomit, and if they suffer liver complications—hepatic lipidosis—that makes fasting dangerous. Cats that do not also have a liver disease should have food withheld for three to four days, and then be slowly introduced to a carbohydrate-rich low-fat diet.

Anecdotal reports indicate that cats with pancreatitis benefit from a transfusion of fresh frozen plasma or fresh whole blood, which contains albumin and other components that help patients suffering from pancreatitis. Selenium, a trace mineral, is required in the diet in tiny amounts to keep the skin and cell membranes healthy. Supplements with this micronutrient have decreased the number of deaths in dogs with pancreatitis. It has not yet been evaluated in cats.

Modern Miracles:
The Holiday Gift

When Debbie De Louise of Hicksville, New York, got married eight years ago, her computer instructor husband, Anthony, worked nights and urged her to get a cat for company. "I had recently lost a gray male cat named Benny, and I wanted another gray boy," she says. A kitten with white socks filled the bill. She named him Floppy, like the computer disks Anthony worked with. The cat's nonstop energy and happy disposition endeared him to the couple, and he became a big part of Debbie's life.

When he was six years old, Floppy developed diabetes. Debbie, a librarian by profession, researched all she could about the disease. For a year and a half she worked with Dr. Mitchell Kornet of Mid-Island Animal Hospital to get her cat regulated on insulin. Then in early May 2000, Floppy's personality changed. "He was normal when I left for work, but when I came home, he was throwing up, listless, and hiding," says Debbie. She spent the night sleeping on the floor halfway under the bed, to be near him. The next day—on Debbie's birthday—Floppy was hospitalized. "I thought he was dying," she says.

He was given emergency intravenous fluids, antibiotics, and insulin for his diabetes. "They ran all sorts of tests, and at first they thought it was a very bad virus," she says. He was so sick that he began vomiting blood. When the vet called, wanting to do a $200 sonogram test, she told him to go ahead.

The sonogram confirmed Floppy had a very severe case of pancreatitis. "I was in tears," says Debbie. Her research told her the outlook was poor, especially for a diabetic cat. "I ordered a casket for him," she says, "then prayed I wouldn't need it."

She scheduled vacation time so she could spend as much time as possible with Floppy at the hospital. She brought him his heart-shaped catnip pillow to remind him of home when she couldn't be there. "I'd call every night and first thing every morning. I couldn't sleep thinking, is he going to be okay in the morning?"

The illness was so severe that Dr. Kornet called several specialists to find out the best way to treat the cat. "My husband, Anthony, knew it would be costly. But if we had to mortgage the house, we were going to do what we could for our cat!" says Debbie.

The specialists said keeping Floppy off all food would help heal his pancreas. "But Floppy was overweight, so I knew fasting could also cause fatty liver disease," says Debbie. "They said prednisone could reduce the inflammation, but it interfered with his insulin. Everything was complicated." Finally, a bland diet—boiled chicken—was prescribed, and Debbie hand-fed her cat to make sure he'd eat and regain his strength.

Floppy had just started to feel better when he turned bright yellow—jaundiced. The skin inside his ears and mouth nearly glowed yellow, which meant his liver was sick. Also, he couldn't shake a fever. By this time, hospitalization was costing about $100 a day. Several sonograms later, Dr. Kornet was still puzzled and suggested a liver biopsy to figure out the problem. It required anesthesia, though, and Debbie refused because she was afraid Floppy wouldn't survive the procedure. He'd gone from a solid nineteen pounds to a frail fourteen-pound cat.

After ten days in the hospital, the fever and yellow faded enough for

Floppy to go home. He needed three medications, three times a day. "Giving insulin injections was a breeze compared to pilling him," says Debbie. Less than a week later, though, he turned yellow again despite the drugs. This time Debbie was referred to Dr. Richard Reid at the Long Island Veterinary Specialists Hospital in Plainview, New York.

Yet another sonogram revealed a brand-new swollen mass on Floppy's liver. The news was grim—Dr. Reid said the swelling had a 90 percent chance of being cancer. A $2,000 surgery to remove the growth was one option, but Floppy was losing a pound a week and now weighed only eleven pounds. The experts agreed he probably couldn't survive an operation. The other choice was massive amounts of prednisone that might reduce the swelling, on the slim chance it wasn't cancer after all.

"Anthony said we had to consider Floppy's quality of life, and what's best for him," says Debbie. "We cried, and talked about euthanasia too, but we decided to try the medication first." Moral support from other owners whose cats had gone through similar problems and recovered kept their hopes alive.

Sadly, the medicine didn't help reduce the size of the mass on his liver. Despite the illness, though, Floppy was still eating, purring, and no longer acted uncomfortable. "I kept praying we'd find something that would work," says Debbie. He'd been deathly ill since May, and by the Fourth of July, he had lost 50 percent of his body weight because his body couldn't process the food he ate. But everyone, even the specialists, thought Floppy seemed stronger. They decided to try one last treatment, and pinned all their hopes on the liver operation that would remove the mysterious mass.

This time Debbie agreed to a biopsy of the swollen spot. Dr. Reid used an ultrasound to guide the needle, which collected a tissue sample to be analyzed. That way they'd know, prior to the surgery, what kind of cancer or liver disease it was so they could plan how to treat it. Debbie had to wait over the long July Fourth holiday weekend, and got the biopsy results two days later.

The test showed that not just the liver, but all of the cat's organs—heart, lungs, pancreas—were enlarged. "I was numb when I heard that," says Debbie. She kept thinking about the tiny casket, still in the box, out in the garage. But she couldn't believe what they said next. "The test was negative for cancer! The mass was a cyst, caused by E-coli." The infectious bacteria often contaminates food.

Debbie feared she'd somehow poisoned her cat's food, but Dr. Kornet explained that small amounts of E-coli live in all pets and people, but our normal immune systems keep us healthy. Floppy's illness made him so sick, though, that even when the pancreatitis went away, his resistance was too low to fight off the bacteria. The biopsy results meant that it was E-coli that had kept him near death's door for three long months.

The doctor said ten days of the antibiotic Baytril would get rid of the infection. "I was skeptical," says Debbie. "I was afraid to feel any hope." Floppy had been so sick for so long, she couldn't believe the cure could be so simple. But only five days after starting the medicine, she was amazed when all the yellow abruptly went away. "The vets were in shock too," says Debbie. "Floppy literally came back from the dead."

By the end of July, and after nearly $4,000 in medical bills, Floppy was cured. "He's eight years old now, and still so sweet," says Debbie. "All the hard decisions turned out to be the right ones." Christmas this past year was extra special. One package, though, remained unopened in the garage—the box with the cat-size casket. Debbie is confident it won't be needed for another eight to ten years at least. "I cry when I think what he went through," she says, "but it was worth every penny. My best holiday gift is having Floppy still with us."

PARALYSIS

The most common spinal cord injury to dogs is a herniated disk. Dachshunds, Beagles, Bassets, Corgis, and sometimes Poodles have a predisposition to dislodge a disk, says Dr. Richard B. Borgens, an anatomy professor at Purdue University. In humans a slipped disk moves outward and away from the spinal cord, and causes pain when it presses on nerve roots, yet it rarely causes spinal cord injury. But because of differences in a dog's anatomy, a slipped disk becomes a projectile that actually crushes the dog's spinal cord.

Also, most disks are forced out of position in people and dogs at the junction of the lumbar (lower back) and thoracic (midback) vertebrae. "That's where a person's spinal cord ends; it stops at L1 [lumbar 1]," says Dr. Borgens, "but in dogs the cord continues all the way down to about L6 [lumbar 6]." Dogs and cats have five extra vertebrae in their back, which helps make them more flexible.

The spinal cord functions like a highway, running north and south, with many entrances and exits along the way. The on- and off-ramps are bundles of nerve fibers on each side of the spinal cord. Those either route signals to the brain or away from the brain to a body part. The northbound lanes are formed by millions of single nerve fibers coming in from the body and carrying the information to the brain. Most of this incoming traffic is sensory information from the world around us. The southbound lane is from the brain to the body. This traffic is largely "motor" information sent to organs and muscles, giving both conscious and unconscious directions to move a foot or make the heart beat.

When the spine is crushed or bent during an accident, the cord is severely bruised. The localized nerve cells and their fibers can suffer injury or death. Too much damage causes a roadblock that stops the nerve impulses from traveling, and leads to paralysis.

Two Faces of the Disease

Dr. Borgens says spinal cord injury must be categorized as two very distinct types of diseases, because impairment of the nerves occurs in a series of phases. The first two to three days—and especially the first six hours—following the injury are the acute phase. "The cord is in better shape one minute after the injury than it is an hour later, and is much worse five hours after the injury than it is at one," says Dr. Borgens. The injury continues to get worse with time until it reaches a plateau three to five days after the initial trauma. In this chronic phrase, the injury won't get worse. But if the nerve cell dies or separates, paralysis occurs. That means a fresh injury should be treated as soon as possible. "Treat them early, and the earlier you treat them, the better," says Dr. Borgens.

Injury to the spinal cord causes it to swell inside the vertebral column, like inflating a balloon inside a water pipe. Essentially, the cord crushes itself and causes even further damage. "The only treatment since World War II has been to give antiinflammatories and follow that with decompression surgery to remove bone, expose the cord, and remove any bone chips," says Dr. Borgens. But a new treatment using a polymer called polyethylene glycol (PEG) offers new hope.

PEG

All cells are semiliquid, halfway between liquid and gel, and floating inside them are the structural parts that make them work. When an injury to the spine pokes a hole in the membrane of the nerve cell, the body either seals the hole so the nerve can keep working, or the membrane—and then the nerve—dies. Injured nerve pathways begin to get worse from the time of the injury. Dr. Borgens's research, though, has developed a treatment that helps stop this process and rescues function.

"The treatment works at the union between neurobiology and chemical engineering," he says. "We use some very large polymers, which are large-molecular-weight compounds that we have found can seal holes in nerve membranes, and even join cells back together." The treatment is like a biological glue gun that allows the cell membranes, lined up like beads on a string, to flow into each other and spontaneously reassemble. "If we can treat within the first day, these particular polymers can actually seal the holes, and rescue huge numbers of nerve fibers that would ordinarily go on to dissolution and death," says Dr. Borgens. Sealing the holes also restores the cells' ability to conduct nerve impulses, so within minutes the nerve can become active again. PEG (polyethylene glycol) works as long as it's used within eight hours of the injury.

PEG is commonly used in medicine and cosmetics. The treatment consists of applying PEG directly onto the exposed, injured portion of the spinal cord for two minutes and then rinsing the polymer away. Preliminary studies in guinea pigs showed that the treatment prompted recovery of nerve conduction in every one of the animals. All of the control group that didn't receive PEG failed to conduct impulses.

Dr. Borgens has recently begun clinical trials in dogs, and the first two dogs treated have done very well. A team from Purdue will work with the Indiana University School of Medicine and their department of neurosurgery to design clinical treatments in dogs ultimately to be used in people. Although the outcome is too early to predict, Dr. Borgens anticipates canine patients will have the same remarkable results as with guinea pigs, where all of the animals responded within the first week and most within the first hour of treatment with PEG. "If you have even five percent of the nerve fibers carrying nerve impulses, you'll get significantly more than five percent back in terms of restored behavior," says Dr. Borgens. Return of bladder control, for example, might be possible.

Because the treatment must be administered within several hours of the injury, most of the twenty dogs for the trial are being referred from veterinary hospitals in the Purdue area. "We only take those dogs with the very worst of the worst injuries that the veterinary neurologists believe have no chance of getting anything back," says Dr. Borgens. "We pay for all the expenses, and the owner does nothing except follow our directions on how to take care of their pet. We even buy them carts to rehab the dogs."

Extraspinal Oscillating Field Stimulator

Studies have proven that very weak, naturally produced electrical fields in the embryo are involved in the development of the nervous system. Scientists have duplicated that process in countless laboratory experiments. "The electrical field is 1,000 times weaker than what's needed to fire a nerve impulse," says Dr. Borgens. Yet with that knowledge in hand, he set out a decade ago to find a way to use electrical fields to regenerate nerve fibers in damaged spinal cords.

The result is a kind of battery-powered nerve-growth pacemaker, called an Extraspinal Oscillating Field Stimulator (OFS). The device is temporarily implanted in injured patients to jump-start the regeneration process. Like the PEG therapy, the OFS technique must begin shortly after the injury takes place.

The OFS unit, about twice the size of a lipstick tube, is implanted in deep muscle. Six platinum-tipped electrodes run from the unit to the outside of the nearby vertebrae in an array of three above and three below the injury. The injured spinal cord experiences the electrical field even without contact with the electrodes. "The surgeons love this because we don't have to touch the [spinal] cord," says Dr. Borgens. "We reverse the electrical field polarity every fifteen minutes, to encourage nerve growth in both directions."

After many published studies proved the stimulator works in guinea pigs, the trials moved to dogs about ten years ago. Prior to launching a human trial, revamped stimulators for human use were implanted in forty-two dogs. Half received the real thing; half were implanted with placebo units.

With OFS, improvement does not occur in hours or even days. Regeneration means growth and growth takes time, and the nerve fibers grow only a short distance. It also takes time for the nervous system to relearn how to conduct impulses, says Dr. Borgens. The unit remains implanted for fourteen weeks, long enough to wake up the body to start the process, and then they are surgically removed. "We usually begin to see improvements in function in a month or two in dogs," says Dr. Borgens, "but we continue to see improvements out to six months, where we usually stop the studies."

The dogs with the units achieved major quality-of-life changes, he says. The dog that did the best came to Purdue with a neurologically complete spinal cord injury and scored zero on all tests of function— complete paralysis below the injury. But after the treatment, even experts couldn't tell the dog had ever been injured at all. "All of the dogs with the stimulator were remarkably improved, and probably 5 percent of dogs you could refer to as truly cured," he says.

Researchers are awaiting FDA approval for OFS trials in up to twenty human patients. "We hope we get 25 percent of the dog success in people!" says Dr. Borgens.

4-AP

"After the cord has been injured and forms a scar, and months or years go by, the character of that injury becomes very different," says Dr. Borgens. This is the second face of spinal disease. Some of the nerves that could have been rescued with early treatment have degenerated and are completely gone, and if the nerve remains, part of its fiber is gone forever. "That's irreversible," he says. "We can't grow back processes that have been lost."

Yet almost all the spinal injuries in people and animals are compression injuries. The cords are crushed, not cut in two pieces. Plus, a lot of nerve fibers remain intact in spinal cord injuries—they just don't work. In pets and humans, the spinal cord dies from the inside out after being crushed. Almost always an outside rind of fibers and nerves is left intact, but nerve impulses are blocked and can't get past the region of the injury.

Dr. Andrew Blight, Dr. Borgens, and veterinary neurosurgeon Dr. James Toombs from Purdue University have worked together to figure out the cause of the nerve blockage. "It turns out, the nerve impulses were linking to an ion called potassium," says Dr. Borgens. When the insulating myelin sheath around an axon (nerve cell fiber) is damaged, potassium channels become exposed and that permits current to leak from the axon. Instead of traveling along the nerve highway, the nerve impulse takes a detour. It jumps to the potassium the way lightning is drawn to a lightning rod.

The scientists decided to try a potassium channel blocker called 4-aminopyridine (4-AP) to see if that would set the impulses back on the right route. "The first time I saw this, I about fell over backward, I knew we were on to something hot," says Dr. Borgen. Blocking the potassium channel restores the ability of the axon to conduct nerve impulses—and that can restore some function.

In 1988 the drug was first tested on Kessa, a longhaired Dachshund who had been paraplegic (no use of rear legs) for some time. Within fifteen minutes of the injection, she was bearing weight, standing, and moving her paws. But two hours later, after the drug had worn off, she relapsed. Recovery lasted only as long as the drug remained in her system.

After the study documenting success in dogs was published in 1995, two human trials conducted by Dr. Robert Handsebout and Dr. Keith Hayes began in two hospitals in Ontario, Canada. They turned out to be a smashing success. The IV injections they used will soon become an oral medication. "We are now in the era where you can take a pill for paraplegia," says Dr. Borgens.

The treatment does not mean a cure, but about half of patients—dogs and people alike—show remarkable improvement. They regain sexual function and continence, the ability to breathe, and various degrees of function in their limbs. It should be noted, though, that an equal number have no response at all or cannot tolerate the drug. The smallest group regains true quality-of-life changes in perhaps one or two areas that are meaningful to them, says Dr. Borgens.

To address the problem of tolerance levels, the researchers have pioneered a new delivery system that places an indwelling pump directly on the spinal cord injury. "We spray the injury with the drug," says Dr. Borgens. He expects that some patients not helped with the shots or oral treatment will benefit from the pump.

Purdue has licensed the patent for 4-AP to a biotech company called Acorda Therapeutics, which has completed Phase I FDA studies and feasibility studies in people. Currently, a time-release oral version of 4-AP called fampridine, made by Elan Corporation, is being tested in ten medical centers around the country.

Leaving Dogs Behind

Unfortunately, as animal trials give way to human studies, oftentimes the pet gets left out in the cold. The treatments made possible by dogs are no longer available to help them. Dr. Borgens and his colleagues are frustrated by this reality of commercial medical development. "These treatments really do work in dogs," he says. So Purdue seeks to become involved with a company specifically involved in veterinary medical development. So far, Dr. Borgens and Purdue have been unable to make such a deal.

The PEG solution, he says, should cost almost nothing for pet owners once it's available. "Some of these things are kind of brilliant biology, but turn out to be fairly simple and inexpensive to implement," he says. "We've just used PEG in a novel way that works." Medical devices like the electric field stimulator or drug pump, though, can cost thousands of dollars.

Until these techniques are approved for veterinary medicine, only Purdue will have them available for injured dogs. Dr. Borgens says his team has designed a lower-cost version of the electric field stimulators. "We will provide a unit free, and pay for half the cost of surgeries to encourage people to bring their dogs to us," he says. "We do that so we can slowly build up a larger population of animals that have recovered significantly, and convince veterinarians to help us. We need veterinarians to help us pressure companies into developing these things."

PARASITES

Parasites feed on other organisms, usually at the expense of that organism. Cats and dogs are hosts to a wide range of both external and internal freeloaders. Fleas, ticks, and mites live on or in the pet's skin and can cause many types of skin diseases. Parasites may even cause systemic (whole body) illness when they transmit microscopic organisms to the pet. Worms, protozoa, and bacteria form colonies in the intestines, blood, heart, or other organs. These can cause chronic to acute disease that may ultimately kill the pet.

The science of parasite control has made great strides. In the past, a variety of insecticides designed to kill parasites such as fleas could also prove toxic to the pet itself. Some flea products were so overused that fleas became resistant. Ten years ago, veterinarians were recommending a three-pronged program for eradicating fleas: treating the pet, the house, and the yard outside. That approach began to change with the advent of IGRs—insect growth regulators—which attack insects but not the cat or dog. IGRs have not only provided safer on-pet control, but have also helped control the parasite where the pet lives.

Methoprene (Siphotrol) was the first IGR. It was initially available for house control and later for on-pet flea control. Later, a once-monthly pill, lufenuron (Program), used an IGR that inhibited the development of chiton, the exoskeleton of the flea. A much more stable IGR, pyriproxifen (Nylar), is now available for indoor and outdoor control in the form of collars, foggers, and on-animal sprays. Pyriproxifen works like methoprene but has increased potency, killing eggs and larvae. Sodium polyborate (contained in borax products) for indoor control has become popular because it lasts a long time in the environment. And today, biological control with nematodes—worms that eat immature fleas—has become popular.

The Next Generation

Parasite-control products of the past targeted one or at most two types of pests. For instance, traditional flea products for dogs often had some effect against ticks as well. But not until the past few years have parasite products become so effective or wide-ranging. They not only kill pests, they sterilize them (so fleas can't reproduce), repel them, and require monthly application rather than daily use. In addition, a better understanding of flea biology has helped in developing molecules that specifically attack the flea nervous system. Because its nervous system is so different from mammals', these products offer effective control with a wide safety margin for pets.

Two topical products changed the way pet owners and veterinarians approached parasite control. Fipronil (TopSpot and Frontline Spray) and imidacloprid (Advantage) are applied once monthly to the pet and are absorbed through the skin. Imadacloprid was developed in the mideighties and used widely in agriculture as a systemic absorbed by the root system, soil, or seeds of plants. As a spot-on pet product, it kills adult fleas with 98 to 100 percent efficacy within twenty-four hours. Fipronil is equally effective against fleas, and has the added advantage of killing ticks.

Dogs in Australia and Switzerland are already benefiting from nitenpyram from Novartis, a compound similar to imidacloprid. Administered as a pill, nitenpyram is pending FDA approval in the United States. It is said to kill fleas that feed on a treated dog within hours. However, it will likely not provide the thirty-day protection available from some other systemic treatments—products like pills or applications that are absorbed into the skin and spread throughout the whole body.

Flea Vaccines

Heska Corporation, based in Fort Collins, Colorado, continues research to make a vaccination against fleas a reality. Studies focus on finding the flea proteins that would be susceptible to vaccine-induced antibodies in the host pet. It's likely that any commercial flea vaccine remains years in the future.

Tick Control

Tick control has become more and more important as a wider range of tick-borne diseases have been identified in people and pets. The tick acts as a vector, or carrier, that can transmit a variety of microscopic disease-causing organisms through its bite. Common illnesses include canine ehrlichiosis, Rocky Mountain spotted fever, and Lyme disease. The tick must be attached for at least twenty-four to thirty-six hours to transmit the infective agent to the cat or dog. Products that repel or kill ticks within this time offer protection against these diseases. Some dogs that live in regions known to have a high rate of Lyme disease benefit from a vaccine.

Modern products have nearly eliminated the need for premise control in your house or yard, but frequent vacuuming is recommended because it removes up to 90 percent of flea eggs and 50 percent of larvae from carpets. Also, there remains a concern that using one or two products to the exclusion of all other types of control may lead insects to develop a resistance. Dr. Michael W. Dryden, a parasite specialist at Kansas State University, has repeatedly warned of the potential for flea resistance. He explains that some pests, including fleas, have the ability to evolve until subsequent generations are able to tolerate doses that would have killed previous generations. For instance, by 1983 eight species of fleas, including the common cat flea, had demonstrated resistance to many of the insecticides then used in flea control. Cat fleas are thought to be resistant to more chemicals than other fleas.

Heartworms

The heartworm *Dirofilaria immitis* is a type of roundworm that lives in the pulmonary arteries and heart of dogs and, less commonly, cats. Feline heartworm disease causes more acute and severe complications, including sudden death. In dogs, adult worms that clog the heart and arteries typically cause chronic progressive illness. Mosquitoes transmit the immature parasite to pets through their bite, so the more mosquitoes there are, the greater the risk for pets. Infected pets often die without treatment, but the treatment may also be stressful or even dangerous for the pet.

Prevention is the best choice, and a variety of drugs are available for dogs. Only recently has heartworm prevention become available for cats, because cats weren't thought to get the disease. Actually, about one cat for every ten dogs gets heartworms. Heartgard for Cats (ivermectin) is a chewable tablet administered once a month that kills the tissue stage of the larvae; it also prevents hookworm.

Recently, selamectin (Revolution) for both dogs and cats has become available. It targets several kinds of parasites, including heartworms. Some experts say it may, in fact, be better categorized as a drug rather than an insecticide, because it acts on the inside of the body. Made by bioengineering techniques, it is derived by the chemical modification of a form of avermectin (another insecticide) and causes neuromuscular paralysis in the target organism. The spot-on topical product is absorbed into the skin to kill ticks, ear mites, and sarcoptic mites as well as adult fleas—it also prevents flea eggs from hatching. From the skin it is rapidly absorbed into the bloodstream, where it prevents heartworm in both dogs and cats. Finally, it is excreted into the intestinal tract, where it kills hookworms and roundworms in cats.

Combination Tests for Parasites

A variety of tests have been made available over the years for diagnosing specific parasite infestations. IDEXX Laboratories, Inc., has launched Snap Canine Combo Heartworm Antigen/*Ehrlichia canis* Antibody Test. Infections from *Ehrlichia canis*, common tick-borne bacteria, cannot be diagnosed on clinical signs alone, and infected dogs often go for months or years after exposure without showing symptoms. Dogs that are at risk for exposure to ticks may especially benefit from such early detection and treatment.

Giardia

A wide range of drugs is available for treating and preventing infestation with intestinal parasites. However, the protozoan *Giardia lamblia*, a single-cell organism that lives in the small intestines of dogs and cats, has been notoriously difficult to diagnose and eradicate. Some surveys indicate that one in eight pets seen by veterinarians harbor the parasite. The organism interferes with digestion and causes intermittent and chronic diarrhea. It can also affect people. Flagyl (metronidazole) has been the treatment of choice.

Tests to detect the organism aren't always accurate, and intermittent shedding of the immature organism in the pet's feces may mean the tests show negative even in the presence of infection. An ELISA test used to diagnose human cases is much more accurate but is rarely available for use in veterinary medicine.

GiardiaVax for dogs, and Fel-O-Vax Giardia for cats, two new vaccines, were launched by Fort Dodge Animal Health in 1998. They prevent the cyst (infective stage) from being shed from infected animals, which can spread the disease. Two vaccinations are required the first year and boosters once a year thereafter. The dog product was launched in Canada in January 1999 and is in the regulatory works in many countries outside the United States.

Fascinating Facts! New Feline Parasite

Scientists from the University of Connecticut-Hartford and the Louisiana State University School of Veterinary Medicine recently identified a new species of skin mite. *Demodex gatoi* lives directly on the skin surface, unlike *Demodex cati*, which lives beneath the skin in the hair follicle. The new mite was found on a cat suffering from feline immunodeficiency virus infection.

Managing Mites

A variety of tiny mites target cat and dog skin. They live on the surface or burrow into the skin itself. Some, like *Demodex canis*, are normal parts of the pet's skin fauna and do not cause problems in normal pets. But this cigar-shaped microscopic mite can cause devastating skin disease—demodecosis or demodectic mange—in immune-deficient dogs. (*Demodex cati* affects cats only rarely.) It is the sixth most common canine skin disease in North America and the third most common in the Southeastern regions of the country.

Effective Treatments for Common Parasites		
Treatment	**Pet**	**Parasites Affected**
Permethrin	Dogs only	Control of fleas, ticks, Cheyletiella, and lice
Imidacloprid	Dogs and cats	Monthly flea control
Fipronil	Dogs and cats	Monthly flea and tick control; also for lice, Cheyletiella, and sarcoptic mange mites
Selamectin	Dogs and cats	Monthly flea control and HW prevention; sarcoptic mange in dogs; ear mites in cats; roundworms and hookworms in cats; tick control in dogs
Milbemycin	Dogs only	Monthly heartworm prevention; control of round, hook, and whipworms; control of demodex and sarcoptic mange
Lufenuron	Dogs and cats	Control of fleas
Milbemycin and Lufenuron	Dogs only	Heartworm prevention and control of round and hookworms
Ivermectin	Dogs and cats	Monthly heartworm prevention
Ivermectin and Pyrantel	Dogs only	Monthly heartworm prevention and control of round and hookworms
Methoprene	Dogs and cats	Control of fleas on the pet and in the environment
Pyriproxifen	Dogs and cats	Control of fleas on the pet and in the environment
Nitenpyram	Dogs only	Treatment for fleas (pending FDA approval)
Amitraz	Dogs only	Treatment for demodex and sarcoptic mange mites

This condition, also referred to as "red mange," has in the past been incredibly difficult to cure. Until recently Mitaban (amitraz), an insecticide applied as a dip, was the most effective treatment. Today, the active ingredients in some heartworm-prevention products—specifically milbemycin and ivermectin—have shown to kill the demodex mite. Moxidectin (Cydectin) is a milbemycin-based product that has been used for several years in Europe. In one study it reportedly cured all eight adult dogs with generalized demodicosis when given as an oral dose each day. Symptoms improved, and decreased mite counts were seen after thirty days. Dogs were cured on average after seventy-five days of treatment.

The mite that causes scabies affects both dogs and cats and is highly contagious. Primarily a parasite of dogs, *Sarcoptes scabei* burrows beneath the skin. Notoedric mange, also called head mange or feline scabies, is caused by the mite *Notoedres cati*, which deposits eggs in burrows it makes in the outer surface of the cat's skin. A number of new treatments are now available, including topical (pour-on) ivermectin; and treatments such as the topicals selamectin, and fipronil and the oral milbemycin, which are used in flea and heartworm treatments.

The most common mite affecting cats is *Otodectes cynotis*, the ear mite; it also affects dogs, and is very contagious. Ear mites live on the surface of the ear canal and are a common cause of ear infections in dogs and cats. Cleaning affected ears with a miticide has been the gold standard of treatment but can be difficult in hard-to-handle pets. New oral medications that prevent heartworm—selamectin—also prevent earmites in cats.

SKIN ALLERGIES

The immune system contains specialized cells called antibodies that protect against foreign invaders such as viruses and bacteria. A hypersensitive reaction, or allergy, occurs when these cells target harmless substances like pollen, proteins in food, or saliva from insect bites. The overreaction of the immune system to these substances, called allergens, can cause an itchy skin reaction in dogs and cats.

Anything can trigger a reaction. The pet must be exposed for a time to the allergen for the immune system to be "primed" and develop a response. The tendency to develop an allergy is inherited, and so skin allergies are much more common in small terriers, especially the West Highland White Terrier, as well as Boxers, Dalmatians, Golden Retrievers, English and Irish Setters, Lhasa Apsos, Miniature Schnauzers, and Shar-Peis.

Flea allergic dermatitis (FAD) is the number one cause of skin disease in cats and dogs. Surveys estimate that 40 percent of the dog and cat population are affected. Allergic pets react to a protein in flea saliva that typically causes all-over seasonal (summer) itching. Only a few flea bites may prompt an allergic reaction lasting a week or more—the more fleas, the worse the reaction. The most common sign is extreme itchiness on the rear half of the dog, particularly the area on the back immediately above the tail. Cats more typically itch all over and may break out in tiny scabby bumps called miliary dermatitis.

Airborne allergens like dust and mold that trigger sneeze and wheeze reactions in allergic people more often prompt skin disease in pets when the substance is inhaled or absorbed through the sensitive skin of the footpads. Called atopy, or inhalant allergy, some allergic cats may also develop asthma.

About 10 percent of dogs develop atopy, and itch on the front half of their body. Scratching of the armpits, feet, face, neck, and chest is typical, and affected dogs also tend to develop recurrent ear infections.

Atopic cats break out in miliary dermatitis. The allergy also may cause cats to develop eosinophilic plaque, an extremely itchy area of bright red, oozy, and elevated sores usually on the inside of the thighs or abdomen. Eosinophilic granulomas, also believed to be allergy-related, are yellow to yellow-pink raised sores that form straight lines usually on the back of both hind legs.

It is nearly impossible to avoid allergens, because dog and cat fur acts like a dust mop to collect and trap allergens. Blood serum tests to identify allergenic substances get mixed reviews from veterinarians and researchers. Intradermal skin tests—similar to those performed in people—still offer the best option for diagnosis. Some newer tests such as the HESKA Flea Allergy Dermatitis Test use flea saliva to measure reactivity in the skin. Tests for a wide range of inhalant allergens generally run about $150 to $200. Suspected allergens are injected into a sedated pet's shaved skin, which becomes swollen and red within five to fifteen minutes if the pet is allergic.

Treatment Options

Flea control is essential for pets suffering from flea allergic dermatitis (FAD). Today's products are very effective. Some products work only when the flea is poisoned by biting the pet and drinking the treated blood, which means that the pet still gets exposed to flea saliva. But even these products control FAD remarkably well.

Management of skin allergies often includes a combination of drugs that help control the inflammation. Dr. Dawn Merton Boothe, from Texas A&M College of Veterinary Medicine, points out some of the newest therapies for allergic skin disease. Misoprostol has recently been studied for treatment of chronic itching, and in one study, 60 percent of the animals improved by 50 percent or more within three weeks. Pentoxyfylline (Trental) has been touted as the "drug of the decade." It is now used to treat itchy skin disease associated with atopy, as well as a wide range of other veterinary skin problems, according to dermatologist Dr. Sandra R. Merchant.

"Of all the components of the environment, nutrition is not only one of the largest, it's one of the few that you can absolutely control," says Dr. Dan Carey, a veterinarian at the Iams Company. "You can't control the weather or pollen count, but you can determine what your pet eats." Although allergies can't necessarily be cured through nutrition, they can be managed. "For instance, dogs suffering from inflammatory conditions and on corticosteroids [steroids] oftentimes can be weaned off or at least reduce dosages if they're fed certain nutrients," says Dr. Carey.

Dietary supplements with the proper balance of omega-6 and omega-3 essential fatty acids help many dogs and cats with allergic skin disease. The essential fatty acid targets membranes in the skin. Rather than using drugs to suppress itchiness, such treatments seek to help the animal's body rebalance itself.

Allergy shots (hyposensitization) may also help in up to 80 percent of pets, if the specific allergen can be identified. The treatment gradually builds up the pet's resistance by increasing exposure with repeat doses of vaccines. The treatment may take months to over a year before the pet shows improvement, and some pets require maintenance injections for life.

SPRAYING

Intact male cats and sometimes females spray objects with urine to mark their territory. Rather than squatting and releasing urine downward as in urination, the spraying cat backs up to the target and stands erect with twitching tail held straight up as he squirts urine against vertical surfaces like walls or trees. The scent of the urine marks boundaries, warning less dominant cats that wander into the area. Intact females spray most often when in heat, to announce their availability to male Romeos.

This normal behavior proves a nuisance to owners when the cat sprays indoors. Tomcat urine has a particularly pungent and offensive odor. Studies have shown that neutering stops male cat territorial spraying in 80 to 90 percent of all cases.

But altered cats of either sex may spray in response to stress. The familiar "self-scent" of urine seems to comfort insecure cats. Most behaviorists prefer to try to identify the trigger that causes the stress and, if possible, eliminate it. For instance, a cat who sprays due to the stress of a visit from the owner's mother-in-law may stop the obnoxious behavior when the unfamiliar human goes home.

In many cases the trigger either cannot be identified or is impossible to eliminate. Households with multiple cats most often suffer from spraying problems, especially when youthful cats reach social maturity at two to four years of age. Prior to that time the cats may get along. Social status changes can then disrupt the balance, and cause spraying by one or more disgruntled cats.

Fascinating Facts! Feline Language Revealed

After five years of research, in 1944 American scientist Mildred Moelk reported that domestic cats make sixteen different sounds of three distinct types; purring and murmurs; vowels or variations of "meow"; and "strained intensity" sounds like screams and hisses. She further verified that cats command nine consonants, five vowels, two dipthongs, and one tripthong.

Drug Therapy

In recent years hard-case cats have sometimes been helped with antianxiety medications like Buspirone, or tranquilizers such as chlordiazepoxide (Librax), alprazolam (Xanax), and diazepam (Valium). Each drug varies slightly in the way the body metabolizes it and how it affects the cat. Some cats do better on one drug than on another.

Spraying behavior can be caused by a combination of factors, so drugs like Valium work on several levels to control the problem. Tranquilizers act on the limbic system to calm anxiety and, as a side effect, prompt more "friendly" behavior between cats. Studies show that Valium stops spraying in 43 percent of cats, and it reduces spraying in 73 percent. Percentages were higher with castrated males and in multicat homes, and lower with spayed females.

A cat's liver must be screened prior to prescribing drugs to be sure the liver is healthy enough to properly metabolize the medicine. Cats frequently walk with a staggering gait for up to the first four days of treatment. After that the side effect spontaneously goes away.

Feline Aromatherapy

The most innovative treatment in recent years is Feliway, says Dr. Myrna M. Milani, an ethologist in New Hampshire. The natural spray, distributed by Farnam Pet Products, contains a synthetic duplicate of feline facial pheromones, chemical substances secreted by animals to communicate by scent with each other. "Pheromones are different than aroma," says Dr. Milani. "Cats have facial pheromones that say, Everything's cool. And the ones in their urine say, Come in here and I'll knock your block off."

Cats use cheek rubbing to mark territory with facial pheromones that leave behind a familiar and comforting scent. Among other things, the presence of facial pheromones will inhibit cats from marking that object with urine. Applying a daily squirt of Feliway onto the places soiled by the cat and on objects he might tend to cheek-rub calms the urge to spray. Product instructions recommend increasing applications to two or three times per day in multicat households. Once the offending feline begins cheek-rubbing the doctored areas, a weekly application continues to reinforce the calming message.

Many, but not all, spraying cats stop with the introduction of Feliway. However, Dr. Milani believes that the product's benefit goes beyond curbing spray behavior. It helps to ease tension in many stressful situations. "It's great for the veterinarian who must deal with frightened cats, or accustoming cats to carriers," she says.

Modern Miracles: Molifying Molly

When Kathy Kettner of Bedford, New Hampshire, made the move from New York three years ago, her family of cats came with her. But once in the new home, the peaceable kingdom became a war zone.

The two six-month-olds, Molly and Lucy, had been exclusively indoor cats and got along famously. They'd also been crate-trained, which gave them a feeling of security, but also kept them segregated from the third cat. Su-Lin, a three-year-old blue point Siamese, had always been allowed in and out at her old home, so the three cats had rarely shared close quarters. But Kathy knew the New Hampshire wildlife wasn't safe for Su-Lin, so the Siamese became an indoor-only cat. The new house was so big,

Kathy thought the extra room would make the crates unnecessary, and so all three cats had free run of the house.

Happy-go-lucky Lucy didn't mind. But steel-blue Molly saw red whenever little Su-Lin appeared. "Molly jumped Su-Lin every chance she got," says Kathy, "but only when Su-Lin wasn't looking." Even though Molly outweighed Su-Lin by five pounds, she seemed to feel intimidated by the older cat. "Molly's behavior was a kind of defensive aggression," says Kathy.

Before long, Kathy saw Molly back up to walls and furniture, shake her tail, and act like she was spraying urine—she was relieved to discover nothing came out. Molly seemed to pantomime marking territory to show off for Su-Lin. Kathy put up with the behavior for months, until she found all-too-real urine marks. Kathy's frustration mounted the more she had to clean. Meanwhile, Su-Lin was a virtual prisoner, darting from shadow to shadow.

Dr. Myrna Milani suggested that Kathy bring back Molly's crate, a familiar and safe retreat that might offer the cat the security and boost in confidence she needed. "Myrna also suggested I separate Molly, because the aggression had become a habit," says Kathy. In fact, cats can develop a reflexive aggression where the mere sight of the other animal prompts an attack.

The third bedroom/computer office was blocked off with a window screen so Molly still could view the rest of the world from the room. Kathy outfitted a large dog kennel with a litter box, cat carrier for a bed, and food and water bowls. "Molly spent the day out in the bedroom but went into the crate at night," says Kathy, "and I spent lots of time in there with her, working on the computer."

The new setup worked like a charm, but made Kathy feel guilty because Molly no longer had the run of the house. So guilty, in fact, that she thought it best if she found Molly a new home where she wouldn't have to compete with other cats. "I thought I'd found her the perfect home," says Kathy. "I even gave them a letter from Molly that said, 'My name is Molly, I'm a good kitty, and I don't scratch the furniture,' says Kathy, still a bit weepy at the memory. "I made them promise to call me if it didn't work out, and I'd come get her."

The new home lasted less than nine days. Molly hid in a closet the whole time. "When I called to her, she said, 'Mew-mew!' and came running out to me," says Kathy, "and I brought her home. We were both so happy!"

Since then Molly has been perfectly happy in her room. Over the next year, Molly learned to tolerate wider access to the rest of the house.

"Molly and Su-Lin still have spats like little kids, and they get a time-out," says Kathy. They don't like each other, but they have learned to tolerate each other, and there's been no more spraying. "Molly goes back to her room and crate willingly, and the other cats don't try to go in. They know that's Molly's room. As long as she has her own room and property, she's happy. She's back where she belongs."

Prediction: Led by the Nose

In the animal kingdom, pheromones trigger all sorts of behavior. Feliway is doubtless the first of many new behavior therapy products designed to offer "mind control" through the nose, says Dr. Milani. Researchers have been fascinated by how mammals, reptiles, and even insects use pheromones in everything from mating behavior and social interaction to feeding themselves.

For instance, a beetle called *Atemeles pubicollis* uses pheromones to induce ants to commit a kind of social suicide. After it finds the ant colony by airborne scent, the beetle shows a worker ant a gland that secretes a calming pheromone. "The chemical tells the ant, Everything's cool, you love me!" says Dr. Milani. Most ants are seduced and carry the beetle into the colony. Once inside the nest, the beetle is fed by the ants, and in turn, the beetle babies feed on ant babies.

The potential for dog and cat behavior medicine seems endless.

TEETH PROBLEMS

Periodontal (dental) disease affects up to 70 percent of all cats and 85 percent of all dogs by age three. Better veterinary care means animals are living longer, and as with people, tooth, gum, and oral bone disorders tend to worsen as the pet ages. "The wolf-type dog of the wild had the perfect size tooth for his perfect size head, but as we bred smaller dogs, their heads became smaller, but the teeth stayed the same size," says Dr. Paul Orsini, a surgeon and dentist at the University of Pennsylvania. That's why dog breeds with crowded mouths, like Yorkshire Terriers, suffer the worst problems. Their tiny jaws don't easily accommodate all their teeth.

Dogs and cats tend not to chew their food, and soft diets that stick to the tooth surface provide the perfect environment for bacterial growth that creates plaque and bad breath. Calculus, or tartar, develops when plaque mineralizes and forms hard yellow or brown deposits. The bacteria in tartar release enzymes that attack the gums and cause inflammation, bleeding, and soreness (gingivitis). It also prompts the gums to pull away from the toxin-producing bacteria that cover the tooth. That forms pockets around the tooth that expose bone. "And because you have loss of bone," says Dr. Orsini, "the root becomes loose, which promotes further periodontal disease, because the moving tooth is destroying the bone because it's moving back and forth. It's a vicious cycle."

Dogs rarely develop cavities, but according to the American Veterinary Dental Society, 28 percent of all cats develop hard-to-detect cervical cavities, or neck lesions, that decay the tooth between the root and the crown of the tooth, where the gum line begins. It may require X-rays to find neck lesions. The entry hole may be tiny even though decay has eaten away the inside of the tooth and left a hollow shell. Mouth infections and tooth disease can impact the pet's overall health because bacteria from the teeth leak into the bloodstream and can damage the lungs, heart, liver, and kidneys.

Dental cleaning requires anesthesia—pets won't "open wide" on command to have their teeth scraped. "General practitioners do nice jobs cleaning teeth and can keep the cost down to maybe $200," says Dr. Orsini. "Specialists will charge more than that, maybe $300 to $400 depending on what's involved."

Because cleaning teeth scratches them and leaves areas where bacteria easily attach, teeth are polished after they're cleaned. "Then it's up to the owner to keep them clean with daily tooth brushing," says Dr. Orsini. Once a week or once a month doesn't do any good, he warns; he feels twice daily is ideal. Today, meat-flavored canine and feline toothpaste and specialized brushes to clean pet teeth are available.

Pets may require antibiotics to treat ongoing infections. Some innovative drug delivery systems actually implant medication into the gum. The timed-release therapy provides antimicrobial activity for several weeks at the site of infection.

The Diet Connection

Wild animals that capture prey for food naturally clean their teeth as they chew raw bone, muscle, and skin, says Dr. Orsini. Although modern commercial foods offer many health benefits, those that provide little "detergent" action, like soft canned diets, may actually predispose pets to dental problems. Dry diets are less likely to promote problems since they don't stick to teeth, but they don't help much either, since cats and dogs don't chew these types of food. They tend to gulp and swallow mouthfuls of kibble at a time.

Some pet food companies have developed "dental diets" to address this problem. For example, Hill's Pet Nutrition has one for dogs and cats called Prescription Diet t/d, and Friskies promotes a dental feline diet. "Dental diets are designed to be more abrasive," says Dr. Orsini, "and they have more fibrous material that actually helps promote clean teeth." Fiber may help scrub teeth as the pet chews, and some dental diets actually add special enzymes that help prevent plaque and tartar from attaching to teeth in the first place. The Hill's diet includes lower levels of calcium and phosphorus to discourage the formation of tartar. Company studies showed that eating the diet resulted in a 29 percent reduction in tartar in dogs and a 47 percent reduction in tartar in cats.

Dr. Orsini says dogs that like to chew can benefit from rawhide toys and safe chew toys, but you have to match the chew to the dog. "Rawhide is the best choice, but be sensible about it," he says. "Take it away before your Labrador swallows a big piece." Aggressive chewers can suffer blocked intestines if they are allowed to eat the rawhide, and the hard plastic chew toys or cow hooves often break teeth.

"For cats, there isn't a lot you can do," he says. Cats don't tend to indulge in recreational chewing. "Cats can use turkey necks," he says. "You can steam it to kill the bugs on it. But we haven't found that it helps much." Cat treats designed to help dental health benefit some cats.

A variety of new dental products designed for convenient use by pet owners continue to be introduced. For instance, neutral-tasting solutions that help reduce the accumulation of plaque and tartar may be added to a pet's drinking water.

Advanced Dental Care

Today, veterinary dental specialists offer everything a human dentist can provide, from fillings and crowns to root canals and even implants. For instance, periodontal disease may be helped by advanced procedures like gingival flaps that save the tooth, says Dr. Orsini. "That's reattaching the gum tissue to a clean root, and covering a root that's exposed," he says. Costs of advanced dental procedures vary, depending on who does them, with root canals costing about $750 to $1,000.

Orthodontics costs in the hundreds to thousands of dollars—the average is around $1,500, depending on what needs to be done—and dogs are the most common patients. "We use orthodontics just like you do with people," says Dr. Orsini. "If you have a tooth going the wrong way and perhaps actually putting a hole in the roof of the mouth when the pet chews, you can put braces on to move that tooth." He notes that abnormalities of teeth are often inherited, and fixing the teeth to look pretty won't prevent passing those traits on to offspring. "At the University of Pennsylvania we're very conservative and use orthodontia only for health reasons," he says. Improved appearance may be a side benefit, but the treatment is used only if the dog benefits medically.

The American Kennel Club and United Kennel Club prohibit showing any dog that has had any artificial alteration of the dog's appearance, and that includes orthodontic work. Owners of conformation show dogs that have had orthodontial correction and continue to show the dog may violate these regulations, and may be fined or even lose the right to show or register dogs and litters. Many veterinary dental organizations have policies that address this matter, and the professional who disregards the policy could risk ethical-code violations, suspensions, or lose accreditation.

Misaligned teeth wear unevenly and predispose the pet to periodontal disease. That's because normal alignment helps clean the teeth as the pet chews, while misdirected teeth catch and hold food particles more easily. Orthodontia may involve retainers, tooth extraction, or restructuring of the tooth with a crown or root canal. Fixed and removable braces, bands, or other devices are often used for the best long-term results. Typically, a mold of the dog's teeth is made once he's anesthetized and is used to design custom dental appliances.

A dog with braces typically visits the canine dentist every one to two weeks for adjustments, and sometimes owners must make adjustments at home every several days. Also, the dog's teeth must be kept clean with daily brushing during the treatment period. Braces are typically kept in place for a minimum of four months.

Computed Dental Radiography

Intraoral X-rays, taken from inside the mouth rather than outside, help reveal the extent of bone loss in periodontal disease, the extent of decay, misaligned teeth, tooth development, and even jaw fractures or oral tumors.

Computed dental radiography (CDR) requires the pet to be anesthetized. A receptor, rather than X-ray film, is placed in the mouth. The receptor is connected by a fiber optic cable to a computer. Instead of storing the image on the receptor as the picture is taken, it's captured by the computer and stored as digitized pixels immediately available for viewing on the monitor.

CDR saves up to five minutes per image that otherwise would be spent developing conventional X-ray film. Also, there is up to a 90 percent reduction in radiation exposure to the pet. Digitized images can be manipulated—enlarged, zoomed, and enhanced—to provide details not available on standard radiographs. They can also be mailed electronically by computer for consultants or referrals with other veterinary dentists.

The cost of the software runs $10,000 and each receptor runs about $5,000, so the technology currently remains limited to university hospitals and large referral practices. As the technology improves, the cost should drop and CDR should become more readily available.

URINARY STONES

Both dogs and cats are prone to crystals and stones in the urinary tract. Cats are known to suffer from a group of disorders, including stones, as a part of lower urinary tract disease, or LUTD, sometimes called feline urinary syndrome (FUS). Urinary bladder stones occur in about 20 percent of all cats suffering from LUTD. About 3 percent of all dogs suffer from urinary stones.

Both animals may develop microscopic to sand-size crystals in the urine, called urolithiasis. Dogs more often than cats develop bladder stones, but even tiny crystals can interfere with the elimination of urine. Some dog breeds are predisposed to the condition. The Miniature Schnauzer, Dachshund, Dalmatian, Pug, Bulldog, Welsh Corgi, Basset Hound, Beagle, and Terrier breeds are at highest risk.

Signs of urinary stones may include any one or combination of the following: a break in housetraining, dribbling urine, straining in the litter box or spending lots of time "posing" in the yard with little result, bloody urine or urine with a strong ammonia smell, crying during urination, or excessively licking the genitals. Dogs of either sex may assume a strange splay-legged position when urination is painful. Partial obstruction in dogs may result in a weak, splattery stream of urine even when the pet shows no other signs of distress. Diagnosis is based on these symptoms, urinalysis, and/or X-rays to reveal stones in the bladder. Without prompt medical attention, the blocked pet will die when toxins build up in the bloodstream, the kidneys stop working, or the bladder ruptures.

Urinary stones are composed of a combination of minerals and organic substances found in the urine. The mineral(s) must be present in the urine in the right concentrations, the urine must have a favorable acid-base balance (pH), and urine must remain in the urinary tract long enough for crystals to precipitate. The formation of stones is influenced by the volume of urine, frequency of urination, genetics—and infection. The causes of some types of stones are known, while others remain a mystery. For instance, canine urate stones are caused by problems with metabolism, while canine struvite stones are associated with urinary tract infections.

While canine bladder stones are almost always caused by urinary tract infections, the cause of crystals in cats often can't be identified. Diet can play a role in the formation of certain types of feline stones. And because up to 70 percent of all cats and a large percentage of dogs have repeated episodes of stones, diet has become the standard way to treat and in some cases prevent them.

The Struvite Solution

In the past, struvite crystals were the most common stones to form. In addition, some types of dietary magnesium decrease the normal acidity of the urine and promote the formation of these crystals. That led to the belief that adjusting dietary magnesium, combined with other measures to increase urine acidity, would prevent the problem.

Cat food manufacturers adjusted formulations accordingly. Nearly every commercial cat food on the market today has been designed to reduce the chance of struvite formation. In the past few years diets specifically marketed to promote the cat's "urinary tract health" have become available in supermarkets.

Veterinarians routinely prescribe therapeutic diets to benefit cats diagnosed with LUTD and urolithiasis. Some of these dissolve existing struvite crystals, while others prevent new crystals from forming. Similarly, therapeutic diets that address the various stones that dogs may develop help prevent canine bladder stones from coming back. Diets that dissolve stones offer a noninvasive alternative to the surgical removal of the mineral deposits. Most large stones, however, must be removed with surgery.

The Calcium Oxalate Conundrum

Ten years ago, 80 percent of all feline bladder stones were struvite, but recent surveys indicate that figure has been cut in half. At the University of Minnesota College of Veterinary Medicine Urolith Center, recent studies show that calcium oxalate is now the most common type of stone. Unfortunately, the change in commercial diet formulations to reduce struvite is likely influencing the rising number of calcium oxalate stones. That's because the increased blood-acid level these diets promote tends to leech calcium from the bones, which is then spilled into the urine, where it can form calcium oxalate stones.

Calcium oxalate stones cannot be dissolved by diet, and must be removed surgically if they're too big to pass with the urine. Although there are no diets available to dissolve calcium oxalate stones, some diets will help to prevent them. Dr. Joseph W. Bartges and his team at the University of Tennessee are near completion of a study funded by the Morris Animal Foundation and Hill's Pet Nutrition that is investigating an alkalinizing diet high in fiber. They theorize that dietary components such as an excess of vitamins D or C, deficiency of vitamin B_6, high sodium, or low fiber may promote the formation of feline calcium oxalate stones. The study is also investigating the possibility of a metabolic factor that causes skeletal diseases in cats, which in turn result in the release of excess calcium from the bones.

A New Direction

An innovative approach targets the relative super saturation (RSS) of the urine instead of worrying about pH. Urine solutes are defined as any one or combination of twelve common "ingredients" in pet urine that come together to form stones or crystals. Undersaturation keeps the pet's urine diluted enough that even when solutes are present, they won't form stones.

Think of Karo Syrup. "Add a little sugar to it, and all kinds of crystals form because you've pushed it to supersaturation and the sugar can no longer stay in solution," says Dr. James H. Sokolowski. Conversely, a tablespoon of Karo Syrup mixed in a gallon of water creates an undersaturated solution. "That's the direction we want to go with the pet's urine," he says. The Waltham Canine Lower Urinary Tract Support Veterinary Diet (canned and dry) and Feline S/O Control pHormula Diet are new diets designed to create urine that's undersaturated for specific ingredients that make struvite and oxalate stones in cats and dogs, and brushite in dogs.

Laser Therapy

Although some bladder stones can be treated successfully with diet or medicine, for many types of stone, surgery is the only alternative. That can require multiple incisions to open the abdomen and bladder, and recovery time can be prolonged. An innovative technique developed by Dr. J. Paul Woods at Oklahoma State University provides an alternative.

Laser-Induced Shock Wave Lithotripsy breaks up the stones into tiny pieces that are able to pass naturally out of the body. An endoscope is guided through the dog's urethra into the bladder so the surgeon can actually see the stone. Then a laser light beam transmitted through fibers in the endoscope shatter the stone into smaller and smaller pieces. "It takes about two seconds," says Dr. Kenneth E. Bartels, a professor of laser surgery at OSU. The technique isn't widely available yet, but it has been used with success on large animals like steers and experimentally in dogs.

P/U Surgery

Cats that become blocked from urethral plugs—crystals mixed with mucus that get stuck in the urinary track—typically are unblocked with catheters to reestablish flow from the bladder. But repeated catheter use may cause scar tissue in the urethra that makes the problem even worse. Perianal urethrostomy (P/U) may be an option for these cats. The surgery shortens the male urethra by removing the penis, which creates a wider conduit for release of urine so the urethra doesn't block as easily even if crystals continue to form.

Modern Miracles:
Red's Rescue

The Japanese Chin Care and Rescue Effort (www.japanesechinrescue.org) makes it their business to find and rehabilitate purebred Chins that have fallen on hard times. So when JCCARE director Dana Baldinger of Renton, Washington, found Red at a pound, she was determined to give the sad, confused seven-year-old a last chance at a happy home.

"He was a sweet dog from the beginning," she says. "Red was very loving. He wanted to be near you." A trip to the veterinarian diagnosed an eye problem and skin infections that took weeks to clear up. Meanwhile, Dana searched for the perfect home where Red could spend the rest of his life.

Then she noticed he had an odd way of using the bathroom. "He'd stand for what seemed like hours with his eyes squeezed closed like he was really concentrating, but nothing would happen."

An X-ray revealed the little dog had a bladder stone. "It was the size of an apricot pit, and without a doubt the biggest one my vet said she'd ever seen," says Dana. "No wonder the poor dog couldn't urinate. It must have killed him, it hurt so badly to try."

Removing the stone was anything but simple. The surgeon discovered the stone had adhered to the bladder wall on two sides, so part of the bladder had to be removed along with the stone. JCCARE funded his $1,100 medical care. Their veterinarian discounted the rates for rescues, and Dana was confident Red was worth the expense.

Despite the discomfort from the surgery, Red acted 100 percent better, says Dana, and he was up and around straightaway. The first time he went outside to use the bathroom was a revelation. "The look on his face was priceless," she says. "He went outside, closed his eyes, and I swear to you, he smiled as he weeed for ages! He was so happy, it was magnificent. He must have felt empty for the first time in years."

Dana feared it would be hard to find the right family for Red, and was delighted when Marilee and John Woodrow fell in love with the little dog. Red was equally pleased at the match. "Red relaxed in John's arms right away," she says. "They were his perfect home and he knew it."

Red has since thrived on a special diet that prevents a recurrence of the stones. "He was so prepared to be well," says Dana. "I knew there was a very healthy dog in there just waiting to get out."

Stones in the Genes

Cystine is an amino acid, one of the building blocks of proteins, and normally it is almost completely reasorbed by the kidneys so it isn't lost in the urine. But dogs can inherit a genetic disorder called cystinuria in which the kidney transporter for cystine is defective, so it ends up in the urine. In acid urine, cystine crystalizes and can form cystine stones in the kidney and bladder. Cystinuria affects many dog breeds, but the severest form affects Newfoundlands. Dogs with cystinuria typically show chronic urinary tract problems that start at nearly any age.

The condition is inherited as an autosomal recessive trait in Newfoundlands—the affected dogs must inherit two mutant genes, one from each carrier parent. Carriers have one mutant gene and don't show signs but can pass on the problem to offspring. In one case, an affected Newfoundland stud sired over a hundred offspring, and all are capable of passing on the trait to their pups.

An AKC Canine Health Foundation grant funded research by Dr. Paula Henthorn of the University of Pennsylvania School of Veterinary Medicine that identified the molecular defect in the Newfoundland and developed a genetic test for carriers. Dr. Henthorn continues to look for the defect in other breeds as well. The Section of Medical Genetics at the University of Pennsylvania offers several tests to detect affected dogs and carrier dogs. The nitroprusside spot test costs about $18, requires only a tiny amount of urine, and can be used to test any dog or cat. The DNA blood test for Newfoundland dogs runs about $75.

Hemalert: Litmus Litter

Cats that have suffered from one episode of LUTD have a 68 percent chance of experiencing repeated episodes. Blood in the urine may be an early sign of trouble, but it can be difficult and time-consuming to collect urine and look for the presence of blood. A new home-use product makes it easier.

Hemalert, a new litter additive, turns the cat's normal litter into a litmus test that detects the presence of blood in the urine. The pink Hemalert particles are mixed with the cat's usual cat box filler and react by changing color to blue if blood is present, alerting owners to a possible health problem.

Hemalert is sold only through veterinarians as part of the Purina CNM Urinary Tract Disease Management Program. The product comes six packets to a box, and costs about $33 for the box. Cats with recurrent problems may benefit from a Hemalert test once or twice a month. "Some veterinarians may just send home one packet," says Dr. Grace Long, as a follow-up test after the cat has been on a therapeutic diet for a couple of weeks.

VACCINATIONS

The immune system provides a protective barrier between illness and good health. Preventative vaccinations build on the foundation of a pet's own natural immunity by programming the body to recognize danger and mount a defense against it. The injections or nasal drops expose the pet to non-disease-causing forms of viruses or bacteria. That stimulates the body's production of immune agents such as antibodies designed to seek out and destroy disease-causing bacteria, viruses, or other pathogens.

Not all pets should receive every single vaccine. People aren't vaccinated against sleeping sickness, for example, unless they might be exposed to it by traveling overseas. Consequently, pets need vaccinations only against diseases they might be exposed to.

Most cats benefit from protection against upper respiratory disease and panleukopenia (feline distemper), and most dogs benefit from vaccination against distemper and parvovirus. A rabies vaccination is often required by law. Today these are called "core" vaccines, recommended for all cats or dogs.

Examples of "noncore" vaccines are those that protect cats against feline leukemia virus, or dogs against Lyme disease or leptospirosis. Pets never exposed to ticks, for instance, would not benefit from the Lyme vaccine, while other vaccinations have questionable effectiveness. "The feline infectious peritonitis vaccine, for example, is marginal in terms of efficacy and is not recommended except in very unique situations," says Dr. Dennis Macy, an internist and vaccine specialist at Colorado State University.

A one-size-fits-all vaccination program has fallen out of favor as researchers learn more about how long the various vaccines provide protection. Researchers also recognize potential risks when the vaccines are overused. More than ever before, vaccination use is balanced with considerations regarding the long-term health of the individual pet.

Very young and very old dogs and cats tend to have less effective immune systems, and so are at higher risk for disease. Exposure to other pets also increases the risk. Show animals and those being boarded or in animal shelters also have higher stress levels, which leave them more susceptible to illness. Cats and dogs kept confined in the house or yard have the least risk, but where they live can influence their risk of exposure. For instance, in some parts of the country pets have a greater risk of catching canine leptospirosis or feline leukemia virus.

Immunity-Boosting Blood

A Morris Animal Foundation grant helps fund research into an innovative immune-boosting therapy for newborn kittens. Kittens depend on colostrum (first milk from Mom) for protection against serious infections. But kittens whose mothers die, or are very ill or have poor-quality milk, may not receive this protection. Other kittens are part of large competitive litters, are weak and unable to nurse, or have blood-group incompatibilities with their mother, and fail to nurse colostrum.

Researchers have shown that antibodies found in the blood of normal adult cats can be transferred to kittens by serum injection either beneath the skin or into the abdomen. The process could be used to save at-risk newborn pet kittens as well as endangered cat species.

Research conducted by Dr. Julie Levy, an assistant professor of small animal medicine at the University of Florida College of Veterinary Medicine, along with Dr. Cynda Crawford, a postdoctoral associate in the department of pathobiology, continue to refine the treatment. They want to establish a convenient dosage and determine the most efficient and effective method of giving the serum.

A pet's immune system doesn't fully mature until about eight weeks of age. Prior to that time, puppies and kittens rely on passive immunity passed to them through their mother's first milk, called colostrum. But this borrowed immunity also interferes with vaccinations, because it attacks and destroys the "foreign" protective agents in the vaccines, just as though they were viruses. Passive immunity may neutralize vaccines until about fourteen weeks of age, although the timing varies. It's nearly impossible to predict the exact time when passive immunity fades and the young pet's own immune system takes over. Therefore, a series of vaccinations are given to young animals to better protect them when this window of opportunity leaves them at risk for disease. Kittens and puppies are typically vaccinated beginning at about six to eight weeks of age, and again every three to four weeks until they are about four months old.

Potential Vaccine Problems

"Twenty years ago we worried about stamping out distemper and rabies, and we've done a good job of reducing the incidence of a number of those diseases," says Dr. Macy. "But now we recognize those vaccine products are not as safe as we thought they were."

Pets often suffer from slight swelling or soreness at the site of injection, and perhaps lethargy or fever for a day or so after vaccination. For instance, temporary reactions from local pain to diarrhea typically occur in 14 percent of all feline patients (mostly kittens) that receive the feline leukemia virus vaccine. More severe allergic reactions (anaphylaxis) that develop within ten to fifteen minutes following the injection are considered rare, but they can cause anything from facial swelling or hives to difficulty breathing, collapse, and death.

Traditionally, most vaccines for dogs and cats have been of two types, depending on the infectious agent—"live" or "killed" vaccines. Live vaccines have been modified to reduce their ability to cause the disease but can still multiply inside the body just like the virus. That stimulates the immune system to fight back more effectively. But extremely virulent agents like rabies are difficult to inactivate to the point where they won't cause the disease they are trying to prevent. Killed vaccines offer a safer alternative, but they need an adjuvent—an additive that helps stimulate immunity—to be sure they get the attention of the immune system.

About ten years ago, a handful of holistic veterinarians began sounding warnings about excessive vaccinations that they felt prompted immune problems in some pets. But the wake-up call to the veterinary industry as a whole came only when cats began to develop cancer at the site of vaccination—usually right between the shoulder blades. The tumors developed in about 20 out of every 100,000 cats vaccinated and seemed to be associated primarily with the feline leukemia virus (FeLV) and rabies vaccinations—but no particular brand. Ongoing studies funded by the Vaccine-Associated Feline Sarcoma Task Force

(VAFSTF) continue to try to pinpoint the causes. It is suspected that the adjuvant—the additive that helps stimulate immunity—in rabies and FeLV killed vaccines may be at least part of the problem. But a genetic component may also be involved, since closely related cats seem more likely to develop sarcomas. New feline vaccination site guidelines specify tracking procedures to better determine information about the tumors.

After the vaccine-sarcoma issue raised safety concerns, a number of adverse side effects were investigated more fully in both cats and dogs. "It appears that the number of vaccines that one gets directly correlates to the increased risk for these adverse events, whether it be polyarthritis [affecting many joints] or sarcomas or autoimmune disease in dogs," says Dr. Macy. The leptospirosis vaccine is notorious for adverse reactions, especially in young pups and toy breeds. More dogs die of the reaction than ever do of leptospirosis.

Such concerns have prompted the vaccine industry to push harder for safety not only in terms of frequency of use, but also in the types of vaccines available. For instance, Dr. Macy says the new Purevax feline rabies vaccine introduced by Merial addresses the sarcoma issue by eliminating the need for an adjuvant; it produces virtually no reactions at all. Instead of being a traditional killed vaccine, the Merial cat rabies vaccine is genetically engineered.

Dr. Macy says the jury is still out on a brand-new leptospirosis vaccine. Part of the frustration with older leptospirosis vaccines was that they often didn't protect against the "real world" strains of the virus, but Duramune from Fort Dodge Animal Health has added the strains called *grippotyphosa* and *pomona*, which are involved in the most recent outbreaks of the disease.

How Long Protection Lasts

No vaccine gives 100 percent protection. Some vaccinations are designed to reduce or treat the symptoms of the disease but not necessarily to prevent the illness. The health of an individual pet's immune system, how often he is exposed and the virulence of the agent, and the type of vaccine all influence how effective it is. How long protection lasts depends on the type of infectious agent and the form of the vaccination. Immunity against viruses lasts longer than bacterial immunity. Killed vaccines don't protect nearly as long as modified live vaccines. Local immunity in the nose or eyes doesn't last as long as protection that includes the whole body.

After the first series of puppy or kitten shots, vaccinations traditionally were repeated every year. "But that protocol has been totally arbitrary," says Dr. Macy. "It's not based on duration of immunity studies." The only exception is rabies. Because of the human health risk, rabies has been required by law to be proven protective for a one- to three-year period. With other vaccinations there is no proof of how long they last. "The public and veterinarians have become oversold on the vaccine as a cure-all," Dr. Macy says.

In reality, pets twelve weeks of age or younger are extremely susceptible to disease, whereas a one-year-old pet is less so. "That suggests," says Dr. Macy, "that if a vaccine has some risk with it, like sarcoma development in cats, you need to vaccinate young animals but maybe don't need to vaccinate the older patient on an annual basis." He believes vaccinations should all be targeted toward the young, just as in human medicine. He recommends vaccinating, with a series of boosters, until the pets are twelve to sixteen weeks of age, one year later, and then every three years. "So far," he says, "about ten of the veterinary schools have adopted that recommendation for both dogs and cats." Studies are underway to determine the actual duration of vaccination protection and the best revaccination schedule.

Immune-Boosting Diets

New research into antioxidants is allowing pet food manufacturers to make food that may reduce the frequency of necessary vaccinations. Whether it involves food or the body, oxidation is, in simplest terms, biological rust caused by contact with oxygen or other components of decay. Pet food preservatives, otherwise known as antioxidants, can be synthetic chemicals (BHA, BHT, ethoxyquin) or "natural" ones such as mixed tocopherol (vitamin E) and ascorbic acid (vitamin C). Research has shown that natural antioxidants improve the immune response, and provide better protection against disease.

The next "wellness diet" line of lifestage products introduced by Waltham, and available through veterinarians, touts single-animal source protein, and a whole meat, like chicken, instead of fractions, like "chicken by-products." It also includes rice, barley, or oats, along with an immune-boosting antioxidant "cocktail" that not only preserves the food naturally but also benefits the pet's health.

Feline Vaccination Recommendations

To further define the cause of vaccine-associated sarcomas and their treatment, veterinarians have been asked to standardize vaccination procedures. That includes keeping a record of where on the cat's body the injection is given and the type of injection (manufacturer, serial number, etc.). That way, if a tumor develops on the cat's body, the veterinarian will know exactly what vaccine caused the problem. Pet owners should also pay attention to what vaccines are given and monitor that area of the body following the injection.

It is recommended that:

1. Panleukopenia (distemper) and upper respiratory vaccines should be given on the right shoulder.
2. Rabies vaccines should be given on the right rear limb, as far down as possible.
3. Feline leukemia virus vaccines should be given on the left rear limb, as far down as possible.

A full report of the recommendations, written by Dr. James R. Richards, of the Cornell Feline Health Center and chairperson of the education/communication subgroup, Vaccine-Associated Feline Sarcoma Task Force, was published by the *Journal of the American Veterinary Medical Association* and is available online at www.avma.org/vafstf/

The cocktail includes vitamins A, C, E, zinc, selenium, taurine, grape pumice, tomato pumice, and marigold. Researchers tested paired litter mates by feeding one the new diet and the other a diet without the antioxidants, and then vaccinating them both. The pet eating the antioxidant cocktail developed higher blood levels of antibodies from the vaccine much earlier. The results suggest that diet could be of significant assistance in allowing pet owners to safely lengthen the interval between revaccinations.

WOUND HEALING

Cats and dogs injure themselves in a variety of ways. The greatest culprit in their failing to heal is infection, so cleanliness continues to be the mainstay of healing wounds. "The tincture of time is always good," says Dr. Giselle Hosgood, a surgeon at Louisiana State University. Injuries don't heal overnight, and patience is key. For instance, a large degloving wound—where the skin is peeled away from a limb—may take three to four weeks before it can be closed.

In the last ten years, knowledge of wound healing has expanded. "We've gone from an understanding of what's going on at the microscopic level to an understanding of what's going on at the biochemical level," says Dr. Hosgood. The general practice veterinarian successfully manages pet wounds all the time. But in certain circumstances, specialty care helps speed recovery and it may even be necessary in the case of burns, massive wounds to the back or abdomen, or injuries to the face or lower leg areas, which have little extra skin to spare.

Some wounds benefit from hyperoxygenation of the wound, accomplished by placing the dog or cat in a diving chamber. "They breathe pressurized oxygen that supersaturates their blood," says Dr. Hosgood. When the blood reaches the wound, it hyperoxygenates the wound and can help speed healing.

Some wounds require a period of time just to clean the wound and to allow the injury to start to generate new tissue that will accept a graft. There are areas of extra skin and tissue that can be used to donate a necessary skin flap.

When possible, skin flaps loosened from any extra skin around the injury pull together to close the wound. "We can also do free skin grafts," says Dr. Hosgood, "where you actually take a piece of skin from another part of the body, then place it on the wound, and it's accepted by the wound. And we do free vascular [blood vessel] grafts, where you take a piece of skin from another part of the body and then connect the artery and vein to an artery and vein in the area of the wound."

In people, partial-thickness grafts are commonplace, particularly for burn victims. "They take an instrument like a cheese slicer and slice off layers and layers of very thin healthy skin and put those on the wound," says Dr. Hosgood. That allows the doctor to obtain lots of donor skin from a relatively small area.

Veterinarians who treat wounds in dogs and cats take advantage of these animals' loose, elastic, and excess skin. "We have the luxury of lots of skin to work with most of the time," says Dr. Hosgood. For instance, a Labrador has much loose skin over the chest, so a full-thickness graft can be harvested to graft onto a leg wound. "That allows us to close up that donor site so it's less painful," she says. "And with that full thickness of skin you also take hair follicles with it, so that graft will then grow hair and you won't have bald patches."

Innovative Wound Protection

The stitches required to repair cuts and lacerations often bother pets more than the injury itself. New wound-closing techniques eliminate the need for irritating sutures, staples, or skin strips. Dermabond Topical Adhesive (Ethicon Inc.), approved by the FDA in 1999, simply glues the sides of the cut back together. It shouldn't be used on very deep or heavily bleeding injuries, but for certain wounds it offers the advantage of avoiding the trauma of stitches or anesthetics.

Similarly, Facilitator Liquid Bandage (hydroxyethylated amylopectin), introduced by Blue Ridge Pharmaceuticals in late 1999, helps heal chronic wounds like acral lick granulomas. Dogs sometimes lick their forelegs so much, due to an itch or boredom, that they develop these hard-to-heal shiny red ulcers. The odorless, nonirritating gel applied to the wound dries quickly and protects the raw, inflamed area as it heals.

Another innovation goes even further. Pets with wounds often lick and chew the sore, or even pull out their stitches as they try to soothe the itch or irritation. Licking interferes with and slows normal healing. Traditional cone-shaped restraints called Elizabethan collars that fit around the pet's neck can prevent teeth and tongue from reaching the area, but these restraints often cause the pet as much stress as the wound itself.

WoundWear introduced the WoundWear Body Suit, a postsurgical garment developed as a stress-free alternative to the Elizabethan collar. The WoundWear Body Suit allows the dog freedom of movement without limiting her ability to eat, sleep, or see. Constructed of tough yet lightweight material, the suit prevents the pet from tearing out stitches or scratching or licking body wounds.

Wound Study Center Researches Healing

The Wound Healing/Reconstructive Surgery Program at the Scott-Ritchey Research Center at Auburn University researches wound healing and prevention for both humans and animals. A variety of cutting-edge techniques are used at the center.

Computer-aided planimetry measures how fast open wounds heal. Scintigraphy uses radionuclide imaging to evaluate the injury. Laser doppler imaging evaluates the blood supply available to the wound, while tensiometry measures wound strength. Electrodiagnostics measures the relationship between wound healing to nerve involvement (enervation). And kinetic pressure evaluation systems study the effectiveness of various bandage and splint materials.

Researchers at Auburn University also study how chemicals derived from insects improve blood circulation to facilitate wound healing, and how magnetic field therapy improves wound healing by stimulating and augmenting the body's own natural magnetism. A magnet on either side of a bone fracture, for instance, has been shown to speed the rate of healing so the ends of the bones grow back together. For the Auburn study, the entire animal is placed in the electromagnetic field. "The pulsed electromagnetic field therapy study evaluated this form of radiation on the healing of soft tissue wounds," says Dr. Steven F. Swaim, a professor and specialist in wound healing at Auburn University.

Biologically active glass is a compound that has been successfully used for years in human medicine to enhance the healing of bone and dental wounds. It's difficult to get bone or tissue to adhere to commonly used metal implants like artificial hips. Tooth loss often leads to bone loss in the jaw, but bioactive glass like PerioGlas (USBiomaterials Corp.) can be sculpted to fill in the deficit. Bone also readily "grows into" bioactive glass, so it can be used to coat metal replacement joints or rods used in fracture repairs, or can be used as a scaffold for new bone to grow. Some types of biologically active glass are compounded to release bone-building components like calcium that stimulate new growth.

Bioglass is an inorganic material that has been shown to bond to a wound and positively influence the rate at which tissues regenerate. Its composition attracts the body's tissue-repairing molecules and proteins, which promotes faster and more efficient healing, says Dr. David Greenspan, vice president and principal scientist for USBiomaterials. "These new compositions [bioglass] give us the potential to place drugs, proteins, or cells into a specific site in the body that will allow for a more predictable result than is currently available."

A new product that incorporates bioglass has shown dramatic healing rates on Hansen's disease (leprosy) when it was tested in humans in China.

Prediction: Growth Factors and Healing

In the past decade researchers have learned more about the complex interaction of factors that are secreted by the different cells involved in healing wounds. These factors are collectively called growth factors, or cytokines.

Current research looks at ways to manipulate growth factors to stimulate wound healing. In a normal wound, adding extra growth factors won't make a difference, but wounds that are deficient in these growth factors stand to benefit. "Everyone wants to heal a wound quicker and faster and better," says Dr. Hosgood. "The future of wound healing in both people and pets potentially lies in applications of the growth factors."

PART THREE

Appendixes

U.S. Veterinary Schools

Veterinarians usually attend a total of eight to ten years of school to receive their doctor of veterinary medicine (DVM) degree. The University of Pennsylvania is the only school that awards a *veterinariae medicinae doctoris* (VMD) degree instead. Veterinarians schooled in other countries may use other designations. For instance, MRCVS means Royal College of Veterinary Surgeons and is a British equivalent to DVM or VMD.

Specialists and cutting-edge research are most often found at veterinary universities. University websites often publish information about their current programs, researchers involved, and whether pet cats and dogs may participate in these studies. Many times, the researchers send announcements about these programs to nearby private veterinary practices. You can ask your veterinarian about these opportunities, or contact the university directly.

ALABAMA

Auburn University
College of Veterinary Medicine
180 Greene Hall
Auburn University, AL 36849
http://www.vetmed.auburn.edu

Tuskegee University
School of Veterinary Medicine
T. S. Williams Veterinary Medical Library/AV-AT Center
Patterson Hall
Tuskegee, AL 36088
http://svmc107.tusk.edu/Tu/svm/svm-toc.html

CALIFORNIA

University of California
School of Veterinary Medicine
Davis, CA 95616-8734
http://www.vetmed.ucdavis.edu

COLORADO

Colorado State University
College of Veterinary Medicine and Biomedical Sciences
W102 Anatomy Building
Fort Collins, CO 80523
http://www.cvmbs.colostate.edu

FLORIDA

University of Florida
College of Veterinary Medicine
PO Box 100125
Gainesville, FL 32610-0125
http://www.vetmed.ufl.edu

GEORGIA

University of Georgia
College of Veterinary Medicine
Athens, GA 30602
http://www.vet.uga.edu

ILLINOIS

University of Illinois
College of Veterinary Medicine
2001 South Lincoln

Urbana, IL 61802
http://www.cvm.uiuc.edu

INDIANA

Purdue University
School of Veterinary Medicine
1240 Lynn Hall
West Lafayette, IN 47907-1240
http://www.vet.purdue.edu

IOWA

Iowa State University
College of Veterinary Medicine
2503 Veterinary Administration
Ames, IA 50011-1250
http://www.vetmed.iastate.edu

KANSAS

Kansas State University
College of Veterinary Medicine
Anderson Hall, Room 9
Manhattan, KS 66506-0117
http://www.vet.ksu.edu

LOUISIANA

Louisiana State University
School of Veterinary Medicine
South Stadium Road
Baton Rouge, LA 70803
http://www.vetmed.lsu.edu

MASSACHUSETTS

Tufts University
School of Veterinary Medicine
200 Westboro Road
North Grafton, MA 01536
http://www.tufts.edu/vet

MICHIGAN

Michigan State University
College of Veterinary Medicine
A-120E East Fee Hall
East Lansing, MI 48824-1316
http://www.cvm.msu.edu

MINNESOTA

The University of Minnesota
College of Veterinary Medicine
1365 Gortner Avenue
St. Paul, MN 55108
http://www.cvm.umn.edu

MISSISSIPPI

Mississippi State University
College of Veterinary Medicine
Box 9825
Mississippi State, MS 39762
http://www.cvm.msstate.edu

MISSOURI

University of Missouri
College of Veterinary Medicine
Columbia, MO 65211
http://www.cvm.missouri.edu

NEW YORK

Cornell University
College of Veterinary Medicine
Box 39, Schurman Hall S3-005
Ithaca, NY 14853-6401
http://www.vet.cornell.edu

NORTH CAROLINA

North Carolina State University
College of Veterinary Medicine

4700 Hillsborough Street
Raleigh, NC 27606
http://www.cvm.ncsu.edu/

OHIO

The Ohio State University
College of Veterinary Medicine
101 Sisson Hall
1900 Coffey Road
Columbus, OH 43210
http://www.vet.ohio-state.edu

OKLAHOMA

Oklahoma State University
College of Veterinary Medicine
Stillwater, OK 74078-2008
http://www.cvm.okstate.edu

OREGON

Oregon State University
College of Veterinary Medicine
200 Magruder Hall
Corvallis, OR 97331-4801
http://www.vet.orst.edu

PENNSYLVANIA

University of Pennsylvania
School of Veterinary Medicine
3800 Spruce Street
Philadelphia, PA 19104-6047
http://www.vet.upenn.edu

TENNESSEE

University of Tennessee
College of Veterinary Medicine
PO Box 1071
Knoxville, TN 37901-1071
http://www.vet.utk.edu

TEXAS

Texas A&M University
College of Veterinary Medicine
College Station, TX 77843-4461
http://www.cvm.tamu.edu

VIRGINIA

Virginia Tech and University of Maryland
Virginia-Maryland Regional
College of Veterinary Medicine
Blacksburg, VA 24061-0442
http://www.vetmed.vt.edu

WASHINGTON

Washington State University
College of Veterinary Medicine
Pullman, WA 99164-7010
http://www.vetmed.wsu.edu

WISCONSIN

The University of Wisconsin-Madison
School of Veterinary Medicine
2015 Linden Drive West
Madison, WI 53711
http://www.vetmed.wisc.edu

Veterinary Specialty Colleges

The American Board of Veterinary Medical Specialties (ABVMS) and the American Veterinary Medical Association (AVMA) publish standards that must be met in order for a veterinarian to be certified in a particular specialty. There are about twenty specialty boards, often referred to as "colleges," currently recognized by the ABVMS and AVMA. Certification means that a "medical specialist" has successfully completed an approved educational program. Requirements generally include:

1. Completion of DVM or VMD degree (or an overseas degree equivalent)
2. Completion of three to seven years of full-time training in an accredited residency program
3. Assessments of individual performance and competence from the residency director
4. Passing a written and/or oral exam given by the senior members of the specialty college

Veterinarians are then awarded the designation "Diplomate" of the particular college specialty, and are certified (or "boarded") as specialists. Generally, the designation follows the DVM or VMD degree. For instance, DACVA means "Diplomate of the American College of Veterinary Anesthesiologists."

Many specialty colleges list their members, by location, on their websites, along with information about continuing education programs and conferences, studies, researchers involved, and whether pet cats and dogs may participate in these studies. Many times, the researchers send announcements about these programs to nearby private veterinary practices. You can ask your veterinarian about a referral to a nearby specialist.

A description of the various specialties follows. Contact information and website addresses are located at the end of this Appendix.

American College of Theriogenologists (ACT)

Theriogenology deals with reproduction, physiology, and pathology of the male and female reproductive systems in all domestic species, including cats and dogs. The practice of veterinary obstetrics, gynecology, and semenology (including advances in artificial insemination) mostly applies to fanciers of pedigreed cats and dogs involved in professional breeding programs.

American College of Veterinary Anesthesiologists (ACVA)

"Anesthesia is really pretty new in medicine in general," says Dr. William Tranquilli, an anesthesiologist at the University of Illinois. "We've only been using relatively safe anesthetic drugs for the last fifty or sixty years." Interest in veterinary anesthesia followed that of the human field and prompted the formation in 1970 of the American Society of Veterinary Anesthesiologists (ASVA). It became recognized as a specialty college in 1975, changing its name to ACVA.

Veterinary anesthesiologists continue to work primarily in universities. Half or more of the boarded anesthesia specialists practice at veterinary teaching hospitals. There are currently only about 150 veterinarians boarded in anesthesiology worldwide. About half of that number have been boarded in just the past six years.

A few large private surgical referral practices have hired a staff anesthesiologist, or a consulting specialist who travels from clinic to clinic. "Over the next five to ten years we'll see pain-management practice start to creep into the private practice arena," says Dr. Tranquilli. "It can be a major growth area for small-animal practitioners."

Part of that slowness in growth reflects the need to perfect safe anesthetic techniques in different animals. Human anesthesiologists deal with only one species. Veterinary anesthesiologists use many techniques that are not routinely available in private practice. Many of these techniques involve modern pain control that speeds healing and improves quality of life for chronic care patients.

American College of Veterinary Behaviorists (ACVB)

One of the hottest areas of veterinary medicine addresses behavior and training for dogs and cats. More than any other disease, bad behavior is the leading cause of death in pets because most problem animals are given up to shelters, where they are put down. Today, more and more owners are seeking specialized help to avoid such drastic measures. Animal behavior specialists study the relationship of animals to their physical environment as well as to other animals. They are concerned with understanding the causes, functions, development, and evolution of behavior, and they use that knowledge to help owners and pets build positive relationships.

"There's a whole realm of people who do behavioral work in animals," says Dr. Myrna M. Milani, an ethologist and behaviorist in New Hampshire. Many have degrees in human psychology or sociology. Others have done extensive work on their own, learning about animal behavior and training. A certification program for animal behaviorists was developed by the Animal Behavior Society in 1991, but not until the ACVB was established in 1993 did board certification become possible. "Probably one main thing that distinguishes the veterinary behaviorists is that they're the only ones licensed to prescribe and dispense controlled drugs," says Dr. Milani.

Many veterinary behaviorists are not boarded Diplomates. That's because the behavior college is so new that only a handful of veterinary schools include behavior medicine in their curriculum, says Dr. Karen Overall, a behaviorist at the University of Pennsylvania. "Opportunities for residency are extremely limited," she adds, "and we get a dozen applicants for each position. Residencies are usually two to four years, and I only took one resident for the entire period because we wanted to make sure we did everything right." As of this writing, there are only twenty-three boarded veterinary behaviorists in the world: nineteen in the United States, three in Canada, and one in Australia. Another half dozen or so a year can be expected to take the exam.

Many veterinary behaviorists learned on their own prior to 1995 by taking graduate courses, going to seminars, and practicing techniques in their own clinics, says Dr. Overall. "You can't penalize people who've already been doing this for the past ten or twenty years without the benefit of a college," she says. So in those circumstances they can become boarded via a "nonconforming residency" that basically fulfills the same criteria (i.e., case reports, publications, board exam), with on-the-job experience taking the place of the university residency.

American College of Veterinary Dermatology (ACVD)

Nearly 150 board-certified members of the ACVD practice in the United States, Canada, and Australia. The dermatology college was established in 1978, and Diplomates have a special expertise in skin diseases of dogs and cats, and many other animal species.

The skin constitutes the largest organ of the pet's body, and a wide array of illnesses express themselves through skin disease, which makes veterinary dermatologists uniquely qualified to diagnose and treat everything from allergy and parasite infections to ear and foot problems, including hormonal and cancer conditions.

American College of Veterinary Internal Medicine (ACVIM)

Called an umbrella organization, the ACVIM board, founded in 1972, certifies members in internal medicine, plus three subspecialties. "We're all internists. But within that there are subcategories of people who actually do internal medicine: cardiology, neurology, and oncology [cancer]," says Dr. Mark D. Kittleson, a cardiologist at the University of California-Davis.

Many times, when a specialist in one of these subspecialties isn't available, an internist is able to address the problem. "There are a number of large urban centers in the U.S. that don't have a veterinary cardiologist that could use one," says Dr. Kittleson.

"Internal medicine is fairly broad," says Dr. David S. Bruyette, an internist in Los Angeles. "We deal with problems related to kidney, intestine, blood, and the endocrine systems." Within internal medicine the specialist may concentrate on a particular area. "For instance," says Dr. Bruyette, "primarily what I do is endocrinology, so that's diabetes, thyroid, adrenal, reproductive, anything that's hormonal."

American College of Veterinary Nutrition (ACVN)

Veterinary nutritionists specialize in dog and cat food at the molecular level, learning how it can promote and maintain pet health. The specialty includes understanding how disease changes the body's metabolism—the way it processes nutrients—and using that knowledge to create diets that treat a variety of diseases. The majority of boarded nutritionists work either in academia or in the pet food industry.

American College of Veterinary Ophthalmologists (ACVO)

Veterinary ophthalmologists do everything their human counterparts do, but there are just over 200 Diplomates of the ACVO, compared to 30,000 human ophthalmologists, says Dr. J. Phillip Pickett, an ophthalmologist at Virginia-Maryland. That's one reason why many eye problems are managed by general veterinarians. Some serious conditions that may require surgical intervention or advanced therapies, such as cataracts, glaucoma, or cancer of the eye, benefit from a specialist's skill. Dogs especially tend to suffer inherited eye problems.

Although in the past, most boarded veterinary ophthalmologists worked only at large veterinary schools, that has changed in recent years, says Dr. Pickett. "Today just about every major metropolitan area in the U.S. has a veterinary ophthalmologist with a referral practice who works with the local veterinarians to take care of the animals' eyes."

American College of Veterinary Radiology (ACVR)

This specialty offers diagnosis and treatment using a variety of imaging technology, from X-rays and sonograms to magnetic resonance imaging (MRI) and computed tomography (CT). The ACVR, founded in 1961, includes over 200 Diplomates in the specialty of radiology. In 1993, a subspecialty within the ACVR was created in radiation oncology—that is, a specialty in cancer treatment using radiology techniques.

American College of Veterinary Surgeons (ACVS)

"The American College of Veterinary Surgeons sets the standards of surgical care in our profession," says Dr. Lillian Aronson, a surgeon at the University of Pennsylvania. Founded in 1965, it has certified nearly a thousand Diplomates. "At one time they nearly all were at academic institutions. But now over half of us are in private practice and referral centers," says Dr. A. D. Elkins, a surgeon practicing in Indianapolis.

Although the ACVS does not have subspecialties, many Diplomates focus on a particular area of surgery. For instance, about 40 percent focus on small-animal general and orthopedic surgeries. "There isn't a specific board for orthopedics, but there aren't enough of us and the demand is very high," says Dr. Paul Gambardella, a surgeon at the University of Pennsylvania. Still, most perform general surgery. Dr. Aronson says, "I do all soft tissue surgery as well as transplantation. I didn't want to just specialize, I wanted to continue doing all kinds of surgery."

American Veterinary Dental College (AVDC)

"There are three professional veterinary dental groups," says Dr. Paul Orsini, a surgeon and dentist at the University of Pennsylania. Thousands of veterinarians with an interest in dentistry belong to the American Society of Veterinary Dentists or the Academy of Veterinary Dentistry. "The American Veterinary Dental College was accredited by the AVMA in 1988," he says. Veterinary dentists are able to provide advanced procedures—everything from root canals or fillings to orthodontics and implants. A two-year residency program, either at a veterinary school or in private practice under the direction of a boarded dentist, is required for AVDC membership. Presently there are only about fifty boarded members in the United States. Most general veterinarians routinely offer teeth-cleaning services for dogs and cats.

VETERINARY SPECIALTY COLLEGES
(Contact Information)

Most but not all include a website listing of Diplomates by state for referral purposes.

American Board of Veterinary Practitioners
530 Church Street, Suite 700
Nashville, TN 37219-2394
http://www.abvp.com

American Board of Veterinary Toxicology
University of Pennsylvania
New Bolton Center
382 West Street Road
Kennet Square, PA 19348
http://www.abvt.org

American College of Laboratory Animal Medicine
96 Chester Street
Chester, NH 03036
603-887-2467
http://www.aclam.org

American College of Theriogenologists
School of Veterinary Medicine
Department of Clinical Science
Baton Rouge, LA 70803
504-346-3183
http://128.192.20.19/ACT/ACT.HTML

American College of Veterinary Anesthesiologists
Department of Small Animal Clinical Sciences
Virginia-Maryland Regional College
Phase II Bldg., Duckpond Drive
Blacksburg, VA 24061-0442
540-231-9268
http://www.acva.org

American College of Veterinary Behaviorists
Department of Small Animal Medicine and Surgery
College of Veterinary Medicine
Texas A&M University
College Station, TX 77843-4474
409-845-2351
http://www.var.vet.uga.edu/behavior/html/acvb.htm

American College of Veterinary Clinical Pharmacology
Department of Veterinary Physiology & Pharmacology
College of Veterinary Medicine
Texas A&M University
College Station, TX 77843-4466
409-845-9368
http://www.acvcp.org

American College of Veterinary Dermatology
Animal Dermatology Clinic
5610 Kearney Mesa Road, Suite B
San Diego, CA 92111
619-560-9393
http://www.dermvet.com

American College of Veterinary Emergency and Critical Care
Department of Clinical Sciences
School of Veterinary Medicine
Tufts University
200 Westboro Road
North Grafton MA 01536
508-839-5395
http://www.veccs.org

American College of Veterinary Internal Medicine
2750 S. Wadsworth Boulevard, Suite C-109
Denver, CO 80227-3400
303-980-7136
http://acvim.org

American College of Veterinary Microbiologists
College of Veterinary Medicine
University of Tennessee
PO Box 1071
Knoxville, TN 37901
423-974-5575
http://cem.vet.utk.edu/acvm.html

American College of Veterinary Nutrition
Department of Large Animal Sciences
Phase II
Virginia-Maryland College of Veterinary Medicine
Blacksburg, VA 24061-0442
540-552-3988
http://acvn.vetmed.vt.edu

American College of Veterinary Ophthalmologists
Department of Veterinary Clinical Sciences
Louisiana State University
Baton Rouge, LA 70803
225-346-3333
http://www.acvo.com

American College of Veterinary Pathologists
875 Kings Highway, Suite 200
Woodbury, NJ 08096-3172
609-848-3172
http://www.afip.org/acvp

American College of Veterinary Preventive Medicine
3126 Morning Creek
San Antonio, TX 78274
http://www.acvpm.org

American College of Veterinary Radiology
PO Box 87
Glencoe, IL 60022
847-251-5517
http://www.acvr.ucdavis.edu

American College of Veterinary Surgeons
4401 East West Highway, Suite 205
Bethesda, MD 20814-4523
301-913-9550
http://www.acvs.org

American Veterinary Dental College
Department of Surgical & Radiological Sciences
University of California
School of Veterinary Medicine
Davis, CA 95616
530-754-8254
http://hometown.aol.com/AMVETDENT

APPENDIX C

Health and Research Associations

A number of professional organizations, health associations, and research foundations provide education, accreditation, and funding in the veterinary arena. Some of these associations, although not "boarded" specialties, serve in similar capacities to train veterinarians in specialized techniques. Others sponsor research or fund studies. Many are at the forefront of cutting-edge veterinary care. You can learn more about each organization by writing to them, or reviewing information posted on their listed websites.

SPECIAL-INTEREST HEALTH ASSOCIATIONS

American Academy of Veterinary Acupuncture
PO Box 419
Hygiene, CO 80533-0419

American Animal Hospital Association
PO Box 150899
Denver, CO 80215-0899
303-986-2800

American Holistic Veterinary Medicine Association
2214 Old Emmorton Road
Bel Air, MD 21014

Association of American Veterinary Medical Colleges
Curt J. Mann, DVM, Executive Director
1101 Vermont Avenue, NW, Suite 710
Washington, DC 20005-3521
202-371-9195
202-842-0773 (fax)
aavmc@aavmc.org (e-mail)

American Association of Feline Practitioners
530 Church Street, Suite 700
Nashville, TN 37219
800-204-3514
615-259-7799
http://www.aafponline.org

American Veterinary Chiropractic Association (AVCA)
623 Main
Hillsdale, IL 61257

PET RESEARCH FOUNDATIONS

AKC Canine Health Foundation
251 West Garfield Road, Suite 160
Aurora, OH 44022
888-682-9696
http://www.akcchf.org

American Veterinary Medical Association
1931 North Meacham Road, Suite 100
Schaumburg, IL 60173-0805
http://www.avma.org

Canine Eye Registration Foundation (CERF)
SCC-A

Purdue University
West Lafayette, IN 47907
317-494-8179
http://vet.purdue.edu/~yshen/cerf.html

Delta Society
289 Perimeter Road East
Renton, WA 98055-1329
425-226-7357
http://www.petsforum.com/deltasociety

GeneSearch
11014 Schuylkill Road
Rockville, MD 20852
301-770-6970

Morris Animal Foundation
45 Inverness Drive East
Engelwood, CO 80112-5480
800-243-2345
303-790-2345
http://www.morrisanimalfoundation.org

OptiGene
Cornell Business and Technology Park
33 Thornwood Drive, Suite 102
Ithaca, NY 14850
607-257-0301

Orthopedic Foundation for Animals
2300 East Nifong Boulevard
Columbia, MO 65201-3856
573-442-0418
http://www.offa.org

PennGen Laboratories
3850 Spruce Street
Philadelphia, PA 19104-6010
215-898-3375

VetGen
3728 Plaza Drive, Suite 1
Ann Arbor, MI 48108
800-483-8436
http://www.vetgen.com

The Winn Feline Foundation, Inc.
1805 Atlantic Avenue
PO Box 1005
Manasquan, NJ 08736-0805
732-528-9797
http://www.winnfelinehealth.org

Glossary

Acupuncture   therapeutic use of needles to effect reversal or relief of medical conditions.

Acute   sudden onset of condition or disease, and/or condition of recent origin.

Adjuvant   substance that stimulates immune response, used in inactivated "killed" vaccines to improve effectiveness of protection.

Allele   one of the forms of a given gene.

Allergen   substance that triggers an allergic reaction.

Allograft   donor tissue obtained from a donor of the same species as the recipient.

Angiogenesis   the ability of cells to prompt outside vessels to supply blood to nurture new tissue growth. Angiogenesis inhibitors are a class of cancer drugs designed to stop this process in tumors.

Arthroscope   an endoscopic tool specific for use within the joints of the body.

BAER Test   brainstem auditory evoked response test, consisting of an electrical recording of the brain's reception of and response to external stimulus, often used to test sensory function such as hearing or nerve impulses.

Balloon Valvuloplasty   a medical procedure using a catheter to insert an inflatable device into the heart to open and correct abnormal narrowing of structures.

Benign   a tumor that doesn't spread, harmless.

Biopsy   a procedure wherein small samples of tissue are obtained for microscopic examination to diagnose a medical condition.

Boron Neutron Capture Therapy   a two-step radiation treatment for cancer that uses the element boron to infiltrate tumors.

Bypass Machine   a medical pump and oxygenation device that temporarily reroutes the blood outside of the body during open heart surgery.

Cachexia   a wasting syndrome, a malnutrition condition that develops despite adequate intake of food, often associated with cancer.

Calcium Channel Blockers   drugs used to treat abnormal heart rates.

Calculolytic   refers to properties that dissolve stones or crystals that have formed in the urinary tract.

Cancellous Bone   bone tissue with a spongy, lattice-like internal structure often used in graft procedures.

Catheter   a tube-like medical device inserted into blood vessels, body cavities, or passageways (i.e., the urethra) to permit injection or withdrawal of fluid.

Central Nervous System (CNS)   the brain and spinal cord.

Chemotherapy   Cytotoxic or cell-poisoning drugs used as systemic (whole body) therapy to attack cancers that have spread throughout the body.

Chromosomes   large, complex molecules of DNA found in every cell that carry genetic information.

Chronic   slow or gradual onset of condition or disease, and/or condition of long duration.

Clicker   a handheld device that produces a "click" as a training cue for shaping behaviors.

Clone   a genetic duplicate created from tissue of the original.

Colostrum   the first milk produced by a mother dog or cat, rich in protective maternal antibodies.

Compounding   refers to the creation of custom-designed prescriptions made more dose-specific and/or easier to administer.

Computed Dental Radiography (CDR)   intraoral X-ray system that stores images on computers rather than traditional X-ray film.

Computed Tomography (CT)   a noninvasive diagnostic test that uses multiple X-rays of "slices" of the internal structure, and then "reconstructs" that object through computer projections into a three-dimensional image of the patient.

Coumadin   an anticoagulant drug that prevents clotting.

Counterconditioning   a behavior modification program that teaches the pet to associate unpleasant experiences with more positive or rewarding situations, and so learn to tolerate them.

Cryosurgery   therapeutic treatment using extreme cold (freezing).

Cyclosporin   an immunosuppressive drug used in organ transplants that helps prevent rejection by the body.

Darthroplasty   surgical grafting procedure that restructures the hip joint in some cases of hip dysplasia. Also called bone graft shelf arthroplasty.

Desensitization   a behavior modification program that uses gradual exposure to unpleasant experiences to build up the pet's tolerance level.

Dialysis   use of an artificial kidney machine to filter waste from the blood.

Echocardiography   a noninvasive diagnostic tool that uses reflection of sound waves from the heart muscle and surrounding tissues and specialized processing of the echoed signals, and then display of this information in a visual or auditory format. Doppler echocardiography is the newest form and adds the detection of direction and velocity of blood flow through the heart.

Electrocardiogram (ECG or EKG)   a diagnostic test that records the electrical activity of the heart during muscle contraction and relaxation.

Electroencephalogram (EEG)   a diagnostic test that records the electrical activity of the brain.

Electroretinogram (ERG)   a specific test for retinal function that measures the mass electrical response of the retina in response to light. It can identify large groups of retinal cells that don't function, to allow a specific diagnosis of retinal dysfunction.

Electrostimulaton (E-STIM)   a rehabilitation therapy that uses electrodes to stimulate specific muscles or muscle groups.

Endoscope   a long, flexible tube employing fiberoptics or other imaging technology able to be inserted through small incisions to view internal structures of the body and then transmit an image of the area to a video screen during surgical procedures.

Euthanasia   humane ending of life.

Extraspinal Oscillating Field Stimulator a battery-powered implant that generates a tiny electrical field to stimulate growth and regeneration of nerve fibers in spinal cord injuries.

Familial appearing in a family line with more frequency than by chance.

Femoral Head Ostectomy a surgical procedure that removes the "ball" portion from the end of the femur (thigh bone) to treat hip dysplasia.

Force-Plate a computerized platform scale set flush in the floor that measures the force/weight placed on a particular limb as the animal moves across it.

Gastrotomy Tube a hollow tube passed into the stomach to feed an ill or recovering patient.

Genes individual units of inheritance made up of stretches of DNA found in chromosomes within each cell.

Gene Therapy involves various techniques that manipulate genes to create medicines or treatments designed to interact with the body on the cellular level and promote healing.

Genome the total genetic information of one individual.

Graft donor tissue.

Halter a training tool that fits over a dog's head in lieu of a training collar.

Hyperthermia Therapy use of heat to kill cancer cells.

Idiopathic no known cause.

IGR (insect growth regulator) a compound often used in flea control preparations that interferes with the development of the flea. Safety margin for pets is high because IGRs do not affect mammals.

Immune System the natural response of the body to fight disease or outside foreign substances. It includes both local (cell-mediated) and systemic (antibody/blood system) immune components.

Immunotherapy treatment designed to stimulate the body's natural immune system to fight disease conditions, specifically cancer.

Intravenous (IV) delivery of therapeutic substances directly into the bloodstream through the veins.

Joint Replacement a surgical technique that removes the natural diseased joint and replaces it with a metal prosthetic joint, most commonly done in the hip.

Laser an instrument that uses photothermal (heat) energy of various kinds of light to vaporize tissue.

Limb Sparing a surgical technique that spares the limb when removing diseased bone and avoids amputation.

Magnetic Resonance Imaging (MRI) a noninvasive diagnostic technique that records radio frequency signals given off by the tissue, using an external magnetic field, and translates the signals into a two-dimensional image.

Malignant a cancer capable of spreading throughout the body beyond the site of origination.

Metastasis the spread of tumor cells from their site of origination.

Myeologram X-ray of the spine using contrast dye.

Necrosis death of cells.

Nerve Conduction Velocity (NCV) studies that measure the electrical impulse and reaction from the nerve to the muscle, using tiny needle electrodes.

NSAIDs nonsteroidal antiinflammatory drugs (like aspirin) commonly used for pain control.

Nuclear Scintigraphy a diagnostic technique that administers radioactive tracers that are preferentially absorbed by certain cells (like thyroid, bone, and certain cancers).

Nutraceuticals nutrients (like vitamins, minerals, certain amino acids, etc.) used as medicine.

Off-Label the use of nonapproved drug therapies, also called "extralabel."

Orthodontics the therapeutic use of intraoral appliances to reconfigure the alignment of the teeth.

Pacemaker electrical device implanted surgically that stimulates heart action with electrical impulses, to treat slow or irregular heart rhythms.

Palliative   a treatment that alleviates the signs of disease without curing the condition.

Phacoemulsification   a surgical technique that breaks up and removes the lens from the eye using ultrasonic vibrations; typically used in cataract surgery.

Phakoemulsification   a surgical tool that uses sound waves to break up and remove cataracts.

Pheromones   chemical "odors" created by the body that prompt specific behavior responses.

Photodynamic Therapy (PDT)   a light-activated chemotherapy using lasers and photosensitizing compounds that targets cancer cells.

Placebo   "pretend" medicine or drug that has no physiologic effect; used in controlled studies to compare and measure against real therapy.

Positive-emission Tomography Scan (PET scan)   a noninvasive diagnostic tool that records electrical activity in the brain.

Radiation Therapy   use of directional X-ray to treat cancer.

Radiograph   the use of gamma rays to view the internal dense structures of the body, also called X-ray.

Retinoscope   a tool that refracts, or measures, the focal point of the eye to determine how well the patient can see.

Schiotz Tonometer   a device used to measure pressure inside the eyeball to diagnose glaucoma.

Socialization   a critical time period, usually very early in life, during which a puppy or kitten learns the proper way to act and react to the world around them.

Subtotal Colectomy   surgical procedure that removes the diseased portion of the intestine in cats suffering from chronic megacolon.

Telemedicine   remote-access diagnosis and consultation from images or test results transmitted by computer or other means.

Therapeutic Diet   a commercial or homemade diet that typically is prescribed by the veterinarian to specifically treat a health condition.

Tibial Plateu Leveling Osteotomy (TPLO)   a surgical technique to restructure and repair injury to a dog's cruciate ligament.

Tonopen   a pen-sized tool for diagnosing glaucoma by measuring pressure inside the eyeball.

Transdermal Delivery   a method in which drugs, often for pain, are able to penetrate the skin and achieve local or systemic therapeutic effect.

Transplant surgical replacement of a diseased organ with a donor organ. In pets, it's most typically the kidney.

Triple Pelvic Osteotomy (TPO) a surgical procedure that cuts the pelvis in three places and rotates the bone to correct hip joint conformation in dogs diagnosed with some forms of hip dysplasia.

Ultrasound noninvasive diagnostic technique that uses reflected sound waves to form an image of internal structures.

Vagal Nerve Stimulator (VNS) a device similar to a cardiac pacemaker surgically implanted in the neck, where it repetitively stimulates the vagus nerve to control epileptic seizures.

Veterinary Orthopedic Manipulation (VOM) a therapy that offers minute adjustments to the nerves and muscles adjacent to the spine using a chiropractic spring-loaded mallet.

X-ray the use of gamma rays to view the internal dense structures of the body, also called radiograph.

Source Notes

PART ONE: 21ST CENTURY MEDICINE

Chapter 1. How We Care for Pets in the New Century

- David S. Bruyette, DVM, DACVIM (internal medicine), is an internist at VCA West Los Angeles Animal Hospital, in Los Angeles.
- Ian Dunbar, PhD, MRCCS, is a veterinarian and dog trainer/behaviorist in Berkeley, California, and the author of *How to Teach a New Dog Old Tricks*.
- Myrna M. Milani, DVM, is a veterinary ethologist and teacher who lives in Charlestown, New Hampshire.
- Maura O'Brien, DVM, DACVS, is a veterinary surgeon at VCA West Los Angeles Hospital in Los Angeles, California.
- Korinn E. Saker, MS, DVM, PhD, is a clinical nutritionist at Virginia-Maryland Regional College of Veterinary Medicine in Blacksburg, Virginia.
- Robert Taylor, DVM, MS, DACVS, is a professor of orthopedic surgery and codirector of Alameda East Veterinary Hospital in Denver.

Chapter 2. Building on Success

- Lillian Aronson, VMD, DACVS, is an assistant professor in surgery at the University of Pennsylvania, School of Veterinary Medicine.

- Kenneth E. Bartels, DVM, MS, is the McCasland professor of laser surgery, and holds the Cohn Chair for animal care at Oklahoma State University.
- Daniel Brockman, BVSc, CVR, CSAO, DACVS, DECVS, MRCVS, is an assistant professor of surgery at the University of Pennsylvania, School of Veterinary Medicine.
- David S. Bruyette, DVM, DACVIM (internal medicine), is an internist at VCA West Los Angeles Animal Hospital, in Los Angeles.
- Dan Carey, DVM, is the director of technical communications for Iams Company.
- Ian Dunbar, PhD, MRCCS, is a veterinarian and dog trainer/behaviorist in Berkeley, California, and the author of *How to Teach a New Dog Old Tricks*.
- A. D. Elkins, DVM, MS, DACVS, is the owner and staff surgeon at Indiana Veterinary Surgical Referral Service in Indianapolis.
- Paul A. Gerding, Jr., DVM, MS, DACVO, is an associate professor and chief of the Ophthalmology Section, Department of Veterinary Clinical Medicine at the University of Illinois.
- Steven Hannah, PhD, is a nutritionist and managing scientist at Ralston Purina Company.
- Nancy Irlbeck, PhD, ACVN, is an associate professor in comparative nutrition at Colorado State University.
- Jeryl C. Jones, DVM, PhD, DACVR, is an assistant professor of radiology in the Department of Small Animal Clinical Sciences at Virginia-Maryland Regional College of Veterinary Medicine.
- Alton Kanak, RPh, is a compounding pharmacist affiliated with www.PeerlessHealth.com from the Katy Compounding Pharmacy sterile products outlet, and Brookshire Brothers Pharmacy in Houston, Texas.
- Mark D. Kittleson, DVM, PhD, DACVIM (cardiology), is a professor in the Department of Medicine and Epidemiology in the School of Veterinary Medicine at University of California-Davis.
- Richard A. LeCouteur, BVSc, PhD, DACVIM (neurology), DECVN, is a professor of neurology and neurosurgery in the Department of Surgical and Radiological Sciences, School of Veterinary Medicine, University of California-Davis.
- Grace Long, DVM, MS, is brand manager for Purina Veterinary Diets.
- Dennis Macy, DVM, DACIM (internal medicine and oncology), is president of the specialty of oncology at Colorado State University School of Veterinary Medicine.
- Myrna M. Milani, DVM, is a veterinary ethologist and teacher who lives in Charlestown, New Hampshire, and the author of *Behavior Problems in Dogs* and many other titles.

- Darryl Millis, DVM, DACVS, is an associate professor and chief of Surgery Services at the University of Tennessee.
- Maura O'Brien, DVM, DACVS, is a veterinary surgeon at VCA West Los Angeles Hospital in Los Angeles, California.
- E. B. Okrasinski, DVM, DACVS, is the owner of Veterinary Surgical Services, a mobile specialty practice in Kirkland, Washington.
- Paul Orsini, DVM, DACVS, DAVDC, is a surgeon and dentist at the University of Pennsylvania School of Veterinary Medicine.
- E. Christopher Orton, DVM, PhD, DACVS, is a professor at the Veterinary Teaching Hospital at Colorado State University School of Veterinary Medicine.
- Karen Overall, VMD, MS, PhD, DACVB, ABS Certified Applied Animal Behaviorist, is a professor of behavior medicine at the University of Pennsylvania School of Veterinary Medicine.
- David Ruslander, DVM, DAVCIM (oncology), DACVR (radiation oncology), is an assistant professor in the Harrington Oncology Program at Tufts University School of Veterinary Medicine.
- Korinn E. Saker, MS, DVM, PhD, is a clinical nutritionist at Virginia-Maryland Regional College of Veterinary Medicine in Blacksburg, Virginia.
- James H. Sokolowski, DVM, PhD, is a marketing manager for Waltham USA.
- Robert Taylor, DVM, MS, DACVS, is a professor of orthopedic surgery and codirector of Alameda East Veterinary Hospital in Denver.
- William Tranquilli, DVM, MS, DACVA, is a veterinary anesthesiologist and professor of veterinary and clinical medicine at the University of Illinois.

Chapter 3. Ethics and New Century Medicine

- Lillian Aronson, VMD, DACVS, is an assistant professor in surgery at University of Pennsylvania School of Veterinary Medicine.
- Kenneth E. Bartels, DVM, MS, is the McCasland professor of laser surgery, and holds the Cohn Chair for animal care at Oklahoma State University.
- Dale E. Bjorling, DVM, MS, is a professor and chair of the Department of Surgical Sciences, School of Veterinary Medicine at the University of Wisconsin-Madison.
- Richard B. Borgens, PhD, is a professor of developmental anatomy at Purdue University, and director of the Center for Paralysis Research.
- William G. Brewer, Jr., DVM, ACVIM, is an assistant professor of internal medicine and oncology and chief of the Section of Small Animal Medicine at Auburn University.

- David S. Bruyette, DVM, DACVIM (internal medicine), is an internist at VCA West Los Angeles Animal Hospital.
- Ruthanne Chun, DVM, DACVIM (oncology), is an assistant professor in oncology at Kansas State University.
- Ian Dunbar, PhD, MRCCS, is a veterinarian and dog trainer/behaviorist in Berkeley, California, and the author of *How to Teach a New Dog Old Tricks*.
- Carolyn Henry, DVM, DACVIM (oncology), is an assistant professor of oncology at the University of Missouri.
- Barbara Kitchell, DVM, PhD, DACVIM (internal medicine and oncology), is an assistant professor of small animal medicine at the University of Illinois.
- Mark D. Kittleson, DVM, PhD, DACVIM (cardiology), is a professor in the Department of Medicine and Epidemiology, School of Veterinary Medicine, University of California-Davis.
- Nancy Irlbeck, PhD, ACVN, is an associate professor in comparative nutrition at Colorado State University.
- Richard A. LeCouteur, BVSc, PhD, DACVIM (neurology), DECVN, is a professor of neurology and neurosurgery in the Department of Surgical and Radiological Sciences, School of Veterinary Medicine, University of California-Davis.
- Dennis Macy, DVM, DACIM (internal medicine and oncology), is president of the specialty of oncology at Colorado State University School of Veterinary Medicine.
- Myrna M. Milani, DVM, is a veterinary ethologist and teacher who lives in Charlestown, New Hampshire, and the author of several books including *The Body Language and Emotions of Dogs*.
- Helen Newman-Gage, PhD, is the owner of Veterinary Transplant Services in Kent, Washington.
- Maura O'Brien, DVM, DACVS, is a veterinary surgeon at VCA West Los Angeles Hospital.
- Karen Overall, VMD, MS, PhD, DACVB, ABS Certified Applied Animal Behaviorist, is a professor of behavior medicine at the University of Pennsylvania School of Veterinary Medicine.
- Charles E. Powell is the communications specialist for Washington State University.
- Gail Smith, VMD, PhD, is a professor in orthopedic surgery and chair of the Department of Clinical Studies at the University of Pennsylvania.
- Jack Stephens, DVM, is founder and president of Veterinary Pet Insurance.
- William Tranquilli, DVM, MS, DACVA, is a veterinary anesthesiologist and professor of veterinary and clinical medicine at the University of Illinois.
- Carmel Travis is the owner of The Lucas House in Pullman, Washington.

- Steve Withrow, DVM, ACVIM (oncology), is the director of the Animal Cancer Center at Colorado State University.

Chapter 4. A Brave New World

- Kirk N. Gelatt, VMD, DACVO, is a professor of comparative ophthalmology in the College of Veterinary Surgery and Medicine at the University of Florida.
- Urs Giger, PD, DrMedVet, MS, FVH, DACVIM, DECVIM, is the Charlotte Newton Sheppard Professor of Medicine and chief of the Section of Medical Genetics at the School of Veterinary Medicine at the University of Pennsylvania.
- Dennis Hacker, DVM, DACVO, is a veterinarian at Animal Eye Specialists in El Cerrito, California.
- Steven Hannah, PhD, is a nutritionist and managing scientist at Ralston Purina Company.
- Stephen J. O'Brien, PhD, is chief of the Laboratory of Genomic Diversity, National Cancer Institute, Frederick Cancer Research and Development Center in Frederick, Maryland.
- J. Phillip Pickett, DVM, DACVO, is a veterinary ophthalmologist and associate professor in the Department of Small Animal Clinical Sciences at Virginia-Maryland Regional College of Veterinary Medicine.

PART TWO: HEALTH AND BEHAVIOR CONDITIONS A TO Z

Aggression

- Ian Dunbar, PhD, MRCCS, of Berkeley, California, is the founder of the Association of Pet Dog Trainers, and author of *How to Teach a New Dog Old Tricks*.
- Myrna M. Milani, DVM, is a Charleston, New Hampshire, veterinary ethologist and author.
- Karen Overall, VMD, MS, PhD, DACVB, ABS Certified Applied Animal Behaviorist, is a professor of behavior at the University of Pennsylvania.

Anemia

- James N. MacLeod, VMD, PhD, is an assistant professor of molecular genetics at Cornell University.
- Charles E. Powell is the communications specialist for Washington State University.
- John F. Randolph, DVM, is an associate professor of theriogenology at Cornell University.

Anorexia

- Andrew Mackin, BVMS, DACVIM, is an associate professor in small animal internal medicine at Mississippi State University.

Arthritis

- LeeAnn McGill, DVM, is a veterinarian at Magnolia Small Animal Clinic in Foley, Alabama.
- Darryl Millis, DVM, DACVS, is an associate professor and chief of surgery services at the University of Tennessee.
- James H. Sokolowski, DVM, PhD, is a marketing manager for Waltham USA.
- Robert Taylor, DVM, MS, DACVS, is a professor of orthopedic surgery and codirector of Alameda East Veterinary Hospital in Denver.

Back Injuries

- Kenneth E. Bartels, DVM, MS, is the McCasland professor of laser surgery, and holds the Cohn Chair for animal care at the University of Oklahoma.
- Roger Clemmons, DVM, PhD, is an associate professor of neurology and neurosurgery in the Department of Small Animal Clinical Sciences at the University of Florida's College of Veterinary Medicine.
- A. D. Elkins, DVM, MS, DACVS, is the owner and staff surgeon at Indiana Veterinary Surgical Referral Service in Indianapolis.
- Matthew Fricke, DVM, is a veterinarian at McKenzie Animal Clinic in Springfield, Oregon.
- Darryl Millis, DVM, DACVS, is an associate professor and chief of surgery services at the University of Tennessee.

Bloat

- Dale E. Bjorling, DVM, MS, is a professor and chair of the Department of Surgical Sciences, School of Veterinary Medicine, University of Wisconsin-Madison.
- Barry Fly, DVM, is a veterinarian at Nolensville Animal Hospital in Nolensville, Tennessee.

Bone Grafts

- William G. Brewer, Jr., DVM, ACVIM (oncology and internal medicine), is an assistant professor of internal medicine and oncology, and chief of the Section of Small Animal Medicine at Auburn University.
- Nichole Ehrhart, VMD, DACVS (oncology), is an assistant professor of small animal surgery, soft tissue surgery, orthopedic surgery, and surgical oncology at the University of Illinois.
- Paul Gambardella, VMD, DACVS, is the chief of staff and an orthopedic surgeon at Angell Memorial Animal Hospital in Boston.
- Helen Newman-Gage, PhD, is the owner of Veterinary Transplant Services in Kent, Washington.
- Maura O'Brien, DVM, DACVS, is a veterinary surgeon at VCA West Los Angeles Hospital.
- Steve Withrow, DVM, ACVIM (oncology), is the director of the Animal Cancer Center at Colorado State University.

Brain Tumors

- Patrick Gavin, DVM, PhD, is a professor at Washington State University in Pullman.
- Richard A. LeCouteur, BVSc, PhD, DACVIM (neurology), DECVN, is a professor of neurology and neurosurgery in the Department of Surgical and Radiological Sciences, School of Veterinary Medicine at the University of California-Davis.

Cancer

- William G. Brewer, Jr., DVM, ACVIM (oncology and internal medicine), is an assistant professor of internal medicine and oncology and chief of the Section of Small Animal Medicine at Auburn University.
- Ruthanne Chun, DVM, DACVIM (oncology), is an assistant professor in oncology at Kansas State University.
- Barbara Kitchell, DVM, PhD, DACVIM (internal medicine and oncol-

ogy), is an assistant professor of small animal medicine at the University of Illinois.

- E. Gregory MacEwen, VMD, ACVIM (internal medicine and oncology), is a professor of oncology in the School of Veterinary Medicine at the University of Wisconsin.
- Dennis Macy, DVM, DACIM (internal medicine and oncology), is president of the specialty of oncology at Colorado State University.
- Gregory K. Ogilvie, DVM, DACVIM, is a professor of oncology and internal medicine, in the College of Veterinary Medicine and Biomedical Sciences at Colorado State University.
- John S. Reif, DVM, is a professor and head of the Department of Environmental Health at Colorado State University.
- David Ruslander, DVM, DAVCIM (oncology), DACVR (radiation oncology), is an assistant professor in the Harrington Oncology Program, Tufts University School of Veterinary Medicine.
- Steve Withrow, DVM, ACVIM (oncology), is director of the Animal Cancer Center at Colorado State University.

Cataracts

- Carmen Colitz, DVM, PhD, DACVO, is an assistant professor of ophthalmology at Louisiana State University School of Veterinary Medicine.
- Paul A. Gerding, Jr., DVM, MS, DACVO, is an associate professor and chief of the Ophthalmology Section in the Department of Veterinary Clinical Medicine at the University of Illinois.
- Christopher J. Murphy, DVM, PhD, DACVO, is a professor of ophthalmology at the School of Veterinary Medicine, University of Wisconsin-Madison.
- J. Phillip Pickett, DVM, DACVO, is a veterinary ophthalmologist and an associate professor in the Department of Small Animal Clinical Sciences at Virginia-Maryland Regional College of Veterinary Medicine.

Clawing

- Kenneth E. Bartels, DVM, MS, is the McCasland professor of laser surgery, and holds the Cohn Chair for animal care at Oklahoma State University.

Cognitive Disorders

- Dawn Merton Boothe, DVM, PhD, DACVIM, DACVCP, is of Texas A&M University, College of Veterinary Medicine.

- David S. Bruyette, DVM, DACVIM (internal medicine), is a veterinarian at VCA West Los Angeles Animal Hospital.
- Richard A. LeCouteur, BVSc, PhD, DACVIM (neurology), DECVN, is a professor of neurology and neurosurgery in the Department of Surgical and Radiological Sciences, School of Veterinary Medicine at University of California-Davis.

Corneal Transplants

- Carmen Colitz, DVM, PhD, DACVO, is an assistant professor of ophthalmology at Louisiana State University School of Veterinary Medicine.
- Christopher J. Murphy, DVM, PhD, DACVO, is a professor of ophthalmology at the School of Veterinary Medicine, University of Wisconsin-Madison.
- Helen Newman-Gage, PhD, is owner of Veterinary Transplant Services in Kent, Washington.
- J. Phillip Pickett, DVM, DACVO, is a veterinary ophthalmologist and an associate professor in the Department of Small Animal Clinical Sciences at Virginia-Maryland Regional College of Veterinary Medicine.

Cystitis

- Dawn Merton Boothe, DVM, PhD, DACVIM, DACVCP, is of Texas A&M University, College of Veterinary Medicine.
- Sarah Stephenson, DVM, is a veterinarian at Valley West Veterinary Hospital in Charleston, West Virginia.

Diabetes

- Dan Carey, DVM, is the director of technical communications for Iams Company.
- Paul A. Cuddon, DVM, DACVIM, is a neurologist at the College of Veterinary Medicine and Biomedical Sciences at Colorado State University.
- Grace Long, DVM, MS, is a brand manager for Purina Veterinary Diets.
- Mark E. Peterson, DVM, is a researcher for the Animal Medical Center in New York.

Elbow Disorders

- A. D. Elkins, DVM, MS, DACVS, is the owner and staff surgeon at Indiana Veterinary Surgical Referral Service in Indianapolis.
- Paul Gambardella, VMD, DACVS, is chief of staff and an orthopedic surgeon at Angell Memorial Animal Hospital in Boston.
- Kurt S. Schulz, DVM, is an assistant professor of surgical and radiological sciences at University of California-Davis.
- Robert Taylor, DVM, MS, DACVS, is a professor of orthopedic surgery and codirector at Alameda East Veterinary Hospital in Denver.

Epilepsy

- Thomas R. Famula, PhD, is a professor in the Department of Animal Science at the University of California-Davis.
- Karen R. Munana, DVM, MS, DACVIM, is a researcher at North Carolina State University at Raleigh.

Fear

- Myrna M. Milani, DVM, is a veterinary ethologist and teacher who lives in Charlestown, New Hampshire.
- Karen Overall, VMD, MS, PhD, DACVB, ABS Certified Applied Animal Behaviorist, is a professor of behavior at the University of Pennsylvania.

Food Allergies

- Steven Hannah, PhD, is a managing scientist and nutritionist at Ralston Purina Company.
- Korinn E. Saker, MS, DVM, PhD, is a clinical nutritionist at Virginia-Maryland Regional College of Veterinary Medicine.

Glaucoma

- Carmen Colitz, DVM, PhD, DACVO, is an assistant professor in ophthalmology at Louisiana State University School of Veterinary Medicine, Department of Veterinary Clinical Sciences.
- Kirk N. Gelatt, VMD, is a professor of comparative ophthalmology in the College of Veterinary Surgery and Medicine at the University of Florida.
- Paul A. Gerding, Jr., DVM, MS, DACVO, is an associate professor and

chief of the Ophthalmology Section in the Department of Veterinary Clinical Medicine at the University of Illinois.

- Dennis Hacker, DVM, DACVO, is a veterinarian at Animal Eye Specialists in El Cerrito, California.
- J. Phillip Pickett, DVM, DACVO, is a veterinary ophthalmologist and an associate professor in the Department of Small Animal Clinical Sciences at Virginia-Maryland College.

Hearing Problems

- Blanche L. Blackington, MACCCA, is a clinical audiologist at San Diego Hearing Center in California.
- George M. Strain, PhD, is a professor of neuroscience at the School of Veterinary Medicine at Louisiana State University.
- Richard Johnson, DVM, and Nancy Hampel, DVM, DACVS, are veterinarians practicing in San Diego.
- Michael Podell, MSc, DVM, DACVIM (neurology), is an assistant professor and director of the comparative neurology service at the Department of Veterinary Clinical Sciences at the College of Veterinary Medicine at Ohio State University in Columbus.

Heart Disease—Canine

- Daniel Brockman, BVSc, CVR, CSAO, DACVS, DECVS, MRCVS, is an assistant professor of surgery in the College of Veterinary Medicine, University of Pennsylvania.
- Mark D. Kittleson, DVM, PhD, DACVIM (cardiology), is a professor in the Department of Medicine and Epidemiology, in the School of Veterinary Medicine at University of California-Davis.
- E. Christopher Orton, DVM, PhD, DACVS, is a professor at the Veterinary Teaching Hospital at Colorado State University.

Heart Disease—Feline

- Christine Cannon, DVM, is a veterinarian at Exclusively Cats in Waterford, Michigan.
- Mark D. Kittleson, DVM, PhD, DACVIM (cardiology), is a professor in the Department of Medicine and Epidemiology, in the School of Veterinary Medicine at University of California-Davis.
- E. Christopher Orton, DVM, PhD, DACVS, is a professor at the Veterinary Teaching Hospital at Colorado State University.

Hip Dysplasia

- A. D. Elkins, DVM, MS, DACVS, is the owner and staff surgeon of Indiana Veterinary Surgical Referral Service in Indianapolis.
- Mark Markel, DVM, PhD, DACVS, is the chair of the Department of Medical Sciences and Professor of Surgery at the University of Wisconsin in Madison.
- Gail Smith, VMD, PhD, is a professor in orthopedic surgery and chair of the Department of Clinical Studies at the University of Pennsylvania.

Hyperthyroidism

- Joseph Taboada, DVM, DACVIM, is a professor in the Department of Veterinary Clinical Sciences at Louisiana State University.

Kidney Disease

- Lillian Aronson, VMD, DACVS, is an assistant professor in surgery at the School of Veterinary Medicine, University of Pennsylvania.
- Larry Cowgill, DVM, PhD, is an associate professor and chair of faculty at the University of California-Davis.
- Clare Gregory, DVM, is the director of the Comparative Transplantation Laboratory at the University of California-Davis.
- Grace Long, DVM, MS, is a brand manager for Purina Veterinary Diets.

Knee Injury

- A. D. Elkins, DVM, MS, DACVS, is the owner and staff surgeon of Indiana Veterinary Surgical Referral Service in Indianapolis.
- Paul Gambardella, VMD, DACVS, is chief of staff and orthopedic surgeon at Angell Memorial Animal Hospital in Boston.
- Helen Newman-Gage, PhD, is the owner of Veterinary Transplant Services in Kent, Washington.

Liver Disease

- Dr. Karen M. Tobias is a veterinary researcher at Washington State University.

Megacolon

- Gary W. Ellison, DVM, MS, DACVS, is a veterinary surgeon at the University of Florida.

Obesity

- Dan Carey, DVM, is director of technical communications for Iams Company.
- Nancy Irlbeck, PhD, ACVN, is an associate professor of comparative nutrition at Colorado State University.
- Grace Long, DVM, MS, is a brand manager for Purina Veterinary Diets.
- Andrew Mackin, BSc, BVMS, MRCVS, DACVIM, is an associate professor of Small Animal Medicine at the College of Veterinary Medicine, Mississippi State University.
- James H. Sokolowski, DVM, PhD, is marketing manager for Waltham USA.

Pain

- Steven L. Marks, BVSc, MS, MRCVS, DACVIM, is an internist at Louisiana State University.
- William Tranquilli, DVM, MS, DACVA, is a veterinary anesthesiologist and professor of veterinary and clinical medicine at the University of Illinois.

Pancreatitis

- David A. Williams, MA, VetMB, PhD, MRCVS, DACVIM, is a veterinary researcher from Texas A&M University.

Paralysis

- Richard B. Borgens, PhD, is a professor of developmental anatomy at Purdue University, and director of the Center for Paralysis Research in the Institute for Applied Neurology (affiliated with Indiana University Medical Center).

Parasites

- Michael W. Dryden, DVM, PhD, is an associate professor at Kansas State University College of Veterinary Medicine.

Skin Allergies

- Dawn Merton Boothe, DVM, PhD, DAVCIM, DACVCP, is a pharmacologist and researcher at Texas A&M College of Veterinary Medicine.
- Dan Carey, DVM, is director of technical communications for Iams Company.
- Sandra R. Merchant, DVM, DACVD, is a professor of dermatology in the Department of Clinical Sciences at Louisiana State University.

Spraying

- Myrna M. Milani, DVM, is a veterinary ethologist and teacher who lives in Charlestown, New Hampshire.

Teeth Problems

- Paul Orsini, DVM, DACVS, DAVDC, is a veterinary dentist and surgeon at the University of Pennsylvania.

Urinary Stones

- Kenneth E. Bartels, DVM, MS, is the McCasland professor of laser surgery, and holds the Cohn chair for animal care at Oklahoma State University.
- Joseph W. Bartges, DVM, PhD, is a veterinary researcher at the University of Tennessee.
- Dr. Paula Henthorn is a researcher at the University of Pennsylvania School of Veterinary Medicine.
- Grace Long, DVM, MS, is brand manager for Purina Veterinary Diets.
- James H. Sokolowski, DVM, PhD, is marketing manager for Waltham USA.
- J. Paul Woods, DVM, is a researcher at Oklahoma State University.

Vaccinations

- Cynda Crawford, DVM, is a postdoctoral associate in the Department of Pathobiology at the University of Florida.
- Julie Levy, DVM, is an assistant professor of small animal medicine at the University of Florida College of Veterinary Medicine.
- Dennis Macy, DVM, DACIM (internal medicine and oncology), is president of the specialty of oncology at Colorado State University.

- James H. Sokolowski, DVM, PhD, is a marketing manager for Waltham USA.

Wound Healing

- Giselle Hosgood, BVSc, MS, DACVS, is a Fellow of the Australian College of Veterinary Scientists and a professor of veterinary surgery at Louisiana State University.

INDEX

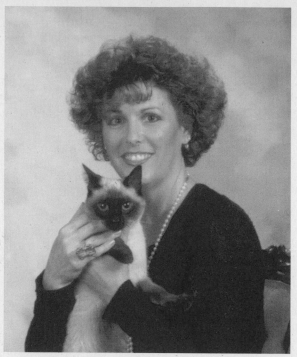

Lavor Quin

Amy D. Shojai is a nationally known authority on pet care and behavior. She is the author of more than a dozen award-winning nonfiction pet books and over 300 articles and columns. Ms. Shojai addresses a wide range of fun to serious issues in her work, covering training, behavior, health care, and medical topics.

Ms. Shojai is a founder and past president of the Cat Writers' Association, and a member of the Dog Writers' Association of America and Association of Pet Dog Trainers. She frequently speaks to groups on a variety of pet-related issues, lectures at writing conferences, and regularly appears on national radio and television in connection with her work. She and her husband live with assorted critters at Rosemont, their thirteen-acre "spread" in north Texas. Ms. Shojai can be reached through her Web site at www.shojai.com.